Chromosome Analysis Protocols

Methods in Molecular Biology

John M. Walker, SERIES EDITOR

Methods in Molecular Biology • 29

Chromosome Analysis Protocols

Edited by

John R. Gosden

Medical Research Council, Edinburgh, Scotland

Humana Press ✳ Totowa, New Jersey

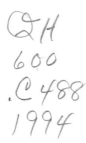

Printed in the United States of America. 10 9 8 7 6 5 4 3 2 1

Library of Congress Cataloging in Publication Data

Main entry under title:

Methods in molecular biology.

Chromosome analysis protocols / edited by John R. Gosden
        p.   cm. —(Methods in molecular biology : 29)
    Includes index.
    ISBN 0-89603-243-4 (comb)
    ISBN 0-89603-289-2 (hard cover)
    1. Chromosomes—Research—Methodology 2. Cytogenetics—Technique 3. Human cytogenetics—Technique I. Gosden, John R. II. Series: Methods in molecular biology (Totowa, NJ) ; 29.
QH600.C488   1994
611'.01816—dc20   93-34459

Preface

Chromosomes, as the genetic vehicles, provide the basic material for a large proportion of genetic investigations, from the construction of gene maps and models of chromosome organization, to the investigation of gene function and dysfunction. The study of chromosomes has developed in parallel with other aspects of molecular genetics, beginning with the first preparations of chromosomes from animal cells, through the development of banding techniques, which permitted the unequivocal identification of each chromosome in a karyotype, to the present analytical methods of molecular cytogenetics.

Although some of these techniques have been in use for many years, and can be learned relatively easily, most published scientific reports—as a result of pressure on space from editors, and the response to that pressure by authors—contain little in the way of technical detail, and thus are rarely adequate for a researcher hoping to find all the necessary information to embark on a method from scratch. A new user needs not only a detailed description of the methods, but also some help with problem solving and sorting out the difficulties encountered in handling any biological system. This was the requirement to which the series *Methods in Molecular Biology* is addressed, and *Chromosome Analysis Protocols* forms a part of this series.

Throughout the book, the primary emphasis is on the application of these methods to human material, since this is where the main thrust of molecular cytogenetics is currently directed. However, in most cases the techniques described are readily applicable to other organisms. Each chapter is written by an author who regularly uses the technique in his or her own laboratory. Most of them describe the very latest developments, but some, particularly the early ones, contain essential, classic methods, with only minor changes to improve their reliability. Each chapter starts with a description of the principle behind the methods to be described. The main thrust of the book,

v

however, is the description of the practical steps necessary to carry out the method successfully. The Methods section, therefore (with one exception), consists of a detailed, step-by-step description of a protocol, that, carefully followed, will result in the successful completion of the method. The Notes section complements the Methods section by indicating possible problem areas and their solutions and emphasizing points where particular care is needed.

The first third of the book describes methods for preparing chromosomes from a number of different cell types, and techniques for producing banded chromosomes and analyzing karyotypes. The remainder of the book focuses on the application of more specifically molecular techniques to those chromosome preparations, and descriptions of techniques for their detailed analysis.

The book is primarily intended for those who, although experienced in general laboratory procedures, have no previous experience of the specific techniques described here. It should appeal particularly to postgraduates, research workers, and those who are establishing new laboratories in the area of molecular cytogenetics.

Acknowledgment

I would like to thank the series editor, John Walker, for his patient advice, constructive criticism, and helpful suggestions to a novice editor.

John R. Gosden

Contents

vii

Contributors

ROBIN C. ALLSHIRE • *Medical Research Council, Human Genetics Unit, Western General Hospital, Edinburgh, Scotland*

PETER F. AMBROS • *Children's Cancer Research Institute, St. Anna Kinderspital, Vienna, Austria*

BENOÎT ARVEILER • *Department Biochimie Medicale, Universite de Bordeaux II, Bourdeaux Cédex, France*

MATTHEW BREEN • *Australian Blood Typing Research Laboratory, University of Queensland, Australia*

STEVEN D. M. BROWN • *Department of Biochemistry and Molecular Genetics, St. Mary's Hospital Medical School, London, UK*

ALYSON H. CAREY • *Department of Biochemistry and Molecular Genetics, St. Mary's Hospital Medical School, London, UK*

NIGEL P. CARTER • *Department of Pathology, University of Cambridge, Cambridge, UK*

ANN C. CHANDLEY • *Medical Research Council, Human Genetics Unit, Western General Hospital, Edinburgh, Scotland*

HOWARD J. COOKE • *Medical Research Council, Human Genetics Unit, Western General Hospital, Edinburgh, Scotland*

J. HANS DE JONG • *Department of Genetics, Agricultural University, Wageningen, The Netherlands*

JOAQUINA DE LA TORRE • *Unidad de Genetica, Universidad Autoademia de Madrid, Spain*

AXEL J. J. DIETRICH • *Institute of Human Genetics, University of Amsterdam, Academic Medical Centre, Amsterdam, The Netherlands*

JUDITH A. FANTES • *Medical Research Council, Human Genetics Unit, Western General Hospital, Edinburgh, Scotland*

JUDY FLETCHER • *Medical Research Council, Human Genetics Unit, Western General Hospital, Edinburgh, Scotland*

ix

JOHN R. GOSDEN • *Medical Research Council, Human Genetics Unit, Western General Hospital, Edinburgh, Scotland*

ELIZABETH GRAHAM • *Medical Research Council, Human Genetics Unit, Western General Hospital, Edinburgh, Scotland*

JIM GRAHAM • *Wolfson Image Analysis Unit, Department of Medical Biophysics, University of Manchester, Manchester, UK*

DARYLL K. GREEN • *Medical Research Council, Human Genetics Unit, Western General Hospital, Edinburgh, Scotland*

BARBARA A. HAMKALO • *Department of Molecular Biology and Biochemistry, University of California, Irvine, CA*

EDGAR HARTSUIKER • *Department of Genetics, Agricultural University, Wageningen, The Netherlands*

CHRISTA HEYTING • *Department of Genetics, Agricultural University, Wageningen, The Netherlands*

STEPHEN P. HUNGER • *Laboratory of Experimental Oncology, Department of Pathology, Stanford University, Stanford, CA*

PETER JEPPESEN • *Medical Research Council, Human Genetics Unit, Western General Hospital, Edinburgh, Scotland*

DIANE LAWSON • *Medical Research Council, Human Genetics Unit, Western General Hospital, Edinburgh, Scotland*

PETER LICHTER • *Forschungsschwerpunkt Angewandte Tumorvirologie, Deutsches Krebsforschungszentrum, Heidelberg, Germany*

KUN MA • *Medical Research Council, Human Genetics Unit, Western General Hospital, Edinburgh, Scotland*

JOHN MAULE • *Medical Research Council, Human Genetics Unit, Western General Hospital, Edinburgh, Scotland*

ARTHUR R. MITCHELL • *Medical Research Council, Human Genetics Unit, Western General Hospital, Edinburgh, Scotland*

SANDYA NARAYANSWAMI • *Department of Molecular Biology and Biochemistry, University of California, Irvine, CA*

JIM PIPER • *Medical Research Council, Human Genetics Unit, Western General Hospital, Edinburgh, UK*

DAVID J. PORTEOUS • *Medical Research Council, Human Genetics Unit, Western General Hospital, Edinburgh, UK*

THOMAS RIED • *Department of Genetics, Yale University School of Medicine, New Haven, CT*

Contributors

Contributors

ANDREW R. ROSS • *Medical Research Council, Human Genetics Unit, Western General Hospital, Edinburgh, Scotland*

FIONA M. ROSS • *Wessex Regional Genetics Laboratory, Salisbury District Hospital, Odstock, Salisbury, UK*

DAVID L. SALTMAN • *Department of Molecular Genetics, Genelabs Incorporated, Redwood City, CA*

DIETER SCHWEIZER • *Department of Cytology and Genetics, Institute of Botany, University of Vienna, Vienna, Austria*

ANDREW SHARKEY • *Department of Obstetrics and Gynecology, Rosie Maternity Hospital, University of Cambridge, Cambridge, UK*

ROBERT M. SPEED • *Medical Research Council, Human Genetics Unit, Western General Hospital, Edinburgh, Scotland*

GEORGE SPOWART • *Medical Research Council, Human Genetics Unit, Western General Hospital, Edinburgh, Scotland*

ADRIAN T. SUMNER • *Medical Research Council, Human Genetics Unit, Western General Hospital, Edinburgh, Scotland*

GILLIAN E. TURNER • *Blood Transfusion and Hematology, Newcastle-upon-Tyne, UK*

VERONICA VAN HEYNINGEN • *Medical Research Council, Human Genetics Unit, Western General Hospital, Edinburgh, Scotland*

CHAPTER 1

Mitotic Metaphase Chromosome Preparation from Peripheral Blood for High Resolution

George Spowart

1. Introduction

The advent of chromosome banding techniques some 20 years ago *(1,2)* allowed the unequivocal identification of every chromosome in the human metaphase and provided a mapping scheme along each chromosome. Subsequently, a great deal of research has centered on preparing longer chromosomes with more bands visible. Chromosomes condense as they move through mitosis, and adjacent bands close up and appear to fuse. The earlier stages are longer with more bands recognized. It is not always possible to define the mitotic stage of a particular cell. International standards have been agreed for various numbers of bands in the haploid set. Thus we have 400-, 550-, and 850-band sets *(3)*. Other workers report the use of even longer chromosomes *(4,5)*. High-resolution banding has undoubted advantages in many fields. As well as allowing greater accuracy in traditional karyotype analysis, there are many reports of microdeletions and other abnormalities detected only on extended chromosomes *(6)*. Likewise, *in situ* hybridization and gene localization techniques are taking advantage of the improved resolution.

The culture technique to prepare human chromosomes still follows the basic scheme laid down by Hungerford *(7)*. Lymphocytes from peripheral blood are stimulated to divide in culture; cells are arrested in mitosis, swollen with hypotonic solution, fixed in an acid–alcohol fix, and spread on microscope slides by air-drying.

From: *Methods in Molecular Biology, Vol. 29: Chromosome Analysis Protocols*
Edited by: J. R. Gosden Copyright ©1994 Humana Press Inc., Totowa, NJ

Published methods on the preparation of elongated chromosomes are abundant. As with banding techniques, different laboratories have preferences for particular methods and have developed their own variations. None of the methods is guaranteed to work with every specimen, being the nature of biological material. There is no doubt that it is very difficult for one laboratory to reproduce exactly all the conditions in another, and it is likely that published methods need some experimentation to optimize them for local conditions. Methods of preparation fall into three general categories. An individual protocol may use one or more of these approaches.

1.1. Induction of Synchrony

Stimulated peripheral blood lymphocytes in culture grow and divide asynchronously, and pass through the prometaphase and early metaphase stages relatively rapidly. Cells are blocked around S-phase *(8)* and, on release, will continue through mitosis in a wave of divisions, thus enhancing the potential yield of early stages. Methotrexate *(9)* and excess thymidine *(10)* are the most successful blocking agents. The timing of the interval between release of the block and harvest is the critical stage in the procedure and depends, in a complex way, on the various culture conditions. This is the main reason that many workers have found it difficult to duplicate successfully published methods or to maintain a high level of success with a particular scheme. To release the cells from the block, the blocking agent is removed, or at least overcome, and cells are encouraged to enter mitosis. The choice of release agent may be determined by the banding technique to be used subsequently.

1.2. Use of Chemicals to Affect the Condensation of the Chromosomes

Chromosomes progressively condense as the cell moves through mitosis. A number of chemicals have been found to counter this *(12–14)*. Care must be taken to balance the reduction in contraction against lowering of mitotic index and/or induction of chromosome aberrations.

1.3. Alteration of Arrest and/or Hypotonic Treatments after Harvest (15–17)

Colcemid is used in most chromosome preparation techniques to destroy spindle formation and arrest cells in metaphase. Wiley et al. *(17)* questioned the necessity for colcemid treatment, but most workers continue to use it in a variety of concentrations and exposure times. Hypotonic treatment with 0.075M KCl still features in the majority of protocols, but many other formulations have been advocated, some with the specified aim of elongating chromosomes.

There are various reasons why a particular method will be preferred for a line of research. However, in general, where time and material permit, it will be good practice to run tandem methods on each specimen. I will detail two protocols that have given good results.

2. Materials

2.1. Method 1

2.1.1. Supplemented Culture Medium

This will usually be prepared in bulk and aliquoted to culture vessels just before cultures are set up. The number of specimens to be processed will determine batch size. A week's supply is typical.

1. RPMI 1640 (Gibco, Gaithersburg, MD), 340 mL.
2. Fetal bovine serum, 60 mL.
3. Phytohemagglutinin (HA15 Wellcome, Dartford, UK), 4 mL.
4. Penicillin and streptomycin (0.1 g and 100,000 U/mL) (Glaxo) mixed solution, 0.4 mL.

Store at 4°C.

2.1.2. Blocking Agent

Methotrexate injection (Lederle #4587-24) is obtained as 25 mg/mL ($5 \times 10^{-2}M$) solution. A working solution ($10^{-5}M$) is prepared by diluting 20 µL with 9.980 mL sterile distilled water. This can be stored at 4°C for several weeks. Methotrexate is a cytotoxic drug, and due care must be taken in handling.

2.1.3. Release Agents

1. Thymidine (Sigma [St. Louis, MO] #T-9250) ($10^{-3}M$) is prepared by dissolving 2.42 mg/mL in sterile distilled water. Store at 4°C.
2. The alternative agent is 5-bromo-2'-deoxyuridine Bdu (Sigma #B-5002): Working solution ($10^{-2}M$) is prepared by dissolving 3 mg/mL in distilled water. Aliquots can be stored frozen for several months. Store vial in use at 4°C. Care must be taken in handling this teratogen and mutagen.

2.1.4. Arresting Agent

Colcemid, 10 µg/mL (Gibco). Store at 4°C.

2.1.5. Hypotonic Solution

KCl (0.075M) (1.4 g in 250 mL deionized water): Make up fresh for each harvest, and heat to 37°C.

2.1.6. Fix

Acetone-free methanol and glacial acetic acid are freshly mixed in the proportion 3:1.

2.2. Method 2

2.2.1. Supplemented Culture Medium

This will usually be prepared in bulk and aliquoted to culture vessels just before cultures are set up. The number of specimens to be processed will determine batch size. A week's supply is typical.

1. RPMI 1640 (Gibco), 340 mL.
2. Fetal bovine serum, 60 mL.
3. Phytohemagglutinin (HA15 Wellcome), 4 mL.
4. Penicillin and streptomycin (0.1 g and 100,000 U/mL) (Glaxo) mixed solution, 0.4 mL.

Store at 4°C.

2.2.2. Inducing Agent

Actinomycin D (Sigma #A-1410) stock solution is prepared by dissolving 10 mg in 1 mL dimethylsulfoxide. Small aliquots are stored at –20°C. Working solution is 50 µg/mL made by diluting thawed stock 200-fold in distilled water. This can be stored at 4°C for up to 2 wk. Actinomycin is poisonous, a known carcinogen and teratogen, and due care must be taken to avoid all contact.

2.2.3. Arresting Agent

Colcemid (Gibco) 10 µg/mL. Store at 4°C.

2.2.4. Hypotonic Solution

KCl (0.075M) 1.4 g in 250 mL deionized water: Make up fresh for each harvest, and heat to 37°C.

2.2.5. Fix

Acetone-free methanol and glacial acetic acid are freshly mixed in the proportion 3:1.

3. Methods

Aseptic laboratory procedures must be observed to avoid microbial contamination during the culture stages. All centrifugations are carried out in centrifuge with swing-out buckets in the rotor.

3.1. Method 1

1. Dispense 9.5 mL of supplemented RPMI 1640 medium (*see* Notes 1–4) into a sterile culture vessel (*see* Note 5), and inoculate with 0.75 mL of whole blood (*see* Note 6).
2. Incubate at 37°C for 72 h.
3. Inject the culture with 100 μL methotrexate solution (*see* Note 7), and reincubate at 37°C.
4. After 17 h, carefully remove the supernatant above the cell layer, preferably with a tube from a suction pump following the meniscus. Pipeting can be used but is more laborious.
5. Flick the flask with the finger to distribute the cells, and resuspend in 9.5 mL supplemented medium.
6. Add 0.2 mL thymidine (*see* Note 8). Reincubate at 37°C for 3.75 h, or add 0.2 mL 5-bromo-2'-deoxyuridine (*see* Note 8). Reincubate at 37°C for 4.25 h.
7. Maintain the culture at 37°C while adding 60 μL colcemid (*see* Note 9), and incubate for a further 10 min.
8. Gently shake the flask, and transfer the culture to a conical-based centrifuge tube.
9. Centrifuge at 150*g* for 10 min.
10. Suck off the supernatant to around 3 mm above the cell pellet.
11. Flick the tube to distribute the cells and pipet in 10 mL of prewarmed KCl (*see* Note 10).
12. Incubate at 37°C for 10 min.
13. Centrifuge at 150*g* for 10 min.
14. Three layers should be visible, a red cell pellet at the bottom, a slightly opaque layer of white cells, and the supernatant. Suck off the supernatant to within 3 mm of the white cell layer.
15. Flick the tube to loosen the cells. Use a vortex mixer to stir the cells more thoroughly while carefully adding a pipetful of fix dropwise to the middle of the vortex (*see* Note 11). Add two more pipetfuls of fix, and allow to stand for at least 30 min.
16. Centrifuge at 150*g* for 10 min, and remove most of the supernatant. Flick tube to resuspend cells, and add 2 pipetfuls of fix.

17. Centrifuge at 150*g* for 10 min, and remove most of the supernatant. Flick tube to resuspend cells, and add 1 pipetful of fix.
18. Centrifuge at 150*g* for 10 min, and remove supernatant to just above cell pellet. Flick tube to resuspend cells, and add fix to give about 0.5 mL suspension.
19. Mix the suspension gently with a pipet and place a drop on a clean polished microscope slide (*see* Note 12). Allow to air-dry and examine under microscope to check cell density, spreading of chromosomes, and so forth. If cells are too densely packed, add more fix. If too sparse, spin down and reduce volume. Different methods of spreading may have to be adopted.

3.2. Method 2

1. Dispense 9.5 mL of supplemented RPMI 1640 medium (*see* Notes 1–4) into a sterile culture vessel (*see* Note 5), and inoculate with 0.75 mL of whole blood (*see* Note 6)
2. Incubate at 37°C for 68 h.
3. Inject the culture with 100 µL actinomycin D solution (*see* Note 13), followed by 60 µL colcemid solution (*see* Note 9), and reincubate at 37°C for 4 h.
4. Transfer to 15 mL conical-based centrifuge tube, and spin at 150*g* for 10 min.
5. Suck off the supernatant to around 3 mm above the cell pellet.
6. Flick the tube to distribute the cells, and pipet in 10 mL of prewarmed KCl (*see* Note 10).
7. Incubate at 37°C for 10 min.
8. Centrifuge at 150*g* for 10 min.
9. Three layers should be visible, a red cell pellet at the bottom, a slightly opaque layer of white cells, and the supernatant. Suck off the supernatant to within 3 mm of the white cell layer.
10. Flick the tube to loosen the cells. Use a vortex mixer to stir the cells more thoroughly while carefully adding a pipetful of fix dropwise (*see* Note 11). Add two more pipetfuls of fix and allow to stand for at least 30 min.
11. Centrifuge at 150*g* for 10 min and remove most of the supernatant. Flick tube to resuspend cells, and add 2 pipetfuls of fix.
12. Centrifuge at 150*g* for 10 min and remove most of the supernatant. Flick tube to resuspend cells, and add 1 pipetful of fix.
13. Centrifuge at 150*g* for 10 min and remove supernatant to just above the cell pellet. Flick tube to resuspend cells, and add fix to give about 0.5 mL suspension.

14. Mix the suspension gently with a pipet and place a drop on a clean polished microscope slide (*see* Note 12). Allow to air-dry, and examine under microscope to check cell density, spreading of chromosomes, and so on. If cells are too dense, add more fix. If too sparse, spin down and reduce volume. Different methods of spreading may have to be adopted.

4. Notes

1. Good results have been obtained with a number of culture media, including RPMI 1640, RPMI 1603, TC199, and McCoy's 5A. I have chosen the readily available RPMI 1640 (Gibco).
2. Published methods suggest a wide range of supplements. Most consider bovine serum the appropriate source of necessary growth factors, but pooled human serum and even artificial supplements have their advocates. There is strong evidence that the serum chosen affects the timing of the mitotic cycle, and since it is difficult to maintain a source of unchanging material, it must be anticipated that regular checks will have to be kept to optimize timings, especially of the interval between release and harvest 15% fetal bovine serum is chosen here.
3. Antibiotics are normally added to avoid microbial infection. Penicillin and streptomycin are the usual choice. The relatively short culture time means that mycoplasma infection is not a problem.
4. Phytohemagglutinin is unrivaled as mitogen to stimulate lymphocytes to divide. Lyophilized HA15 (Wellcome) is reconstitued with distilled water and added to the culture medium in the proportion 1:100. With a few hematological conditions, it may be necessary to use pokeweed mitogen as well.
5. Heparinized peripheral venous blood is the most readily available and convenient material to produce chromosome preparations. Some workers prefer to enrich the proportion of leukocytes in the inoculum by centrifugation and taking plasma and white cell layers along with some of the red cell layer. I do not do this routinely, but if the medical history of the donor suggests high red cell or low white cell count, it could be advantageous. Specimens from patients on drug therapy or that have taken several days to reach the laboratory often benefit from having plasma replaced by pooled human serum. Blood from neonates normally contains a very high number of leukocytes, and a smaller inoculum will suffice.
6. Several types of culture vessel give good results, and choice may be determined by budget and availability. There is a complex relationship among various dimensions of culture vessel in whole blood culture. In general, glass or plastic can be used, although it is safer to use plasticware

that is designed for tissue culture. The ratio of cell volume of culture to area of base of the vessel is important, and so is the volume of the gas phase above the culture. Plastic or glass Universal containers with a base area 4–5 sq cm are excellent for the recommended 10 mL culture. Tissue culture flasks with similar area of end wall can be used standing on end. If available specimen volume demands smaller culture, then 15 mL glass McCartney bottles give good results with 5-mL cultures using 0.5 mL blood. Plastic Universals with conical base are not suitable.

7. Methotrexate is the most widely used reagent in blocking cells to encourage synchronization to enrich the harvest of chromosomes in early metaphase. Most reliable is Methotrexate injection (Lederle) equivalent to 25 mg in 1 mL. This is diluted to a working solution of $10^{-5}M$ and used to give a final concentration of $10^{-7}M$.

8. Cells are released from the S-phase block by removing the blocking agent and resuspending the cells in medium enriched in thymidine or its analog 5-bromo-2'-deoxyuridine. Some published methods require the blocking agent to be washed from the cells, but I prefer to minimize the handling of the culture, which may result in cell loss or damage and also requires more time and labor. The medium is simply sucked from above the cells, and the cell are resuspended in fresh medium with the release agent. Thymidine is used as release agent for cultures that will be banded to show G-bands, whereas bromodeoxyuridine incorporation is far better for staining of R-bands. Although different laboratories may prefer one type of banding, most agree that it is better to have preparations available from both for confirmatory analysis. I run two sets of cultures, one to be released with thymidine and the other with bromodeoxyuridine.

9. There is some debate over the role and efficacy of colcemid used to arrest cells. However, there is no doubt that if it is not used, then the mitotic index drops dramatically, although the proportion of early stages is increased. On balance, I prefer to use 60 µL of 10 µg/mL for a 10 mL culture.

10. The hypotonic stage of the harvest is crucial. Many formulations are published, but the most popular is still $0.075M$ potassium chloride. In my experience, it is better if this solution is made up in deionized rather than distilled water.

11. The first fixation stage is the most important. The red cells will fuse into insoluble clumps entrapping the lymphocytes if the cells are not vortexed and the fix added dropwise to the middle of the vortex. Acetone-free methanol may require to be filtered before use. Three parts methanol and one part glacial acetic acid should be mixed in quantity required just before use.

12. The spreading of cells on the slide depends on the size of the drop of cell suspension, cell density, slide surface, ambient temperature, humidity, and so on. If spreading is not satisfactory on a dry polished slide, the following can be tried:
    a. Breathing on the slide just before placing the drop.
    b. Suspending slide above an open 60°C water bath.
    c. Chilling slide.
    d. Reducing or increasing size of drop.
    e. Altering the height above the slide from which to drop the cells.
13. I agree with Wiley et al. *(17)* that actinomycin D and colcemid together give a high mitotic index. Although actinomycin alone gives a higher proportion of early stages, I prefer to have more cells of all stages to chose from. I agree also that lower concentration of actinomycin is superior.

References

1. Caspersson, T., Lomakka, G., and Zech, L. (1971) The 24 fluorescence patterns of the human metaphase chromosomes—distinguishing characters and variability. *Hereditas* **67,** 89–102.
2. Sumner, A. T., Evans, H. J., and Buckland, R. A. (1971) New technique for distinguishing between human chromosomes. *Nature New Biol.* **232,** 31–32.
3. ISCN, (1985) *An International System for Human Chromosome Nomenclature* (Harnden, D. G. and Klinger, H. P., eds.) S. Karger, Basel.
4. Yunis, J. J. (1981) Mid prophase human chromosomes; the attainment of 2000 bands. *Hum. Genet.* **56,** 295–298.
5. Drouin, R., Lemieux, N., and Richer, C.-L. (1988) High-resolution R-banding at the 1250-band level. II Schematic representation and nomenclature of human RBG-banded chromosomes. *Cytobios* **56,** 425–439.
6. Schinzel, A. (1988) Microdeletion syndromes, balanced translocations, and gene mapping. *J. Med. Genet.* **25,** 454–462.
7. Hungerford, D. A. (1965) Leukocytes cultured from small inocula of whole blood and the preparation of metaphase chromosomes by treatment with hypotonic KCl. *Stain Technol.* **40,** 333–338.
8. Camargo, M. and Cervenka, J. (1980) Pattern of chromosomal replication in synchronised lymphocytes. I. Evaluation of the methotrexate block. *Hum. Genet.* **54,** 47–53.
9. Yunis, J. J., (1976) High resolution of human chromosomes. *Science* **191,** 1268–1269.
10. Viegas-Pequignot, E. and Dutrillaux, B. (1978) Une méthode simple pour obtenir des prophases et des prométaphases. *Ann. Génét.* **21,** 122–125.
11. Schwartz S., and Palmer, C. G. (1984) High-resolution chromosome analysis: I. Applications and limitations. *Am. J. Med. Genet.* **19,** 291–299.
12. Rybak, J., Tharapel, A., Robinett, S., Garcia, M., Mankinen, C., and Freeman, M. (1982) A simple reproducible method for prometaphase chromosome analysis. *Hum. Genet.* **60,** 328–333.

13. Matsubara, T. and Nakagone, Y. (1983) High-resolution banding by treating cells with acridine orange before fixation. *Cytogenet. Cell Genet.* **35,** 148–151.
14. Ikeuchi, T. (1984) Inhibitory effect of ethidium bromide on mitotic chromosome condensation and its application to high-resolution chromosome banding. *Cytogenet. Cell Genet.* **38,** 56–61.
15. Bigger, T. R. L. and Savage, J. R. K. (1975) Mapping G-bands on human prophase chromosomes. *Cytogenet. Cell Genet.* **15,** 112–121.
16. Rønne, M., Neilsen, K. V., and Erlandsen, M. (1979) Effect of controlled colcemid exposure on human metaphase chromosome structure. *Hereditas* **91,** 49–52.
17. Wiley, J. E., Sargent, L. M., Inhorn, S. L., and Meisner, L. F. (1984) Comparison of prometaphase chromosome techniques with emphasis on the role of colcemid. *In Vitro* **20,** 937–941.

Chapter 2

Chromosome Preparation from Hematological Malignancies

Fiona M. Ross

1. Introduction

Hematological malignancies encompass a wide variety of diseases. To a certain extent the same basic method can be used to prepare chromosomes from all these diseases, largely because they all yield single-cell cultures relatively easily. Nevertheless, the fact that the different malignant cells have different properties is reflected in the differential success of their chromosome preparation; the acute myeloid leukemias are now relatively well understood and, in general, give fairly consistent results. The acute lymphoid leukemias still have major problems with the quality of the abnormal chromosomes, and some diseases, such as Hodgkin's disease, still do not have reliable methods to produce any abnormal metaphases.

The general standard of chromosome preparations from most hematological malignancies has undoubtedly improved greatly during the 1980s. It is not entirely clear, however, just why this improvement has occurred. Certainly, many laboratories have found that the use of synchronizing agents, such as methotrexate or FdU, improves both the length of the chromosomes obtained and the quality of the subsequent banding (1,2). However, this has not been a universal finding, and there is no other single technique available that can be proved to have any significant effect. It seems probable that much of the improvement is simply owing to accumulated experience and considerable attention to detail.

From: *Methods in Molecular Biology, Vol. 29: Chromosome Analysis Protocols*
Edited by: J. R. Gosden Copyright ©1994 Humana Press Inc., Totowa, NJ

The main problems with attempting to prepare chromosomes from malignant tissue are the frequent low mitotic indices and the poor quality of the chromosomes. A variety of conditioned media or potential mitogens have been employed in an attempt to increase the mitotic indices, but apart from the use of polyclonal B-cell mitogens, such as TPA or EBV in B-cell CLL *(3,4),* nothing has been shown to have a good enough effect to become generally accepted. Indeed, great care must be taken when using any potential mitogen since several agents can improve the mitotic index, but they do this by stimulating the normal cells in preference to the abnormal cells *(5).*

An alternative approach to stimulating division is to remove cells that are incapable of dividing. Myeloproliferative disorders, particularly CML, are characterized by the accumulation of large numbers of mature neutrophils, cells that cannot divide under any circumstances. Thus, although these cells are part of the abnormal clone, it makes sense to remove them before culturing the cells for chromosome analysis. Fortunately, a large reduction in neutrophil numbers can be very simply achieved by standard lymphocyte separation techniques. The quality of the chromosome preparations from such cultures is often better than in conventional CML cultures, and it is thought that this may be the result of the reduction in neutrophil enzymes released into the culture by the dying cells.

The most commonly used tissue for the study of chromosomes in hematological malignancies is the bone marrow, which is usually the primary site of disease. However, peripheral blood can be treated as if it were bone marrow in many leukemias, wherever there is a significant proportion of malignant cells capable of spontaneous or stimulated division present. The bone marrow is not the primary site of disease in lymphomas, and is frequently not involved at all. Even where there is lymphoma in the marrow, it is often localized to the peritrabecular areas, and very few of the relevant cells will be found in the aspirate. Lymph node, spleen, or other solid lymphoid deposits give a much better yield of abnormal cells, at least in non-Hodgkin's lymphoma. The problems with these tissues tend to be more in the logistics of getting them to the cytogenetics laboratory. The vast majority of published cases are from single centers where there is good liaison among the operating theater staff, the pathologists, and the cytogeneticists, so that very rapid processing is possible. I have had considerable success, however, with samples sent in from outlying hospitals. The viability of high-grade lymphomas does usually decrease quite rapidly after removal from the body, so that the failure rate will increase with time in transit, but there is little evidence for any such effect in the low-grade lymphomas. Consistent results are not yet appearing for Hodgkin's disease, but it seems probable that such samples will need very rapid processing if any abnormal mitoses are to be found.

The abnormality rates for different leukemias, like the success rates, vary. At one time, it was thought that improvements in techniques would eventually lead to a 100% abnormality rate, at least in the acute leukemias *(6)*. It is now recognized, however, that in at least some cases, all genetic changes in the malignant cells can occur at the submicroscopic level. The most notable example of this is in CML, where the same molecular rearrangement can be achieved by a visible translocation between chromosomes 9 and 22 or a submicroscopic insertion of part of the c-ABL gene from chromosome 9 into the BCR gene on chromosome 22 *(7)*. Whether similar events will be shown to account for all the cases of acute leukemia where no abnormality can be detected (presently around 20–30% in most centers *[8]*) or whether there are also classes of disease where the relevant cells do not divide under current culture conditions will have to await further advances in our understanding of the molecular events in the leukemic process.

2. Materials

All hematological material should be considered potentially dangerous, and therefore, should be handled in sterile safety cabinets; gloves and laboratory coats should be worn by the cytogeneticist. Sterile graduated plastic pastets or Gilson automatic pipets with sterile tips can be used in all situations in preference to needles.

1. Transport medium: Any medium containing heparin and serum can be used if bone marrow or lymphoid tissue samples are to be sent through the post. We use Leibovitz L-15 medium, because it retains a neutral pH for longer than our standard culture medium. To each 500-mL bottle of medium, add 100 mL serum FCS 30,000 IU penicillin + streptomycin, 10 mL 200 mM L-glutamine, and 6000 U preservative-free heparin. The complete medium should be made up fresh every month and thereafter stored at 4°C. If only very short times are involved between collection and processing of samples, a simple saline heparin solution is

adequate. This can be stored for long periods at 4°C. Peripheral blood samples should be sent in lithium heparin tubes.

2. Culture medium: Although a variety of media have been used successfully to culture leukemic cells, the most popular medium is RPMI 1640. The levels of fetal calf serum supplements vary, but I find that 20% is best since this allows some leeway for poorer batches of serum. The medium should also be supplemented with 10 mM L-glutamine and 5000 IU penicillin + streptomycin/mL. Make up the complete medium as required, but use quantities that will ensure that it is all used within 2 wk. Store at 4°C. Unseparated bone marrow and peripheral blood samples will do well in ungassed incubators in this medium. If separated samples and lymph node tissue are being cultured in ungassed incubators, it is advisable to use the HEPES buffered version of RPMI.

3. Culture tubes: The majority of laboratories use 10-mL culture volumes in Universal tubes. I have found considerable benefit, however, from moving down to 5-mL volumes and culturing in flat-sided plastic test tubes. This gives improved gas exchange, which increases the mitotic index, and it has the added advantage that more cultures can be set up from small samples.

4. Mitotic arrest agent: colcemid at 10 μg/mL.

5. Synchronization and release agents: $10^{-5}M$ FdU in PBS; $4 \times 10^{-4}M$ uridine in PBS; $10^{-3}M$ thymidine in PBS. All these solutions can be kept for years at –20°C. Once thawed, store at 4°C, and use within 1 mo. Although the FdU and uridine are always used together, we have found that they are more effective if stored separately.

6. Mitogens: TPA*—store frozen at 1 μg/mL in dimethyl sulfoxide. It is helpful to store very small quantities in Eppendorf tubes to prevent excessive thawing and refreezing. PHA—reagent grade. Store at 4°C after reconstitution, and use within 2 wk.

7. Lymphocyte separation medium: Various commercial preparations are available. The density should be 1.077 g/mL. The method described in Section 3. is for Lymphoprep. If any other preparation is used, follow the manufacturer's instructions for the ratio of separation medium to sample and for optimum centrifuge speed.

8. Hypotonic solution: 0.075M potassium chloride. We prefer to make up only small quantities and use within 2 d (*See* Note 2).

9. Fix: 3 parts methanol to 1 part glacial acetic acid. Fix should be made up immediately before use.

---

*Potential carcinogen. Rinse all containers with methanol.

10. Wright's stain: 2.5 g Wright's stain in 1 L methanol. Stir for 1 h, and then filter through a double thickness of Whatman no. 1 filter paper into a brown bottle. Store for at least 2 wk before use. The bottle must be kept tightly capped between use; otherwise the staining time will become unpredictable.
11. Buffers: Wright's buffer—0.06*M* Sorensen's phosphate buffer, pH 6.8. Add 0.06*M* disodium hydrogen orthophosphate to 0.06*M* potassium dihydrogen orthophosphate to give required pH. The approximate quantities will be 99 and 101 mL, respectively. (Ready prepared Sorensen's phosphate buffer is also available commercially.) Buffer for trypsin staining is the same, but 10 times more dilute.
12. Destaining alcohols, (2 min/alcohol):
    a. 70% Ethanol.
    b. 70% Ethanol.
    c. 95% Ethanol containing 1% HCl.
    d. Methanol. Slides need not be thoroughly dried between alcohols.
13. Trypsin: 5% Bacto-Trypsin in saline made up immediately before use.
14. Slides: Frosted end slides are easiest to label. Commercially precleaned slides may be clean enough for direct use, but it is helpful to clean them further either by rubbing with muslin (taking care not to transfer grease from the hands to the muslin and thence to the slides) or by soaking in acid alcohol (dilute HCl in ethanol).
15. Nigrosin: 0.45%. Once sterilized this will keep for prolonged periods at room temperature.
16. Ammonium chloride: 1.5 m*M,* sterile, stored at room temperature.
17. H_2O_2: 30% in tap water. Store at room temperature, and make up fresh whenever it stops fizzing actively when put on the slides.

3. Method

The precise details of leukemic cytogenetic techniques tend to be laboratory specific. I list here a general outline, but it will be necessary to experiment with some of the steps to determine what is most effective under the given conditions. Certain steps, particularly the actual slide making, may vary from day to day, because chromosome preparation is very sensitive to both ambient temperature and humidity.

3.1. Standard Bone Marrow Culture

3.1.1. Counting and Setting Up
Bone Marrow Samples

The number of cells in a bone marrow sample may differ by three orders of magnitude depending on the cellularity of the marrow, the degree of fibrosis, the competence of the hematologist, and the proportion of the sample required for other investigations. It is thus essential to count the number of nucleated cells in the specimen if consistently high success rates are to be achieved.

1. Mix a small quantity of marrow in transport medium (e.g., 0.1 mL) with an equal quantity of 1% acetic acid containing a little methylene blue. Count in a hemacytometer. If phase-contrast optics are available, the methylene blue is unnecessary.
2. Meanwhile, spin down the marrow cells at 200g for 5 min. Resuspend in culture medium to give 10^7 cells/mL.
3. Add 0.5 mL cell suspension to 4.5 mL culture medium in a flat-sided test tube for each culture required (i.e., final concentration 10^6 cells/mL). Incubate at 37°C. For the choice of cultures to set up, *see* Section 3.6.

3.1.2. Harvesting Standard Cultures

1. Add 0.05 mL colcemid to the culture. Mix and reincubate at 37°C for 30 min.
2. Spin at 200g for 5 min.
3. Remove supernatant and resuspend in 8–10 mL hypotonic solution. Incubate at 37°C for an appropriate length of time. This varies in different laboratories from the minute or two that it takes to resuspend all cultures being harvested together up to 30 min incubation. In general, leukemic cells are likely to require a slightly longer time in hypotonic than PHA-stimulated lymphocytes.
4. Spin at 200g for 5 min.
5. Resuspend in 8–10 mL fix, adding the first 1 mL dropwise while agitating the suspension on a whirlimix. This step is critical to successful chromosome preparation.
6. Leave in refrigerator or freezer for a minimum of 1 h. It will often be convenient to leave cultures in first fix overnight.

3.1.3. Slide Making

1. Change the fix four times by spinning at 200g for 5 min each time.
2. At the final resuspension, add only enough fix to make the suspension slightly turbid.
3. Drop one or two drops of suspension onto a thoroughly clean slide from about 2 cm above the slide. Allow to air-dry.
4. If phase-contrast optics are available, check for suitable cell concentration and metaphase spreading under phase with a 10× lens. If this is not possible, stain the slide for 30 s in 5% Geimsa, and examine with standard optics.

5. If necessary, adjust the cell concentration or method of making the slide (*see* Note 1). When satisfied, make the required number of slides from each culture. (We generally make 4 slides/culture to allow for problems with banding or for additional banding techniques. If the mitotic index is exceptionally low, more than four slides may be required.)

3.1.4. Banding

Two G-banding methods are described here. Wright's banding has two major advantages: It does not bloat the chromosomes as much as trypsin, and therefore analysis of poorly spread metaphases is easier, and poor quality banding from under- or overstaining can be rectified. It is not always possible, however, to produce very sharp bands with good contrast using Wright's stain, and therefore it can be useful to have the trypsin technique available. When this works well, it gives extremely good definition, but the enzymatic treatment of the chromosomes means that mistakes of timing in trypsin cannot be rectified.

3.1.4.1. G-BANDING WITH WRIGHT'S STAIN

1. Place two slides horizontally on a rack over the sink.
2. Add 1 mL Wright's stain to 3 mL buffer in a bijou. Mix rapidly with a pastet, and pipet evenly onto the two slides.
3. Leave for 2–5 min according to the batch of stain.
4. Rinse off the stain in gently running tap water for 5 s.
5. Dry rapidly in a warm air flow. Wright's stain is water-soluble, so that the drying must be rapid and consistent if a uniform effect is to be achieved.
6. Examine under a high dry lens (preferably 63×, but 40× is adequate with practice). If the staining is underdone (chromosomes slightly bloated and pale with only landmark bands visible), simply repeat the staining procedure for an appropriate length of time. If it is overdone (chromosomes dark and approaching block staining), destain the slide by leaving it in each of the destaining alcohols described in Section 2. Dry the slide and stain it again for a shorter period.
7. Mount with DPX or Histomount.

3.1.4.2. G-BANDING WITH TRYPSIN

1. Pipet H_2O_2 onto a horizontal slide. Leave for 30 s to 2 min, depending on the age of the slide (longer for younger slides). Meanwhile, prepare the stain by adding 1 mL Leishman's stain to 2 mL buffer in a Universal.
2. Wash peroxide off with buffer and blot dry.

3. Dip the slide in saline and then very briefly in trypsin.
4. Place the slide on a rack, and immediately flood with stain. Leave until a goldish sheen covers the surface of the stain. Rinse off with buffer. Dry and examine under a high dry lens. Understaining can be corrected by repeating the staining procedure. Overstaining can be corrected by further rinsing with buffer.
5. Mount with DPX or Histomount.

3.1.5. Chromosome Analysis

Since it is usually necessary to analyze large numbers of cells to be sure of detecting clones that form only a small proportion of the dividing cells, it is not generally practicable to analyze from photokaryotypes. With practice, it is possible to analyze most cases down the microscope, the exceptions usually being those with very high chromosome counts or very extensive rearrangement. Wherever possible, I would recommend the construction of at least one hard copy karyotype from all abnormal cases, but in many laboratories, time constraints mean that this is only possible with the aid of an automatic karyotyper.

Care must be taken in the choice of cells to analyze from hematological malignancies, since abnormal cells are often of poorer morphology than their normal counterparts. In general, I recommend scanning the slides very systematically and examining the first 30 metaphases that are found. In most cases, full analysis should be done on at least 10 cells and preferably 15. The remaining 15 should be counted and briefly examined for any obvious anomaly. The standard of chromosome preparations should be such that even quite small unexpected abnormalities should be picked up while counting the cells in this way. If this is not the case, then a higher proportion of the cells must be fully analyzed. An abnormal clone is defined by ISCN (9) as two cells with the same rearrangement or additional chromosome, or three cells with loss of the same chromosome. Care needs to be taken with the latter definition if many cells have been broken during preparation. Thirty cells are ridiculously few in terms of marrow turnover, but the time involved in chromosome analysis usually precludes anything more. Where patients are being followed up after therapy, however, when there was an abnormal clone found at diagnosis, it is relatively quick just to scan 60–100 cells for that abnormality. Again the quality of the banding should be such that all but the smallest additional abnormality will also be detected.

The vast majority of cases can be adequately analyzed from G-banded slides. Occasionally, more specialist staining techniques are required in order to clarify particular rearrangements. Most staining techniques for PHA-stimulated lymphocytes work in the same way on leukemic chromosomes.

3.2. Alternative Cultures

Various modifications of the basic culture technique can help in different situations. Here I list only those methods that I find most useful for routine cultures in a busy diagnostic laboratory.

3.2.1. Synchronization

This may be attempted over any of the first three nights in culture. The methods are identical except for the prior time in culture. If the cells are to be blocked over the first night in culture, it tends to be more successful if they have had 2–4 h to adjust to the culture medium before the blocking agent is added. A recent paper *(10)* suggests that the maximum number of abnormal metaphases are found in cultures harvested after 48 h. Thus, synchronization over the second night in culture is probably the preferred option. In practice, the intervention of weekends often means that cultures have to be blocked over the first night.

1. Add 0.05 mL FdU + 0.05 mL uridine to the culture sometime between 11 AM and 4 PM. Reincubate at 37°C.
2. Add 0.05 mL thymidine 17–22 h later. Reincubate for 5 h 50 min.
3. Add 0.05 mL colcemid and reincubate for 10 min.
4. Harvest as in Section 3.1.2. steps 2–6.

3.2.2. TPA Stimulation

1. Add 0.01 mL TPA to the culture at the time of setting up.
2. Place in a box or wrap in silver foil to exclude light, and incubate at 37°C for either 72 or 120 h.
3. Harvest as in Section 3.1.2. steps 1–6.

3.2.3. PHA Stimulation

1. Add 0.05 mL PHA to the culture at the time of setting up.
2. Incubate for 72 h.
3. Harvest as in Section 3.1.2. steps 1–6.

3.2.4. Cell Separation
for High Neutrophil Count Samples

1. Pipet 10 mL Lymphoprep into a plastic Universal. Carefully layer 10 mL marrow in medium on top of the lymphoprep.
2. Spin at 400g for 15 min.
3. Remove the interface layer into a test tube, and top up to 10 mL with medium.
4. Spin at 200g for 5 min.
5. Discard supernatant, and resuspend in fresh medium. Spin again as before.
6. Resuspend in 5 mL culture medium. Count the number of cells in a hemacytometer (*see* Section 3.1.1.).
7. Set up 5 × 10^6 cells/culture, and treat exactly as unseparated cultures, except that all resuspensions should be carried out by gentle flicking of the tube with a finger rather than by whirlimixing, since the cells tend to be more fragile.

3.3. Leukemic Blood Samples

Many hematological malignancies will have significant numbers of immature cells, normally only found in the bone marrow, in the peripheral circulation. If this is the case, they can be cultured in exactly the same way as bone marrow cells. Although peripheral blood can be counted in a hemacytometer, the vastly greater numbers of red cells compared to bone marrow tend to cause problems. Full blood counts will nearly always have been done by the hematology laboratory on the sample that is sent for cytogenetic analysis; therefore, request that this information be sent with the sample. If the white count is in the normal range (4–10 × 10^9/L), add 0.4 mL/5 mL culture. Reduce the amount added if the count is higher. If the white count is very low, it may be possible to obtain dividing cells, but it is inadvisable to add more than 0.5 mL blood, since the increased numbers of red cells cause problems with the fixation (*see* Note 6).

In CLL, there are vast numbers of relevant cells in the peripheral blood, but these need to be stimulated to divide. I have had most consistent success using TPA stimulation for B-CLL. If specialist studies of CLL are contemplated, however, it may be helpful to use a variety of polyclonal B-cell mitogens (*3,4*).

3.4. Lymph Nodes or Other Solid
Hematological Tissue

The basic techniques for dealing with solid lymphoid tissue are very similar to those for blood and bone marrow once the cells have been put into suspension culture. Lymph nodes should be placed in medium containing serum as soon as possible after removal from the body. This should be done in the pathology laboratory if the cytogenetics laboratory is located in a different hospital. In general, the application of mitogens to lymph node cultures simply results in large numbers of normal metaphases, and therefore, it is not worth setting up such cultures. The exception to this is in well differentiated lymphocytic lymphoma, the solid tissue equivalent of CLL, where TPA is reasonably effective and the unstimulated mitotic index is often very low.

These techniques can also be used for solid myeloid malignancies, such as chloromas or spleen from patients with CML.

1. If a whole lymph node is received, cut through the sample with sterile scissors. If the node is already cut, move straight to step 2.
2. Break up the node by macerating between two sterile defibrilating sticks (*see* Note 7).
3. Add three drops of the cell suspension to three drops of nigrosin, and perform a viable cell count using a hemocytometer.
4. Set up 5-mL cultures similar to those in Section 3.1.1. with 10^6 viable cells/mL.
5. Harvest all lymph node cultures in the same way as marrows, except that a whirlimix should never be used. Do all resuspensions by gentle finger flicking.
6. Slide making is also the same as in Section 3.1.3., except that it may be necessary to put the cells through one or two extra fix changes in order to produce crisper chromosomes.

3.5. Pleural Effusions, Ascitic Fluid, and Other Exudates

These exudates may occur in many types of malignancy, and may contain neoplastic cells or may simply be reactive. They often also contain a lot of fat, dead cells, or otherwise undesirable material that must be discarded before culture.

1. Spin down and resuspend in fresh medium two or three times until the supernatant appears clear.
2. Count the resulting suspension using nigrosin to obtain a viable cell count and thereafter treat as lymph node tissue.

3.6. Choice of Cultures

In order to ensure success, more than one culture must be set up wherever possible. With unlimited time and resources, it would probably be helpful to set up four or five cultures from each specimen, but

Table 1
Culture Priorities by Diagnosis

Diagnosis	Preferred tissue	Direct	On	FdU	TPA	PHA
ANLL, CML[a]						
MDS, MPD	BM		2	1		
ALL	BM	2	1	4	3	3
B-CLL	Blood				1[b]	
T-CLL	Blood				1	1
NHL low-grade	LN		1	2	3[c]	
NHL high-grade	LN		3	2		
HD[d]	LN	1	2	3		
MM	BM		2	1	3	

[a]Blood often adequate in CML, particularly at diagnosis.
[b]Both 3 and 5 d.
[c]Potential CLL-type lymphoma only.
[d]Adequate reliable methods not yet certain.

in a busy routine laboratory, I can usually make do with 2 cultures/
sample (with a third set up, but not harvested unless there are problems with the other two). If there are enough cells available, there is
not usually any difficulty in deciding which cultures to set up, even
when the diagnosis is uncertain. The problems arise when there are
only enough cells for a single culture. In Table 1, I list my priorities
for the different diseases. Direct preps are not recommended for
ANLL, since the abnormal clone is often undetectable. This is thought
to be because the predominant dividing population in direct harvests
is erythroid, and these cells may not be part of the abnormal clone
(11). In contrast, a direct harvest is essential in samples whose cells
are likely to have poor viability in culture. Although synchronization
techniques work well in many disorders, such that they are my first
choice for the vast majority of specimens that I deal with, they are
not as good in ALL *(1)*, where they tend to promote the normal cells
at the expense of the abnormal.

4. Notes

1. It is always worth putting more effort into the steps up to and including
   making the slides (Sections 3.1.1.–3.1.3.). Once poor slides have been made,
   nothing can rescue them. If the chromosomes appear fuzzy, it may help
   to change the fix another two or three times before making more slides.

If the chromosomes do not spread adequately, check first that the slides are clean enough; a drop of fixed material placed on a dry slide should spread out absolutely evenly with a smooth edge. Beyond this, each lab has its own methods of attempting to improve spreading. Some of these include breathing on the slide immediately before dropping on the cell suspension, breathing gently on the spreading drop, adding another drop of fix before or after the drop of suspension, dropping from a greater height above the slide, using slides fresh from the refrigerator, or using warm slides. In childhood ALLs, which are notoriously difficult to spread, there is considerable support for the edge-flaming technique–allowing the fix to ignite by bringing the edge of the slide momentarily in contact with a naked flame *(13)*.

2. Some labs find that the water used to make up the hypotonic is critical; deionized water works well, but distilled is disastrous. If distilled water is a problem, the metaphases will fail to spread properly, and the quality will get worse with successive fix changes (Section 2. step 8).

3. In samples from MPDs where there are too few cells to permit separation, it may be helpful to use a low dose of colcemid for a longer time, e.g., 0.01 mL colcemid for 3–16 h. This technique may be useful in any sample expected to have a low mitotic index. Because the chromosomes can become excessively condensed under these conditions if the rate of cell turnover is not as low as anticipated, it is advisable to use this technique on an extra culture rather than as a replacement for a standard culture (Section 3.6).

4. If Wright's stain does not produce enough contrast in the banding, a brief pretreatment with H_2O_2 as for trypsin banding may well help (Section 3.1.4.).

5. If CLL samples arrive at a time that would be inconvenient for a harvest later, it is perfectly acceptable to set them up but leave them in the refrigerator for up to 24 h before incubating. This may even improve the mitotic index (Section 3.6.).

6. If the ratio of red cells to white cells is excessively high (e.g., blood samples or marrow blood from pancytopenic patients), it may be possible to improve the preparations by lysing the red cells with sterile ammonium chloride *(14)* (Section 3.3.). Add ammonium chloride to the marrow or blood sample (up to 5 mm) to make up to 14 mL. Stand at room temperature for 30 min. Spin at 200g for 5 min. Remove supernatant and resuspend in fresh ammonium chloride for another 30 min. Spin as before. Resuspend in culture medium, and set up as standard.

7. Macerating lymph nodes, spleens, and so forth, between defibrilating sticks (Section 3.4.) produces a single cell suspension very easily if the

node has NHL involvement. If scalpels or scissors need to be used, the diagnosis is almost certainly not NHL. HD nodes can be quite difficult and will often require fine chopping with scalpels. Myeloid malignancies tend to give firmer tissues, but they should still break up relatively easily without the use of scalpels.

5. Abbreviations

PHA, Phytohemagglutins; FdU, Fluorodeoxyuridine; TPA, 12-0-Tetradecanoylphorbol-13-acetate; EBV, Epstein-Barr virus; FCS, Fetal calf serum; PBS, Phosphate buffered saline; CML, Chronic myeloid leukemia; CLL, Chronic lymphocytic leukemia; ANLL, Acute nonlymphocytic leukemia; ALL, Acute lymphocytic leukemia; MDS, Myelodysplastic syndrome; MPD, Myeloproliferative disorder; NHL, Non-Hodgkin's lymphoma; HD, Hodgkin's disease; MM, Multiple myeloma.

References

1. Yunis, J. J. (1981) New chromosome techniques in the study of human neoplasia. *Human Pathol.* **12,** 540–549.
2. Webber, L. M. and Garson, O. M. (1983) Fluorodeoxyuridine synchronization of bone marrow cultures. *Cancer Genet. Cytogenet.* **8,** 123–132.
3. Gahrton, G., Robert, K.-H., Friberg, K., Zech, L., and Bird, A. (1980) Nonrandom chromosomal aberrations in chronic lymphocytic leukaemia revealed by polyclonal B-cell mitogen stimulation. *Blood* **56,** 640–647.
4. Morita, M., Minowada, J., and Sandberg, A. A. (1981) Chromosomes and causation of human cancer and leukaemia. XLV Chromosome patterns in stimulated lymphocytes of chronic lymphocytic leukaemia. *Cancer Genet. Cytogenet.* **3,** 298–306.
5. Sun, G., Koeffier, H. P., Gale, R. P., Sparkes, R. S., and Schreck, R. R. (1990) Use of conditioned media in cell culture can mask cytogenetic abnormalities in acute leukaemia. *Cancer Genet. Cytogenet.* **46,** 107–113.
6. Yunis, J. J., Bloomfield, C. D., and Ensrud, K. (1981) All patients with acute nonlymphocytic leukaemia may have a chromosomal defect. *New Engl. J. Med.* **305,** 135–139.
7. Kurzrock, R., Gutterman, J. U., and Talpaz, M. (1988) Molecular genetics of Philadelphia chromosome-positive leukemias. *New Engl. J. Med.* **319,** 990–998.
8. Heim, S. and Mitelman, F. (1987) *Cancer Cytogenetics.* Liss, New York.
9. ISCN (1978) An international system for human cytogenetic nomenclature. Birth Defects: original article series, XIV, No. 8, New York, The National Foundation.
10. Li, Y.-S., Le Beau, M. M., Mick, R., and Rowly, J. D. (1991) The proportion of abnormal karyotypes in acute leukaemia samples related to method of preparation. *Cancer Genet. Cytogenet.* **52,** 92–100.

11. Keinanen, M., Knuutila, S., Bloomfield, C. D., Elonen, E., and de la Chapelle, A. (1986) The proportion of mitoses in different cell lineages changes during short-term culture of normal human bone marrow. *Blood* **67,** 1240–1243.
12. Garipidou, V. and Secker-Walker, L. M. (1991) The use of fluorodeoxyuridine synchronization for cytogenetic investigation of acute lymphoblastic leukaemia. *Cancer Genet. Cytogenet.* **52,** 107–111.
13. Williams, D. L., Harris, A., Williams, K. J., Brosius, M. J., and Lemonds, W. (1984) A direct bone marrow chromosome technique for acute lymphoblastic leukaemia. *Cancer Genet. Cytogenet.* **13,** 239–257.
14. Macera, M. J., Szabo, P., and Verma, R. S. (1989) A simple method for short term culturing of bone marrow and unstimulated blood from acute leukemias. *Leuk. Res.* **13,** 729–734.

CHAPTER 3

Meiotic Chromosome Preparation

Ann C. Chandley, Robert M. Speed, and Kun Ma

1. Introduction

The study of chromosomes at meiosis in humans commenced in 1956, when Ford and Hamerton (1) published the first pictures of metaphase I complements of human spermatocytes prepared by "squashing," the only technique available to the meiotic cytogeneticist at that time. A major advance in technique took place, however, when "air-drying" of fixed spermatocytes in suspension superseded squashing *(2),* and this remains the preferred method for preparing human chromosomes for analysis at metaphase I (MI) and metaphase II (MII). The method gives enhanced spreading of the meiotic bivalents at MI, enabling chiasmata to be analyzed and counted, and with the application of C- or Q-banding methods, identification of specific bivalents is made possible. This is also a stage at which structural rearrangements or numerical anomalies can be identified by the univalent, trivalent, quadrivalent, or other multivalent configurations produced. Again, this process of identification being greatly aided by the application of C- or Q- banding techniques. In more recent times, studies have been carried out in which *in situ* hybridization of specific probes to MI bivalents has been used *(3)* and *in situ* nick translation procedures have been applied, for studies of the XY bivalent in particular *(4).*

From: *Methods in Molecular Biology, Vol. 29: Chromosome Analysis Protocols*
Edited by: J. R. Gosden Copyright ©1994 Humana Press Inc., Totowa, NJ

In the 1970s, "microspreading," which had originally been developed to examine the synaptonemal complexes formed between paired chromosomes at meiotic prophase in insect spermatocytes *(5)*, was adapted by Moses et al. *(6)* for use on human spermatocytes. Microspreading provides a simple and quick technique by which a large number of prophase cells can be analyzed from any individual, and meiotic pairing abnormalities, chromosome rearrangements, or numerical anomalies can readily be viewed at this stage. These studies complement those made at MI, and can be especially useful in situations where gametogenic breakdown occurs at the end of the prophase stage (e.g., in X-autosome translocations in males) *(7)* and few, if any, MI divisions are present on the slides. The method has also been successfully applied to human oocytes at the prophase stage, obtained from the ovaries of aborted fetuses *(8–10)*. Depending on the particular analytical requirement, examination of the synaptonemal complexes can be carried out at light microscope (LM) or electron microscope (EM) level. For collection of human oocytes in MI or MII, considerable practical difficulties are encountered, and although a number of attempts to prepare chromosomes in these stages for analysis by air-drying have been made *(11,12)*, high-quality preparations that would allow accurate analysis of, for example, chiasma counts at MI have never really been produced. For further information on this topic and the technical procedures that have been developed, the reader is therefore referred to ref. *13*. The topic will not be covered in this chapter.

Finally, a special air-drying technique using extended hypotonic treatments of spermatocytes has been devised for the production of extended pachytene chromosomes, which can be used for mapping of individual bivalents by the "chromomere" patterns *(14)*. Chromomere preparations have been used to aid the mapping of genes by *in situ* hybridization along the arms of human chromosomes *(15)*, as an alternative to the use of banded somatic chromosomes. In general, accessibility to the *in situ* hybridization procedures appears enhanced in meiotic chromosomes, probe signals being stronger because, it is believed, of the more open DNA conformation of chromatin at meiosis compared with that found at mitosis.

2. Materials

2.1. Method 1: Prophase Analysis of Oocytes Prepared by Microspreading

The following materials are used for Method 1.

1. Dulbecco's phosphate buffered saline (PBS).
2. Fine scalpel (Swann-Morten, Oxoid, UK) Size 20.
3. Microscope slides precleaned in acid–alchohol (two to three drops conc. HCl added to 250 mL methanol).
4. 0.2M Sucrose (filtered).
5. Paraformaldehyde 4% in 0.1M sucrose.
6. NaOH.
7. Borate buffer, pH 9.
8. Photoflo 0.4% (Kodak "Photoflo 600").
9. Gelatin.
10. Formic acid.
11. $AgNO_3$.

If EM analysis is required:

12. Diamond marker.
13. Orange stick.
14. Optilux (Falcon).
15. Chloroform.
16. Rubber adhesive ("Pang" super solution, West Germany).
17. EM grids (G200 HS Cu [Gilder]).

2.2. Method 2: Prophase Analysis of Spermatocytes Prepared by Microspreading

The materials for Method 2 are exactly the same as for Method 1 above.

2.3. Method 3: Prophase Analysis of Spermatocytes (Pachytene) by the "Chromomere" Technique

The following materials are used for Method 3.

1. 0.88% KCl.
2. Methanol.
3. Glacial acetic acid.

4. Giemsa solution (Gurr's phosphate buffered, pH 6.8).
5. 1*M* HCl.
6. 5% Barium hydroxide.
7. 0.3*M* NaCl · 0.03*M* Na$_3$ citrate.

2.4. Method 4: Metaphase I and II Analysis of Spermatocytes by Air-Drying

1. 1% Sodium citrate.
2. Methanol.
3. Glacial acetic acid.
4. Giemsa solution (Gurr's phosphate buffered, pH 6.8).
5. 0.2*M* HCl.
6. 5% Barium hydroxide.
7. 2X SSC.
8. Giemsa solution (Gurr's phosphate buffered, pH 6.8).
9. Distamycin A (Sigma, St. Louis, MO).
10. McIlvaine's citric acid—Na$_2$HPO$_4$ buffer, pH 7.0.
11. DAPI (Sigma).
12. Rubber solution (Pang, Suffolk, UK)

3. Methods

3.1. Method 1: Prophase Analysis of Oocytes Prepared by Microspreading

1. Collect the ovary in Dulbecco's PBS, and cut into small pieces about 2 mm^3 using a fine scalpel (*see* Note 1).
2. Place one piece of tissue onto a clean slide in two to three drops of 0.2*M* (4.5%) sucrose, made up in distilled water and filtered before use.
3. Tease the material apart using the blunt edge of the scalpel and a dissecting needle. Remove large debris, and disperse the cells in the sucrose by gently stirring with the needle. Oocytes will sink through the sucrose and adhere to the slide (*see* Note 2).
4. If cells are required for LM examination only, leave the slide to dry for a minimum of 30 min and even overnight. If EM analysis is required, transfer the cells in sucrose to a plastic-coated slide, and carefully spread over an area 1–1.5 cm^2 without touching the coating. To make the plastic coating, prepare a 0.5% solution of Optilux (Falcon, Los Angeles, CA) plastic in chloroform. Use a Coplin jar for dipping, and then stand the slides on end in a rack to dry in dust-free atmosphere. This procedure is best carried out in a fume cupboard. When dry, seal the plastic

coating to the edges of the slide with rubber adhesive (e.g., Pang) (*see* Note 3).

3.1.1. Fixing

Fix the cells in paraformaldehyde for 5–10 min. Drain off all excess fix and wash the slide for 30 s in 0.4% photoflo from a wash bottle. Allow the slide to dry on the bench at room temperature.

3.1.2. Staining

1. Prepare a colloidal developer solution by dissolving 2 g of powdered gelatin in 100 mL of deionized water and 1 mL of pure formic acid. Stir constantly for 10 min in order to dissolve the gelatin. The solution is stable for 2 wk.
2. Prepare an aqueous silver nitrate solution by dissolving 4 g of $AgNO_3$ in 8 mL of deionized water. This solution is stable. Store both the colloidal developer and silver solution in capped, amber-glass bottles (*see* Note 5).
3. Pipet two drops of colloidal developer and four drops of $AgNO_3$ onto the surface of the slide containing the spread oocytes. Mix the solutions and cover with a coverslip.
4. Place the slide on the surface of a slide warmer (hot plate) that has been stabilized at 70°C.
5. Within 30 s, the silver staining mixture will turn yellow, and within 2 min, it will turn golden brown. Remove the slide and coverslip, and rinse off the staining mixture using deionized water from a wash bottle.
6. Blot the slide dry immediately, and examine at LM level.

3.1.3. Preparation of Grids for EM Analysis

1. Locate good silver-stained spreads under low power (25X) with the LM. Using a Leitz diamond slide marker, score a circle in the plastic coating around the cells required for EM analysis.
2. When all desired cells on a slide are located, float off the round disks of plastic onto the surface of distilled water contained in a large square glass staining dish. This is achieved by gently lowering the slide at an angle into the water, where the surface tension will pull the disks of plastic away from the slide.
3. Pick up disks one by one as follows. Using watchmaker's forceps, carefully lower an EM grid (G200 HS Cu [Gilder]), to a position under the disk. Gently hold the disk in place on the surface of a grid by means of a strong eyelash mounted to the end of a thin wooden (orange) stick,

and pick up the disk by bringing the grid up under the disk and out of the water. Allow the grids to dry before EM examination.

3.2. Method 2: Prophase Analysis of Spermatocytes Prepared by Microspreading

1. Collect testicular biopsies in Dulbecco's PBS, and chop immediately with fine scissors. Agitate the cells and tubule fragments using a stirring bar and magnetic stirrer for about 15 min (*see* Note 4).
2. Draw off the cell suspension, and centrifuge at 150g for 10 min in a conical centrifuge tube.
3. Discard the supernatant, and resuspend the cells in fresh PBS.
4. Wash the cells three times, and leave in a small volume of PBS.
5. Draw up a small amount of the cell suspension into a Pasteur pipet and allow one drop (~0.02 mL) to hang from its tip. Gently touch this onto the surface of the spreading solution (0.2M sucrose in distilled water). Disperse the cells in the sucrose by gently stirring with a dissecting needle. Spermatocytes will sink through the sucrose and adhere to the slide.
6. The fixation, staining, and preparation of grids for EM analysis are exactly as described for oocytes in Sections 3.1.1.–3.1.3. (*see* Note 5).

3.3. Method 3: Prophase Analysis of Spermatocytes (Pachytene) by the "Chromomere" Technique (14)

1. Immerse testicular fragments in 10 mL of 0.88% KCl and keep at room temperature for 8–10 h.
2. Transfer to fixative (3:1 methanol:glacial acetic acid), and leave overnight at room temperature.
3. On the next day, shred the fragments in the fix.
4. Pipet the cell suspension into a conical vial, and centrifuge at 150g for 7 min.
5. Resuspend the pellet in 5 mL of 45% glacial acetic acid, and then immediately centrifuge at 150g for 5 min.
6. Make preparations by dropping suspension from a Pasteur pipet on clean precooled slides, and gently blow dry over a low gas flame.
7. Stain with phosphate-buffered Giemsa solution (pH 6.8).
8. To visualize centromeres, remove the Giemsa using methanol and place the slides in 1M HCl for 5 min at room temperature. Wash in water and treat for 3 min in 5% barium hydroxide solution at 58°C. After washing, place the slides for 20 min in 2X SSC at 58°C, and adjust the pH to 7.0.
9. The same cells photographed for chromomeres at the end of step 7 can be rephotographed after step 8 (*see* Note 9).

3.4. Method 4: Metaphase I and II Analysis of Spermatocytes by Air-Drying (2)

1. Collect testicular biopsy in 1% hypotonic sodium citrate (*see* Note 8).
2. After about 20 min, chop the seminiferous tubules very finely with scissors in a glass Petri dish tilted slightly, allowing large pieces of tubule to settle to the bottom.
3. Draw off the cell suspension with a pipet and spin down for 8 min at 450*g* (1500 rpm).
4. Discard most of the supernatant leaving behind just enough sodium citrate covering the cells to flick the cells into a suspension by gently flicking or tapping the sides of the tube.
5. Add fix (3:1 methanol:glacial acetic acid) slowly down the sides of the tube until the volume of cell suspension is about trebled. Then pipet gently but firmly, breaking up any clumps of cells that may be formed. Add more fix to a volume of about 5 mL. Spin down for 8 min at 450*g* (*see* Note 6).
6. Discard supernatant. Add about 5 mL of fix, and allow the suspension to stand at room temperature for about 1 h, or even overnight at 4°C. (*see* Note 7).
7. Spin down for 8 min at 450*g*.
8. Add about 1 mL of fix (freshly prepared) until a slightly cloudy suspension is obtained.
9. Allow clumps to settle to the bottom, and then make a trial preparation by allowing one drop to evaporate onto a clean dry microscope slide. Breathing on the slide immediately prior to dropping the cells may aid spreading, particularly when humidity in the air is low. Examine under phase microscope, and adjust fix if cell suspension appears too thick or too thin (*see* Note 9).

3.4.1. Conventional Staining

A simple and reliable stain for routine analysis of MI (including chiasma counting) and MII chromosomes is freshly prepared Giemsa. Stain for 5–10 min in a Coplin jar. Rinse off with deionized water.

3.4.2. C-Banding

For further and more accurate identification of meiotic bivalents, or in the interpretations of abnormal configurations, C-banding will be helpful (Fig. 1).

1. Place the slides in 0.2*M* HCl at room temperature for 1 h.
2. Rinse with deionized water.

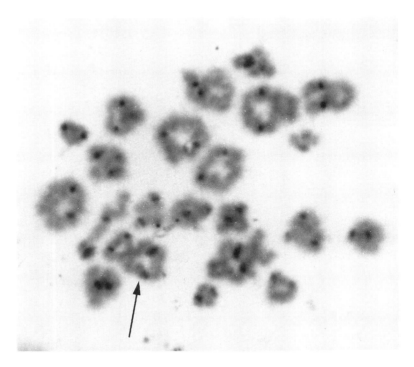

Fig. 1. C-banded air-dried MI preparation from a man with a *t*(9;20) reciprocal translocation. The quadrivalent (arrowed) shows four centromeres, including the prominent C-blocks of chromosome 9. Bivalents show two each. The heterochromatic blocks of bivalents 1,16 and the Y are also prominent. (From ref. *18* with permission).

3. Place the slides in 5% barium hydroxide at 50°C for 30 s.
4. Rinse with deionized water.
5. Place slides with 2X standard saline citrate (SSC) at 60°C for 1 h.
6. Rinse with deionized water.
7. Stain in Giemsa for 45 min to 1 h.
8. Rinse with deionized water, leave for a few minutes to dry thoroughly, soak in xylene, and mount.

3.4.3. Q-Banding

Recent use of the AT-specific peptide antibiotic distamycin A, in combination with the AT-specific fluorescent dye 4',6'-diamidino-2-phenylindole, DAPI (9), on human meiotic bivalents has shown, like

C-banding, that chromosome regions containing constitutive heterochromatin are highlighted. Bright fluorescence is found on pair nos. 1, 9, 16, and the Y chromosome as well as, occasionally, bivalent no. 15 (Fig. 2A). The technique is as follows.

1. Flood the slide with distamycin A (Sigma) solution (0.1–0.2 mg/mL in McIlvaine's citric acid—Na_2HPO_4 buffer, pH 7.0), enough to float a coverslip. Incubate at room temperature for 15 min in the dark in a wet chamber.
2. Wash the coverslip off using a wash bottle containing deionized water.
3. Apply one large drop of DAPI (Sigma) solution (0.2–0.4 g/mL in McIlvaine's buffer, pH 7.0), and lower a fresh coverslip onto the drop. Return the slide to the damp chamber in the dark for 30 min.
4. Wash off again using deionized water.
5. Mount the slide in two drops of McIlvaine's buffer.
6. Blot gently with filter paper until no more buffer comes out.
7. Seal around the coverslip with rubber solution (e.g., Pang).

Distamycin A tends to lack stability in aqueous solution, and it is not recommended to store it in solution. Stained preparations may fade rapidly when first examined, but usually stabilize after a day or so stored in the dark at 4°C. (*see* Note 9).

4. Notes

4.1. Method 1

1. For the collection of human oocytes in various stages of meiotic prophase, fetal ovaries between 16 and 23 wk gestational age are the best. In chromosomally normal fetuses, these should show abundant pachytene cells, with leptotene, zygotene, and some diplotene stages also being present. Chromosomally anomalous fetuses (e.g., XO, trisomic, triploid) may show greatly reduced numbers of oocytes.
2. If storage of slides containing spread oocytes is desired, this can be done in the cold at 4°C after spreading in sucrose. Proceed then by fixing, staining, and so forth, as described.
3. The advantage of analyzing spread oocytes at LM level lies in the ease of identification of the various meiotic prophase stages for rapid ascertainment of the cell stage distribution in a population of, for example, 100 cells. EM level analysis is required for accurate examination of asynapsed and synapsed axes (Fig. 3), and for assessment of abnormal configurations in structural and numerical anomaly (*see* ref. 8).

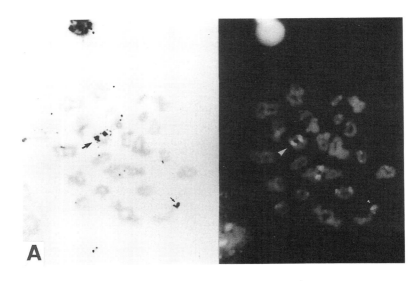

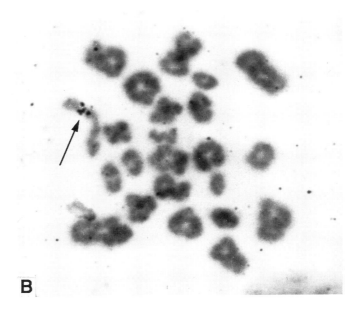

Fig. 2. Isotopic *in situ* hybridization to human MI preparations: (**A**) chromosome 9-specific probe Xb₁, which labels the long-arm heterochromatin. Prior identification of the No. 9 bivalent has been made using Distamycin/DAPI. (From ref. *3* with permission). (**B**) Pseudoautosomal probe 29C1 labeling the XpYp pairing region of the XY bivalent.

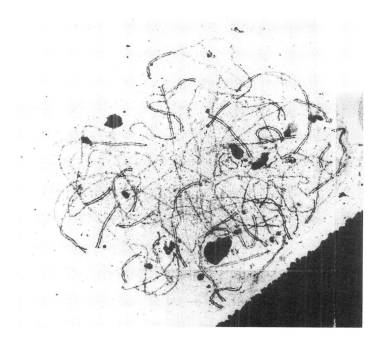

Fig. 3. EM microspread preparation of human oocyte at the zygotene stage when pairing is completed in terminal segments but is still incomplete interstitially. (From ref. *9*, with permission.)

4.2. Method 2

4. To obtain human testicular material, it is necessary to seek the assistance of a cooperative clinical urologist. Usually, the kinds of patients undergoing operations to remove testicular biopsies are those men seeking advice with infertility problems. Much older men with carcinoma of the prostate also sometimes undergo unilateral or bilateral orchidectomy.

5. Because the central element of the tripartite synaptonemal complex is usually not visible when AgNO$_3$ staining is applied to oocytes or spermatocytes, an alternative staining method can be tried using phosphotungstic acid (PTA), although this too may prove temperamental on occasions. The stain is a 1:3 dilution in 95% ethanol of a 4% solution of PTA freshly made up and filtered just before use. Staining can be carried out on EM grids, holding the grid face down on the surface of the ethanol PTA for 1 min with gentle agitation. Drain and transfer to the

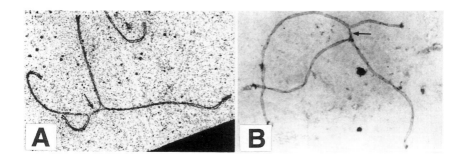

Fig. 4. EM microspread preparation of human spermatocytes at the pachytene stage showing the four-armed quadrivalent of a $t(3;5)$ reciprocal translocation: **(A)** AgNO$_3$ staining, **(B)** PTA staining, which also shows the central element of the synaptonemal complex. (From ref. *17*, with permission.)

surface of 95% ethanol to rinse for 15–30 s. Drain on filter paper and allow to air-dry.

Microspread pachytene spermatocytes from a $t(3:5)$ translocation heterozygote stained (a) with AgNO$_3$ and b) with PTA are shown in Fig. 4. The arrow denotes the interchange segments of the quadrivalent.

4.3. Method 4

6. Primary spermatocytes are large cells that, when swollen by the hypotonic treatment, are very susceptibile to damage. It is very important, therefore, when adding the first fix to the cell suspension, to avoid agitating or bubbling too much. Fix should be added drop by drop down the side of the tube and mixed with the cells by gentle pipeting.

7. The air-drying method can be temporarily stopped after the addition of the second fix. An overnight stop at 4°C followed by centrifugation and refixation for the third and final time can produce much better spreading of the bivalents in MI. If spreading is still poor, additional changes of fix can be tried. C banding applied to an MI cell is shown in Fig. 3.

8. It is important to prepare fresh hypotonic each time a biopsy is collected.

9. Air-dried preparations of human meiotic cells have been successfully used for *in situ* hybridization studies both with isotopic (Fig. 4), and nonisotopic (Fig. 5) methods. The isotopic *in situ* hybridization technique used successfully on meiotic MI bivalents is given in ref. *16*. Fig. 4A illustrates how distamycin A, DAPI staining prior to *in situ* hybridization has been used to make unambiguous identification of bivalent No. 9 in order to localize the probe signal to the proximal long arm segment of fluorescent heterochromatin. Good probe signals using isotopic *in*

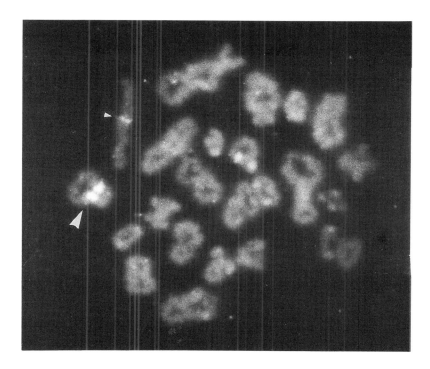

Fig. 5. Nonisotopic *in situ* hybridization to human MI preparation. Alphoid probe pH553 used to label the chromosome 11 centromeres. The X centromere is also prominently labeled (small arrowhead).

situ hybridization have also been obtained *(15)* using Method 3. For nonisotopic *in situ* hybridization to meiotic preparations, the technique described in Chapter 26 can be used.

References

1. Ford, C. E. and Hamerton, J. L. (1956) The chromosomes of man. *Nature,* **178,** 1020–1023.
2. Evans, E. P., Breckon, G., and Ford, C. E. (1964) An air-drying method for meiotic preparations from mammalian testes. *Cytogenetics* **3,** 289–294.
3. Mitchell, A. R., Ambros, P., McBeath, S., and Chandley, A. C. (1986) Molecular hybridization to meiotic chromosomes in man reveals sequence arrangement on the No. 9 chromosome and provides clues to the nature of "parameres." *Cytogenet. Cell Genet.* **41,** 89–95.
4. Chandley, A. C. and McBeath, S. (1987) DNase I hypersensitive sites along the XY bivalent at meiosis in man include the XpYp pairing region. *Cytogenet. Cell Genet.* **44,** 22–31.

5. Counce, S. J. and Meyer, G. F. (1973) Differentiation of the synaptenemal complex and the kinetochore in *Locusta* spermatocytes studied by whole mount electron microscopy. *Chromosoma* **44,** 231–253.
6. Moses, M. J., Counce, S. J., and Paulson, D. F. (1975) Synaptonemal complex complement of man in spreads of spermatocytes, with details of the sex chromosome pair. *Science* **187,** 363–365.
7. Quack, B., Speed, R. M., Luciani, J. M., Noel, B., Guichaoua, M., and Chandley, A. C. (1988) Meiotic analysis of two human reciprocal X-autosome translocations. *Cytogenet. Cell Genet.* **48,** 43–47.
8. Speed, R. M. (1985) The prophase stages in human foetal oocytes studied by light and electron microscopy. *Hum. Genet.* **69,** 69–75.
9. Speed, R. M. (1988) The possible role of meiotic pairing anomalies in the atresia of human fetal oocytes. *Hum. Genet.* **78,** 260–266.
10. Speed, R. M. (1984) Meiotic configurations in female trisomy 21 foetuses. *Hum. Genet.* **66,** 176–180.
11. Yuncken, C. (1968) Meiosis in the human female. *Cytogenetics* **7,** 234–238.
12. Jagiello, G. M., Karnicki, J., and Ryan, R. J. (1968) Superovulation with pituatory gonadotrophins. Method for obtaining meiotic metaphase figures in human ova. *Lancet* **i,** 178–180.
13. Chandley, A. C. (1987) Meiotic analysis in germ cells of man and the mouse. In *Mammalian Development. A Practical Approach.* (Monk, M., ed.) pp. 71–91. IRL, Oxford, UK p. 71–91.
14. Luciani, J. M., Morazzani, M. R., and Stahl, A. (1975) Identification of pachytene bivalents in human male meiosis using G-banding technique. *Chromosoma* **52,** 275–282.
15. Chaganti, R. S. K., Thanwar, S. C., Antonorakis, S. E., and Haward, W. S. (1985) Germ-line chromosomal localization of genes in chromosome 11p linkage: parathyroid hormone, β-globin, c-Ha, *ras*-1, and insulin. *Somat. Cell. Molec. Genet.* **11,** 197–202.
16. Gosden, J. R. (1990) Gene mapping to chromosomes by hybridization *in situ,* in *Methods in Molecular Biology, vol. 5, Animal Cell Culture* (Pollard, J. W., and Walker, J. M., ed.) Humana, Clifton, NJ, pp. 487–500.
17. Guichaoua, M. R., Speed, R. M., Luciani, J. M., Delafontaine, D., and Chandley, A. C. (1992) Infertility in human males with autosomal translocations. II Meiotic studies in three reciprocal rearrangements, one showing tertiary monosomy in a 45-chromosome individual and his father. *Cytogenet. Cell Genet.* **60,** 96–101.
18. Chandley, A. C., Speed, R. M., McBeath, S., and Hargreave, T. B. (1986) A human 9;20 reciprocal translocation associated with male infertility, analysed at prophase and metaphase I of meiosis. *Cytogenet. Cell. Genet.* **41,** 145–153.

CHAPTER 4

Preparation of Chromosomes for Scanning Electron Microscopy

Adrian T. Sumner, Andrew R. Ross, and Elizabeth Graham

1. Introduction

Use of scanning electron microscopy (SEM) to study chromosomes permits their observation at higher resolution than is possible by light microscopy and, at the same time, provides aesthetically pleasing images. Chromosome preparations made for SEM in the three different ways described in this chapter are illustrated in Figs. 1–3. As can be seen, there is a general resemblance among chromosomes prepared by the three different techniques, but also some differences in detailed structure. At present, it is not possible to say which, if any, bears the closest resemblance to the in vivo state.

The methanol–acetic acid fixed chromosomes are probably most convenient for routine morphological studies, because they combine a familiar image with a relatively high degree of preparative success. As well as being used for straightforward morphological studies of mitotic chromosomes at a much higher level of resolution than is possible by light microscopy (*1–3*), such preparations have been used for studies of mechanisms of chromosome banding (*4*) and investigations of chromosome abnormalities, including fragile sites (*5*). It has also been suggested that SEM could be employed usefully for the study of chromosomal heteromorphisms (*6*). Meiotic chromosomes have also been studied (*7*), as well as mitotic, the only practical dif-

From: *Methods in Molecular Biology, Vol. 29: Chromosome Analysis Protocols*
Edited by: J. R. Gosden Copyright ©1994 Humana Press Inc., Totowa, NJ

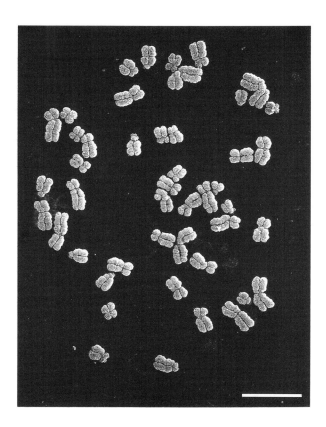

Fig. 1. SEM of human metaphase chromosomes, fixed with methanol–acetic acid. Scale bar = 10 μm.

ferences being in the initial preparation of the chromosomes (*see* Chapter 3). Plant *(8)* and insect (K. Wolf, et al., submitted) chromosomes can also be prepared using similar methods.

Preliminary experiments have also been carried out to combine *in situ* hybridization with SEM of chromosomes. DAB was used as the label for *in situ* hybridization (*see* Chapters 18, 25, and 26), and this becomes strongly impregnated when the chromosomes are osmicated, resulting in a strong hybridization signal, especially using backscattered electrons (Fig. 4). The potential advantage of this approach is the more precise localization of the hybridization signal in relation to morphological features of the chromosomes, although it has not yet

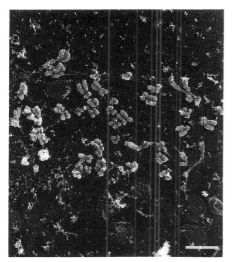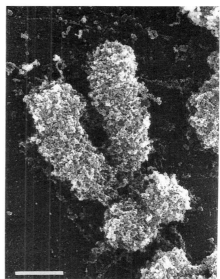

Fig. 2. SEMs of human metaphase chromosomes prepared using the cytocentrifuge method. Left: a metaphase plate. Scale bar =10 μm. Right: a single chromosome from the same metaphase. Scale bar = 1 μm.

been possible to combine *in situ* hybridization with high-quality morphological preservation.

As well as providing alternative approaches to chromosome morphology, the methods using cytocentrifuge preparation and isolated chromosomes have the advantage of using little or no fixation prior to the osmium impregnation procedure. They are, therefore, well suited to the study of chromosomal antigens that might be destroyed or extracted by methanol–acetic acid fixation (Fig. 5).

The principal method used for preparing chromosomes for SEM involves a process of impregnation with osmium tetroxide. This not only appears to stabilize the structure of the chromosomes, but also results in strong secondary electron and backscattered electron signals, which enhance the SEM image. Other treatments, such as mild trypsin digestion, which among other things helps to clear a surface layer of nonchromosomal material from the chromosomes, *in situ* hybridization, and immunocytochemistry, must be carried out before the osmium impregnation.

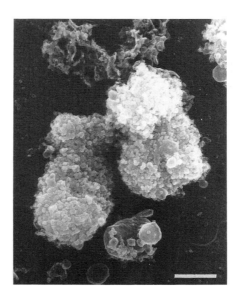

Fig. 3. SEM of an isolated human chromosome. Scale bar = 1 μm.

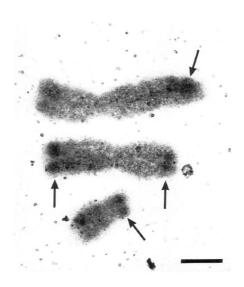

Fig. 4. *In situ* hybridization of a telomeric probe to human chromosomes, viewed using backscattered electrons. Sites of hybridization arrowed. Scale bar = 2 μm.

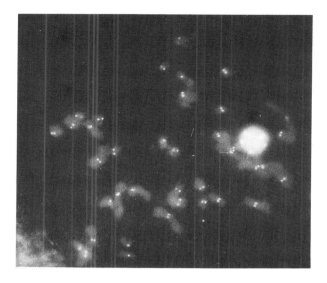

Fig. 5. Cytocentrifuge preparation labeled with CREST serum and horseradish peroxidase-conjugated second antibody, detected using diaminobenzedine and silver intensification. Back-scattered electron image showing paired dots at the centromeres.

2. Materials

1. Difco Bacto trypsin, reconstituted according to the manufacturer's instructions, and then diluted 100X further with distilled water. Use this solution freshly made up.
2. Stenman et al.'s hypotonic solution *(9):* 10 mM HEPES Na (N-2-Hydroxyethyl piperazine-N'-2-ethanesulfonic acid monosodium salt) (2.603 g/L) (pH 7.0), 30 mM glycerol (2.1944 mL/L) 1.0 mM calcium chloride (CaCl$_2$ · 6H$_2$O, 0.2191 g/L), 0.8 mM magnesium chloride (MgCl$_2$ · 6H$_2$O, 0.1626 g/L). Store and use in the refrigerator.
3. Triton X-100: 0.1% in phosphate buffered saline (PBS, Dulbecco "A," tablets obtainable from Oxoid Ltd, Basingstoke, UK).
4. PBS: Dulbecco "A" tablets, Oxoid Ltd., dissolved according to manufacturer's instructions.
5. Glutaraldehyde: 2.5% in 0.1M cacodylate buffer, pH 7.4, containing 0.1M sucrose (34.23g/L) (*see* Note 1).
6. Osmium tetroxide: 1% in distilled water. Use as soon as possible (*see* Note 1).
7. Thiocarbohydrazide (TCH): 0.5% in distilled water. Dissolve at room temperature on the day of use (*see* Note 1).

8. Shandon Cytospin cytocentrifuge (Shandon Southern Products Ltd., Runcorn, Cheshire WA7 1PR, UK).

3. Methods
3.1. Chromosome Preparation

Three distinct procedures have been used to make chromosome preparations for subsequent processing for SEM. Two of these produce metaphase spreads, either fixed conventionally in methanol–acetic acid, or spun down on to a slide or coverslip using a cytocentrifuge. The third method uses isolated chromosomes and, therefore, does not provide the sort of information that can be obtained by examining a whole metaphase; in particular, chromosome identification by relative size is not possible.

In this section, the basic methods of preparing chromosomes are described. Subsequently all three types of preparation go through essentially the same osmium impregnation process, as described in Section 3.2.

3.1.1. Methanol–Acetic Acid Fixation and Spreading

Cultures of dividing cells are fixed in suspension using methanol–acetic acid in the conventional way (Chapter 1). Apart from a requirement that the spread preparations should be as free from cytoplasm as possible, there are no special requirements for SEM. Chromosome spreads are made either on slides, or better, on 22-mm square coverslips. The latter are easier to break up into small enough pieces to attach to the stub of the SEM, although because of the small area, spreading of the chromosomes may be more restricted. If necessary, the fixed cell suspension should be diluted rather more than would be required for spreading on a slide.

The slides or coverslips bearing the spread chromosomes should be allowed to dry and subsequent processing carried out within the next few days. In practice, the chromosome spreads can be made one day, and all the subsequent processing done the next day.

Before osmium impregnation, methanol–acetic acid fixed chromosome spreads are normally treated briefly with trypsin to remove overlying cytoplasmic proteins, although this may be unnecessary with very clean spreads.

1. Digest the chromosome preparations with trypsin for 5 s.
2. Wash thoroughly with distilled water.
3. Transfer to glutaraldehyde (Section 3.2.1.) for subsequent processing.

If the chromosome spreads are covered with a particularly heavy layer of material, the time of trypsin digestion may be increased, even up to 30 s. In general, however, prolonged trypsin digestion causes noticeable swelling of the chromosomes, followed by their morphological destruction. It is always better to start with clean chromosome spreads than to attempt to clean up bad preparations using prolonged trypsin treatment.

3.1.2. Preparation of Metaphases with a Cytocentrifuge

Metaphase chromosome spreads are made by centrifuging cells onto a slide with a cytocentrifuge and extracting the cytoplasm with detergent, before proceeding to the osmium impregnation.

1. Pellet the cells from a human blood culture, and decant off the supernatant.
2. Resuspend the pellet in 10 mL of Stenman's hypotonic, and leave for 10 min in the refrigerator (*see* Note 3).
3. Shake up the cells, and add aliquots of 0.3 mL to the centrifugation chambers of a Shandon Cytospin cytocentrifuge. Spin the cells down on the slides at 1500 rpm for 10 min.
4. Allow the preparations to dry out. They may be left overnight at this stage or transferred to the next stage as soon as they are dry.
5. Treat with Triton X-100 solution, 5–30 min at room temperature. (*see* Note 4).
6. Wash for 5 min in each of three lots of PBS.
7. Transfer to glutaraldehyde (Section 3.2.1.) for subsequent processing.

If the preparations are to be used for immunocytochemistry, this should be carried out immediately following the PBS washes after the Triton treatment. If necessary, the preparations can be given mild fixation (1% formaldehyde in PBS, or 0.05–0.1% glutaraldehyde in PBS, for 10 min at room temperature) before immunolabeling. This procedure works well for light microscopy, but so far has not been perfected for SEM (but *see* Fig. 5).

3.1.3. Isolated Chromosomes

Isolated chromosomes may be prepared using the polyamine method of Sillar and Young *(11)* (*see* Chapter 12) or, in principle, any other method. However, only the polyamine method has been tested for preparing specimens for SEM.

The chromosome suspension is diluted approximately fivefold with PBS (or chromosome isolation buffer). Coverslips of 13-mm diameter are loaded into wells of a multiwell plate (Falcon 24-well plate, catalog no. 3047, Becton Dickinson, Oxnard, CA), and approx 0.5 mL of the chromosome suspension added. The multiwell plates are then centrifuged for 10 min at 1000 rpm in a Sorvall ST 6000 refrigerated centrifuge at 0–4°C.

Without drying, the coverslips are transferred to glutaraldehyde (Section 3.2.1.) for subsequent processing. This may be done in the multiwell plate by pipeting off the supernatant and replacing it with the glutaraldehyde.

3.2. Osmium Impregnation

This part of the preparation is the same regardless of the method of preparing the chromosomes. It consists of a preliminary treatment with glutaraldehyde, followed by alternating treatments with osmium tetroxide and thiocarbohydrazide.

3.2.1. Method (See Note 2)

1. Fix with glutaraldehyde for 30 min or overnight, whichever is more convenient.
2. Wash thoroughly with tap water.
3. Treat with osmium tetroxide, 5 min.
4. Wash thoroughly with tap water (*see* Note 5).
5. Treat with thiocarbohydrazide (TCH) 5 min.
6. Wash thoroughly with tap water (*see* Note 5).
7. Repeat stages 3–6 as often as needed, until the chromosomes are well blackened (up to 10 more times). (*see* Note 6).
8. Treat with osmium tetroxide, 5 min.
9. Wash thoroughly with tap water.
10. Dehydrate through graded acetone solutions (25, 50, 75, and 100%) and critical point dry from liquid carbon dioxide.
11. Cut the slides or coverslips into small enough pieces, and attach them to the stubs with double-sided adhesive tape.
12. Sputter coat the specimen lightly with platinum.

4. Notes

1. All the solutions used in the osmium impregnation procedure are hazardous; the procedure should be carried out in a fume cupboard, and suitable protective gloves should be worn. Making up and disposing of solutions must also be done with proper precautions, according to local regulations.

2. For handling multiple specimens, it is very convenient to use a holder, such as that supplied by Balzers Union (Balzers High Vacuum Ltd., Milton Keynes, UK) (catalog no. BU 011 124-T) for holding coverslips in a critical point drier. Alternatively, holders may be constructed in the laboratory. PTFE is a suitable material, although it soon becomes blackened by the osmium tetroxide. To economize, containers to hold the osmium tetroxide solution may be machined out of PTFE to fit closely the size of the coverslip holder.

3. The hypotonic solution described here gives good results with human lymphocyte cultures and with various cell lines, but alternative hypotonic solutions *(9,11)* may be more appropriate for different types of cells.

4. The optimal length of treatment with Triton X-100 must be found by experience. Even in the best preparations, there may be parts where the cytoplasm has not been removed sufficiently to reveal the chromosomes. However, there is no evidence that prolonged Triton treatment causes any serious damage to the gross morphology of the chromosomes, although it is conceivable that it would extract chromosomal antigens.

5. It is vital that chromosome preparations are washed very thoroughly between treatments with osmium tetroxide and TCH; otherwise, the two compounds will react and form precipitates all over the specimens.

6. The quality of the results depends on the degree of osmium impregnation, which may be varied by altering the number of alternating treatments with osmium tetroxide and TCH. We routinely use nine stages (i.e., nine of osmium tetroxide and eight of TCH). In some cases, fewer stages may be needed. Excessive osmication is rare, but can produce grossly swollen nuclei and chromosomes, or even obscure cell detail.

References

1. Harrison, C. J., Britch, M., Allen, T. D., and Harris, R. (1981) Scanning electron microscopy of the G-banded human karyotype. *Exp. Cell Res.* **134,** 141–153.
2. Mullinger, A. M. and Johnson, R. T. (1987) Disassembly of the mammalian metaphase chromosome into its subunits: studies with ultraviolet light and repair synthesis inhibitors. *J. Cell Sci.* **87,** 55–69.
3. Sumner, A. T. (1991) Scanning electron microscopy of mammalian chromosomes from prophase to telophase. *Chromosoma* **100,** 410–418.
4. Harrison, C. J., Jack, E. M., and Allen, T. D., (1987) Light and scanning electron microscopy of the same metaphase chromosomes, in *Correlative Microscopy in Biology: Instrumentation and Methods* (Hayat, M. A., ed.) Academic, New York, pp. 189–248.
5. Harrison, C. J., Jack, E. M., Allen, T. D., and Harris, R. (1983) The fragile X: a scanning electron microscope study. *J. Med. Genet.* **20,** 280–285.

50   *Sumner, Ross, and Graham*

6. Harrison, C. J., Jack, E. M., Allen, T. D., and Harris, R. (1985) Investigation of human chromosome polymorphisms by scanning electron microscopy. *J. Med. Genet.* **22,** 16–23.
7. Sumner, A. T. (1986) Electron microscopy of the parameres formed by the centromeric heterochromatin of human chromosome 9 at pachytene. *Chromosoma,* **94,** 199–204.
8. Wanner, G., Formanek, H., Martin, R., and Herrmann, R. G. (1991) High resolution scanning electron microscopy of plant chromosomes. *Chromosoma,* **100,** 103–109.
9. Stenman, S., Rosenqvist, M., and Ringertz, N. R. (1975) Preparation and spread of unfixed metaphase chromosomes for immunofluorescence staining of nuclear antigens. *Exp. Cell Res.* **90,** 87–94.
10. Sillar, R. and Young, B. D. (1981) A new method for the preparation of metaphase chromosomes for flow analysis. *J. Histochem. Cytochem.* **29,** 74–78.
11. Perry, P. E. and Thomson, E. J. (1986) Immunogold labelling of metaphase cells. *Cytogenet. Cell Genet.* **41,** 121–125.

CHAPTER 5

Immortalized Cell Lines

Chromosome Preparation and Banding

Judy Fletcher

1. Introduction

The principle of producing mitotic chromosome preparations for analysis by banding techniques and by *in situ* hybridization is to synchronize the cells by blocking them at cell cycle stages preceding mitosis (G1 or S phase), then releasing the block, and allowing the maximum number of cells to reach the desired stage of mitosis, where the cell is again halted by use of mitotic poisons, usually colcemid, which arrest cells in metaphase by blocking cytokinesis. Clearly, the timing of these stages is cell-type dependent, and therefore a matter for trial and error, once the main principles of the process are understood. The timing of addition of colcemid and the duration of exposure to colcemid will also influence the length of the chromosomes obtained.

Making chromosome preparations from cell lines has become an increasingly complicated business. This is partly because of the ever-increasing number of techniques available to choose from. Each individual cytogeneticist will have his/her own preference on this matter, based on what works best for him or her. In this chapter, I describe the three techniques designed for different cell types, which in my hands routinely give good quality, repeatable chromosome preparations. The one point on which I am sure all cytogeneticists will agree

From: *Methods in Molecular Biology, Vol. 29: Chromosome Analysis Protocols*
Edited by: J. R. Gosden Copyright ©1994 Humana Press Inc., Totowa, NJ

is that to obtain good quality chromosome preparations, it is essential to have a population of healthy well-growing cells. Very careful nurturing of cell lines is therefore necessary to ensure success.

2. Materials

1. Culture medium: RPMI 1640, 10% fetal calf serum, 12.5 mM Mops, 100 µ/mL penicillin, 100 µ/mL streptomycin.
2. Phosphate buffered saline (PBS): Dulbecco A Ca^{2+} and Mg^{2+} free from Oxoid. NaCl 8.0 g/L, KCl 0.2 g/L, Na_2HPO4 1.15 g/L, KH_2PO_4 0.2 g/L. Filter sterilize and store at 4°C.
3. Trypsin: 0.2% 1:250 trypsin in PBS. Trypsin 2.0 g/L, 0.2% phenol red 10.0 mL/L, penicillin 0.06 g/L, streptomycin 0.13 g/L. Filter sterilize and store at 4°C.
4. Versene: Disodium EDTA 0.48 g/L, 0.2% phenol red 12.0 mL/L. Filter sterilize and store at 4°C.
5. Fluorodeoxyuridine (FdU): $10^{-5}M$ in distilled water. Filter sterilize and store in the dark at 4°C.
6. Uridine: $4 \times 10^{-4}M$ in distilled water. Filter sterilize and store at 4°C.
7. Bromodeoxyuridine (BdU): $0.2M$ in distilled water. Filter sterilize and store in the dark at 4°C.
8. Ethidium bromide: 1 mg/mL in distilled water. Filter sterilize and store in the dark at 4°C.
9. Colcemid: 0.01 mg/mL in distilled water. Filter sterilize and store at 4°C.
10. Potassium chloride: $0.075M$ KCl in deionized water. This hypotonic solution is made up immediately prior to use.
11. Fix: 3:1 methanol: acetic acid. Made up immediately prior to use because the mixture esterifies.
12. Bacto Trypsin: From Difco Labs (Detroit, MI). Comes as a freeze-dried vial and is made up to 10.0 mL with sterile distilled water and stored at 4°C.
13. Phosphate buffer: Dissolve Gurr's buffer tablets for pH 6.8, as directed. Store at room temperature.
14. Gurr's R66 Giemsa.
15. Sodium hydroxide: $0.7M$ NaOH in distilled water. Store at room temperature.
16. 2X SSC: Sodium chloride 17.53 g, trisodium citrate 8.82 g; make up to 1 L with distilled water. Store at room temperature.
17. Fischer's Giemsa stock: Fischer's Giemsa stain 1.0 g, glycerol 66 mL, absolute alcohol 66 mL. Preparation: Place the powdered Giemsa stain in a pestle and mortar with 5–10 mL of the glycerol and grind to a paste (10–15 min). Add the rest of the glycerol and stir on a magnetic stirrer at 60°C for 6–8 h. Remove from the heat, and add the 66 mL of ethanol,

and stir on a magnetic stirrer overnight at room temperature. The stain is now ready for use; it should be stored in a tightly stoppered bottle in the dark at room temperature.

18. Centrifuge: Bench centrifuge, e.g., WIFUG 500E.

3. Methods

3.1. Culture Conditions

1. To obtain good chromosome preparations, it is essential to have healthy, well-growing cell populations. For this reason, cells are routinely fed 3 times per week. The better you know the growth rate of your cells at this stage, the easier it is to predict the subsequent timings for chromosome preparations.

2. Splitting cells for chromosomes: The cell lines fall into three major categories.

   a. Suspension-type cultures, e.g., lymphoblastoid cell lines (LCL). These are split by gently pipeting the cell suspension to disperse the clumps, and then diluting the cells by the required amount. A stationary phase flask split 1:3 will normally give good results. If the cells are growing very rapidly, then it is advisable to split the flask 1:5; it is just as bad to have too many cells as too few.

   b. Loosely adherent cells, e.g., cell hybrids with mouse myeloma parentage: These cells require quite gentle treatment. Transfer the culture medium to a sterile Universal, and gently wash the flask with PBS. Harvest the cells using 1:1 v/v versene:PBS. Wash the cells off the flask using the original culture medium, and then dilute appropriately. A confluent flask split 1:5 will normally give good results. If the cells are growing very rapidly, then it is necessary to split the flask 1:8.

   c. Adherent cells, i.e., fibroblast-like cells. Transfer the culture medium to a sterile Universal and wash the flask twice with PBS. Harvest the cells using 1:10 v/v trypsin:versene. Wash the cells off the flask using the original culture medium, and dilute appropriately. It is better to allow the cells to float off themselves; mechanical dispersal often results in the cells coming off in sheets, and the resulting clumps are often very difficult to disperse. However, careful watch must be kept to avoid leaving cells too long in trypsin:versene. A confluent flask split in exactly the same way as the myeloma-type cells will give good results.

3.2. Chromosome Preparation

When splitting flasks for chromosomes, I always use 25 cm^2 flasks, and the final volume should be 10.0 mL.

3.2.1. FdU Technique (Originally Described by Webber and Garson [1]).

1. Blocking the cells: 20–24 h after splitting the flask of cells, add 100 μL of FdU (final concentration 0.1 μ*M*) and 100 μL of uridine (final concentration 4 μ*M*).
2. Releasing the block: 17–20 h later, add 100 μL of BdU (final concentration 20 μ*M*). Timing of this stage is critical: Human cell lines and mouse/human hybrids require 7.5–8 h to obtain good results. Hamster cell lines and hamster/human hybrids require 4.5–5 h.
3. Add 100 μL of colcemid for the final 15–30 min to arrest the cells in metaphase (*see* Note 1).

3.2.2. Ethidium Bromide Technique (Originally Described by Ikeuchi [2]).

1. When maintaining cells for making chromosomes by this method, the cells are kept in a semiconfluent state and only split when the flask is fully confluent (stationary phase). This will give a very crude but reasonably effective means of synchronizing rapidly growing cells. However, the chromosomes are in a more nearly "native" state after this.
2. Seventeen to 20 h after splitting the flask, add 100 μL of ethidium bromide and 100 μL of colcemid.
3. Harvest the cells for chromosomes 2–2.5 h later (*see* Note 2).

3.2.3. Colcemid

1. Synchronize the cells in the same way as for the ethidium bromide technique (Section 3.2.2.).
2. Seventeen to 24 h after splitting the flask, add 100 μL of colcemid.
3. Harvest the cells for chromosome preparation 15–45 min later.

3.3. Harvesting

The cells are harvested in exactly the same way as described previously depending on the cell type (Section 3.1.).

1. Transfer the cells to a 10-mL conical bottom tube, and gently pipet the cell suspension to disperse any clumps. It is important to have a near single cell suspension (*see* Note 3).
2. Spin the cells at 1200 rpm for 5 min at room temperature.
3. Discard the supernatant, and tap the cells into suspension (*see* Note 4).
4. Hypotonic treatment: Resuspend the cells in 7–10 mL of KCl, and leave at room temperature for 8 min. It is best to avoid any clumping at this stage also. If necessary, disperse any clumps by gently pipeting the cell suspension.

5. Spin at 1200 rpm for 5 min at room temperature.
6. Discard the supernatant, and tap the cells into suspension.
7. Fixation: Very slowly and mixing constantly, add 7–10 mL of 3:1 v/v methanol:acetic acid down the side of the tube. It is very important to take great care with this first fixation step, because this will determine the quality of the chromosome preparations.
8. Spin at 1200 rpm for 5 min at room temperature.
9. Discard the supernatant and tap the cells into suspension.
10. Add 7–10 mL of fresh fix. Wash the cells this way three times with fresh fix. After the final spin, tap the cells into suspension and add a small volume of fresh fix; the resulting suspension should be slightly cloudy.
11. Slide making: Slides are soaked in ethanol and polished before use. One drop of cell suspension from a fine-tipped plastic Pasteur pipet is dropped onto the slide and allowed to air-dry. Sometimes breathing on the slide to make the surface moist will assist the spreading. The prevailing atmospheric humidity often influences the need for this.
12. The cell suspensions can be stored for fairly long periods of time at –20°C. Slides can then be made as required by leaving the suspension at room temperature for approx 30 min, and then washing the cells twice with fresh fix and making the slides as described above.

3.4. Staining

3.4.1. Giemsa Banding

The technique routinely used is an adaptation of the Gallimore and Richardson technique *(3):* The slides should be allowed to age for 3–4 d before staining.

1. Incubate the slides in 2X SSC at 60°C for 1–3 h.
2. Wash the slides with distilled water.
3. Incubate the slides in 1% Bacto trypsin in distilled water at room temperature for 20–30 s.
4. Wash the slides with distilled water.
5. Stain the slides in 5% Gurr's R66 Giemsa in buffered distilled water, pH 6.8, at room temperature for 7–8 min.
6. Wash the slides with distilled water and blot dry.
7. Soak in xylene and mount in DPX.

If the slides are to be subsequently stained with the G11 (Section 3.4.2.) technique to identify the human chromosomes, then they should not be mounted at this stage. They should be scanned with the microscope oil put directly onto the surface of the slide. Slides are scanned, and analyzable cells are recorded. This involves either: (1) photographing suitable cells and recording the coordinates to enable you to go back to the same cell after G11 staining, or (2) using the cytoscan automatic karyotyping system (*see* Chapter 11) to record cells and then doing the G11 staining. This facility has dramatically reduced the time taken to analyze hybrids, since it eliminates the need for the time-consuming photography. The image enhancement and chromosome enlargement facilities are also very helpful when analyzing both hybrids and LCLs.

*3.4.2. Destaining and G11 Staining (*See *Note 5)*

1. Place the slides in 3:1 methanol:acetic acid fix at room temperature for 5–10 min. The microscope oil will wash off the slide at this stage.
2. Discard the fix, and wash the slides twice with fresh fix, leaving them in the final wash for approx 1 h.
3. Remove the slides from the fix, and allow to air-dry.

The slides are now ready to stain with the G11 technique. This is an adaptation of the technique described by Alhadeff et al. *(4)*.

1. Place the slides in 2X SSC at 60°C for 10 min.
2. Wash the slides with distilled water.
3. While the slides are in 2X SSC, prewarm 19.0 mL of 0.007*M* NaOH to 37°C. Immediately before use, add 1.0 mL of Fischer's Giemsa stock.
4. Place the slides in the staining solution at 37°C for 10 min.
5. Wash the slides thoroughly in running tap water.
6. Dry in warm air, clear in xylene, and mount in DPX.

If the staining is too red/pink, then increase the staining time or decrease the concentration of NaOH. If the staining is too blue, then decrease the staining time or increase the concentration of NaOH. The mouse or hamster chromosomes should be red/pink with blue centromere regions, and the human chromosomes should be blue.

4. Notes

1. Chromosomes made using the FdU technique will not stain with the G11 technique.
2. Chromosomes made using the ethidium bromide technique will not give good results for *in situ* analysis, but will give excellent Giemsa banding of chromosomes on both LCLs and hybrids. It will also give good subsequent G11 results.
3. It is essential when making chromosome preparations to have a near to single-cell suspension; otherwise you will have very clumped preparations that are difficult to spread.

4. Always handle cells gently. Tap the cell pellets into suspension; never vortex them, or you will have very broken cells. It is then very difficult to find intact cells to analyze.

5. There are several problem areas with the G11 technique. After selecting the G-banded cells, do not leave the microscope oil on the slides for longer than 24 h. The oil leaches the stain out of the cells. Subsequent G11 staining will give either chromosomes with a ghost-like appearance, i.e., the edges stain, but the chromosomes look hollow, or the cells do not take up the stain at all. You can destain the slides and then store them on the bench before doing the G11 staining. Never use xylene to remove the stain, since this leaves a film on the surface of the slide, and the subsequent staining results are unsatisfactory.

6. The Fischer's Giemsa stain does deteriorate over a period of time, and if the staining results suddenly go off, then the first thing to try is to stain slides that have never been banded to check this.

References

1. Webber, L. M. and Garson, O. M. (1983) Fluorodeoyuridine synchronisation of bone marrow cultures. *Cancer Genet. and Cytogenet.* **8,** 123–132.
2. Ikeuchi, T. (1984) Inhibitory effect of ethidium bromide on mitotic chromosome condensation and its application to high resolution chromosome banding. *Cytogenet Cell Genet.* **38,** 56–61.
3. Gallimore, P. H. and Richardson, C. R. (1973) An improved banding technique exemplified in the karyotype analysis of two strains of rat. *Chromosoma (Berl.)* **41,** 259–263.
4. Alhadeff, B., Velivasakis, M., and Siniscalco, M. (1977) Simultaneous identification of chromatid replication and of human chromosomes in metaphases of man–mouse somatic cell hybrids. *Cytogenet. Cell Genet.* **19,** 236–239.

CHAPTER 6

Chromosome Banding and Identification Absorption Staining

Adrian T. Sumner

1. Introduction

Chromosome banding is the use of special staining procedures to induce patterns of longitudinal differentiation along chromosomes, in the absence of any structural differentiation *(1,2)*. Specific chromosomes have characteristic patterns that permit their identification throughout a species and even in related species. Some types of banding, however, draw attention to restricted regions of chromosomes and give indications of the functional properties of those regions: for example, nucleolar organizers (NORs) and kinetochores. Other types of bands show differences in size or staining properties between homologous chromosomes. Thus, although in many cases chromosome banding is used purely or primarily as a means of identifying chromosomes, both normal and abnormal, it can also be used to study chromosomal variation or certain aspects of chromosomal function. In addition, banding is a reflection of certain aspects of chromosome organization that are worthy of study in their own right *(2,3)*.

The functional classification of chromosome bands is dealt with in the next section, and applications of the different types of banding are discussed following the description of each banding method. From the purely technical aspect, however, chromosome banding methods may be divided into those that use absorption staining (described in

From: *Methods in Molecular Biology, Vol. 29: Chromosome Analysis Protocols*
Edited by: J. R. Gosden Copyright ©1994 Humana Press Inc., Totowa, NJ

this chapter), and those that use fluorescence (described in Chapter 7). This is not simply a matter of the type of microscope used to examine the chromosomes, important though this is from a technical point of view. Whereas the great majority of fluorescence banding methods simply involve staining with a fluorochrome (which is different in each method), the banding techniques that use absorption staining, described in the present chapter, all involve some sort of pretreatment before staining, and in most cases, staining is with the Giemsa dye mixture, which is not specific to any particular method.

1.1. The Different Classes of Chromosome Bands

Four different classes of chromosome bands have been recognized (*1,2;* Table 1). Heterochromatic bands are localized as discrete blocks on chromosomes and are almost always present at centromeres, but sometimes also at terminal and interstitial sites. They are believed to correspond to heterochromatin, classically defined as failing to decondense in interphase, commonly (but apparently not invariably) contain highly repeated DNA sequences, and lack conventional genes. Evidence is beginning to emerge that heterochromatic bands may contain distinctive proteins, and these may contribute to their compactness. C-banding demonstrates almost all heterochromatic bands (although one or two exceptions have been reported; ref. 2), whereas other methods that stain heterochromatic bands only stain subsets of the total heterochromatin, thereby permitting distinction between different classes of heterochromatin. Note that all the methods for heterochromatic bands stain only constitutive heterochromatin distinctively. Facultative heterochromatin does not stain distinctively with these methods, although a staining method for facultative heterochromatin has been described (*4*).

Euchromatic bands consist of a series of positively and negatively stained bands throughout the nonheterochromatic parts of the chromosomes. The euchromatic bands that can be stained by such methods as G-banding, R-banding, or various fluorochromes are largely confined to higher vertebrates (reptiles, birds, and mammals), although replication bands that generally show patterns corresponding to those produced by the methods just mentioned may well be universal (*2*). It is still not clear whether the lack of euchromatic bands in the chromosomes of almost all plants, invertebrates, and lower vertebrates genu-

Table 1
The Different Classes of Chromosome Bands
and Techniques for Their Recognition

Class	Principal banding methods (the chapter in which they are described is given in parentheses)
Heterochromatic bands	C-banding (this chapter) G-11 banding (this chapter) Q-banding (Chapter 7) Distamycin/DAPI fluorescence (Chapter 7 and 8)
Euchromatic bands	G-banding (this chapter) Q-banding (Chapter 7) R-banding (this chapter and Chapter 7) T-banding (this chapter) Replication banding
NORs	Ag-NOR staining (this chapter)
Kinetochores	Immunofluorescence staining with CREST serum (Chapter 15 and 16)

Table 2
Properties of Euchromatic Bands

Positive G-bands	Negative G-bands
Positive Q-bands	Negative Q-bands
Negative R-bands	Positive R-bands
Pachytene chromomeres	Interchromomeric regions
Early condensation	Late condensation
Late replicating DNA	Early replicating DNA
A + T-rich DNA	G + C-rich DNA
Tissue-specific genes	"Housekeeping" genes
Long intermediate repetitive DNA sequences (LINEs)	Short intermediate repetitive DNA sequences (SINEs)

inely represents a difference in the organization of the chromosomes in these organisms or whether their absence is owing to technical problems that have not yet been solved. Properties of euchromatic bands are summarized in Table 2; a more extensive listing is given by Holmquist *(5)*. Another property of G-bands, at any rate (it is not clear to what extent the bands shown by other methods behave similarly), is that during chromosome condensation the dark bands fuse together, obliterating the pale bands between them. Thus, a particular chromosome will show fewer bands at metaphase than at prophase. The important practical feature of euchromatic bands is that, since they are not all the same size, they form distinctive patterns characteristic of each chromosome pair of a species and can be used to identify that chromosome, even when translocated or rearranged.

The other two categories of bands are more or less self-explanatory. The nucleolar organizer regions (NORs) are those segments of the chromosomes that contain the genes for ribosomal RNA and on which the nucleoli are formed. The NORs, which contain hundreds or even thousands of copies of the ribosomal genes, commonly appear as constrictions of the chromosomes. The nucleoli are the organelles in which the ribosomal RNA transcribed from the genes in the NORs is processed into preribosomal particles. The final class of band is the kinetochores, the sites of attachment of the spindle microtubules to the chromosomes.

2. Solutions
2.1. C-Banding

1. $0.2N$ Hydrochloric acid (17.2 mL of concentrated acid/L).
2. 5% Barium hydroxide octahydrate in distilled water at 50°C. (Warm 40 mL of distilled water in a Coplin jar in a 50°C water bath; a few minutes before use, add 2 g $Ba(OH)_2 \cdot 8H_2O$, and stir well to dissolve. The scum of barium carbonate that forms on the surface is rarely troublesome, but may be skimmed off if necessary. Discard the solution after an hour or so.)
3. 2X SSC at 60°C: $0.3M$ sodium chloride + $0.03M$ trisodium citrate, made by dissolving 17.53 g of NaCl and 8.82 g of trisodium citrate in 1 L of distilled water. Discard the heated working solution after an hour or two.
4. Giemsa: Add 1 mL of Gurr's Giemsa Improved R66 (BDH) to 50 mL of buffer, pH 6.8, made with Gurr's buffer tablets. Discard after an hour or two, since the dye precipitates after dilution.

2.2. G11 Banding

1. Eosin Y, 2.5 mg/mL in distilled water.
2. Azure B, 10 mg/mL in distilled water.
3. Oxidized methylene blue, 10 mg/mL, with potassium dichromate, 2.5 mg/mL in distilled water. Filter these three stock solutions and protect from light.
4. Phosphate buffer: 50 mM disodium hydrogen phosphate (Na_2HPO_4, 7.098 g/L), brought to pH 11.3 with sodium hydroxide.

5. Staining solution: To 100 mL of the phosphate buffer, pH 11.3, add 1.0 mL of eosin Y stock solution, 1.3 mL of azure B stock solution, and 1.1 mL of oxidized methylene blue stock solution. Stir well and warm to 37°C. Remove surface film of insoluble dye complexes before use. Do not use for more than six slides at once, and discard after use.

2.3. G-Banding: ASG Method

1. 2X SSC at 60°C: 0.3M sodium chloride, 0.03M trisodium citrate, made by dissolving 17.53 g of NaCl and 8.82 g of trisodium citrate in distilled water. Discard the heated working solution after an hour or two.
2. Giemsa: Add 1 mL of Gurr's Giemsa Improved R66 (BDH) to 50 mL of buffer, pH 6.8, made with Gurr's buffer tablets.

2.4. G-Banding: Trypsin Method

1. Trypsin: Reconstitute a phial of Difco Bacto Trypsin (catalog no. 0153-59) with 10 mL distilled water. Dilute approx 100-fold with phosphate buffered saline (PBS), prepared with tablets obtained from Oxoid Ltd., (Basingstoke, UK). Prepare and use this solution fresh, and discard as soon as the quality of banding obtained deteriorates.
2. Giemsa: As for the ASG method, above.

2.5. R-Banding

1. Sodium dihydrogen orthophosphate: 1M solution, made by dissolving 156.01 g of $NaH_2PO_4 \cdot 2H_2O$ in 1 L of distilled water. Preheat to 88°C.
2. Giemsa: 5% Gurr's Improved R66 (BDH) in distilled water. Dilute immediately before use, and discard after an hour or two.

2.6. T-Banding

1. PBS made from buffer tablets (Oxoid Ltd., Dulbecco "A"), and adjusted to pH 5.1 with hydrochloric acid or sodium hydroxide. Preheat to 87°C.
2. Phosphate buffer (10 mM), pH 5.1, preheated to 87°C.
3. Giemsa, 3% in either 10 mM phosphate buffer or PBS.

2.7. NOR Staining

1. Silver nitrate: Dissolve 4 g of $AgNO_3$ in 8 mL of distilled water. This solution is stable if kept in the dark, but must be replaced if any blackening occurs.
2. Colloidal developer: Add 2 g of gelatin to 100 mL of distilled water. Stir continuously with gentle warming to dissolve, and add 1 mL of pure formic acid. This solution should be discarded after about 2 wk.
3. Giemsa: 5% Gurr's Improved R66 (BDH) in Gurr's buffer (pH 6.8) made with Gurr's buffer tablets (BDH).

3. Methods
3.1. Methods for Heterochromatin
3.1.1. C-Banding

The BSG method of Sumner *(6)* is, with variations, the standard method for demonstrating virtually all heterochromatic bands in the chromosomes of plants and of animals, both invertebrates and vertebrates. Chromosome preparations, made in the standard ways for the species concerned (Chapters 1–3,5,7, and 12, ref. *7*), are treated successively with dilute acid, warm barium hydroxide solution, warm saline, and Giemsa stain. These procedures degrade the chromosomal DNA and selectively extract it from the euchromatic parts of the chromosomes, leaving the heterochromatin to be stained more strongly by the Giemsa dye.

C-banding is the universal technique for demonstrating heterochromatin in chromosomes. As such, it remains the primary method for identifying chromosomes in those organisms (plants, invertebrates, and lower vertebrates) that lack euchromatic bands on their chromosomes. In higher vertebrates, C-banding is important for distinguishing the heterochromatin and, thereby, contributing to the complete characterization of the karyotype. Euchromatic bands cannot be demonstrated satisfactorily in meiotic chromosomes, even in higher vertebrates, and here again, C-banding is useful for chromosome identification. C-bands can be demonstrated in nuclei and have been used to study chromosomal distribution at interphase *(8,9)*.

Heterochromatic C-bands characteristically show heteromorphism, that is, they vary in size between homologs in the same individual and between different individuals of the same species *(2)*. Different strains of inbred mice show characteristic patterns of C-band heteromorphism *(10),* and extensive variation in C-band size occurs among different races of a species, as for example in certain grasshoppers *(11)*. In humans, attempts have been made to link C-band heteromorphisms with various clinical conditions, such as infertility, congenital abnormality, and mental retardation, without any significant connection being established, however *(2,12)*. There does, nevertheless, appear to be some correlation between heteromorphisms and various cancers *(13)*. Heteromorphisms have also been used to identify the parental origin of extra chromosomes in trisomic and polyploid cells *(14)* for determining paternity, and for identifying the origin of individual cells, as for example in bone marrow transplants *(15)*.

The chromosome preparations should be allowed to age for about a week before C-banding.

1. Immerse the slides bearing the chromosome preparations in 0.2*N* hydrochloric acid for 1 h at room temperature.
2. Rinse briefly with distilled water.
3. Place in the prewarmed barium hydroxide solution for 1–5 min at 50°C.
4. Rinse thoroughly with distilled water to remove as much barium carbonate scum as possible.
5. Immerse the slides in 2X SSC at 60°C for 1 h.
6. Rinse with distilled water.
7. Stain with Giemsa for 45 min.
8. Rinse surplus dye solution off with distilled water, and carefully blot the slides dry.
9. Allow the slide to dry thoroughly for several minutes at room temperature, and then mount in a synthetic neutral mountant (e.g., DPX). Do not use Canada balsam, which is acidic and causes fading.

A C-banded mammalian metaphase spread is illustrated in Fig. 1 (*See* Note 4.1.).

3.1.2. G11 Banding

G11 banding involves, essentially, staining chromosome preparations with an alkaline solution of Giemsa. This produces distinctive staining of a subset of heterochromatic bands in humans and the great apes. Characteristically, the paracentric heterochromatin of human chromosome 9 is stained a magenta color, whereas the chromosome arms are blue. G11 positive segments also occur on other chromosomes, particularly chromosome 1 *(16)* and the Y chromosome *(17);* these segments, as well as that on chromosome 9 *(18),* comprise only part of the heterochromatin of these chromosomes, and vary in size independently of the total heterochromatin. G11 banding is therefore an important part of the characterization of heterochromatin and the study of its heteromorphisms in humans (and in the great apes). Apparently no other organisms show G11 bands.

The most important application of G11 staining is in distinguishing between primate and rodent chromosomes in cell hybrids. Whereas the primate chromosomes stain blue, with limited regions of magenta

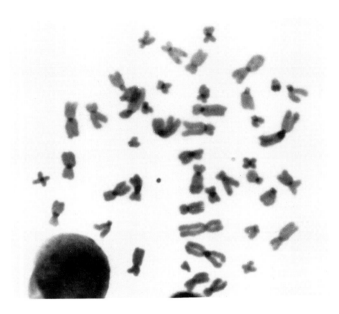

Fig. 1. A C-banded human metaphase spread.

heterochromatin, rodent chromosomes (for example, those of mouse) stain magenta along the arms, with blue heterochromatin *(19,20)*. A partial metaphase of a mouse–human hybrid cell stained in this way is shown in Fig. 2. The G11 staining method is now an essential tool in somatic cell genetics.

The original G11 methods *(21,22)* were rather capricious, and several attempts have been made to devise a more reliable procedure. The one given here is that described by Buys et al. *(19)*.

1. Allow the chromosome preparations to age for 2–3 d before use. Older preparations can be "rejuvenated" by immersion in fresh methanol–acetic acid (3:1) fix.
2. Incubate slides in phosphate buffer, pH 11.3, prewarmed to 37°C, for 1.5 min.
3. Stain for 7–15 min at 37°C in freshly prepared staining solution. Do not stain more than six slides/100 mL of solution.
4. Rinse thoroughly with distilled water.
5. Carefully blot the slides dry, allow to dry thoroughly in air, and mount in a synthetic neutral mountant (e.g., DPX).

A human metaphase chromosome spread-stained by the G11 method is shown in Fig. 3 *(See* Note 4.2.).

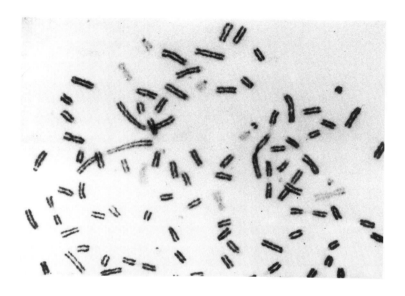

Fig 2.. G11 staining of a mouse–human hybrid cell. Mouse chromosomes appear dark (magenta staining) with pale centromeres (blue staining), whereas human chromosomes are pale except for dark centromeric bands in some cases. Reproduced from Buys et al. (1984) *(19)*, by permission of the authors and Springer-Verlag.

3.2. Methods for Euchromatic Bands

3.2.1. G-Banding

G-banding is the principal method for identifying chromosomes in higher vertebrates and, as such, is probably the most extensively used group of banding techniques. G-banding is an essential part of the characterization of the karyotype of a species. Many species have several chromosome pairs that cannot be distinguished on morphological grounds alone, but are clearly distinct by G-banding.

G-banding patterns remain unaltered when chromosomes are modified, and the techniques are therefore invaluable in numerous clinical situations, such as determining syndromes associated with aneuploidy, deletions, or translocations. Chromosomes involved in Robertsonian translocations can be identified, as well as the complex rearrangements that occur in cultured cells and in cancers. For a more extensive review of the applications of G-banding, *see* Sumner (Section 5.5. of ref. *2*).

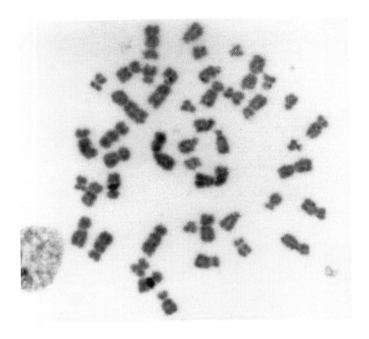

Fig. 3. A G11-banded human metaphase spread.

Two principal methods are in use for G-banding chromosomes, although numerous other procedures have been developed over the years *(2)* and may be useful in particular situations. The ASG method *(23)* generally gives better morphology of the banded chromosomes, although trypsin G-banding methods, based on the procedures of Seabright *(24),* are undoubtedly more widely used.

3.2.1.1. ASG Method *(22)*

Allow the chromosome preparations to age for about a week (acceptable results can probably be obtained between 3 and 14 d, or sometimes much longer).

1. Incubate slides in 2X SSC at 60°C for 1 h.
2. Rinse with distilled water.
3. Stain for 45 min.
4. Rinse thoroughly with distilled water.
5. Blot carefully, allow to dry thoroughly, and mount in a synthetic neutral mountant (e.g., DPX).

A human metaphase and karyotype banded by this procedure are illustrated in Fig. 4 *(See* Note 4.3.).

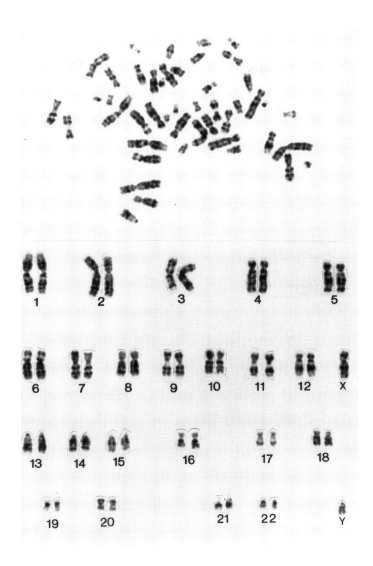

Fig. 4. A human metaphase chromosome spread and karyotype G-banded by the ASG technique. Reproduced from *Nature New Biology,* vol. 232, pp. 31–32. Copyright© 1971 Macmillan Magazines, Ltd.

3.2.1.2. Trypsin-Giemsa Method (after Seabright, Ref. *24*)

1. Digest chromosome preparations with trypsin at room temperature for 5–15 s, by flooding the horizontal slide with the trypsin solution.

2. Rinse slides with distilled water.
3. Stain with Giemsa, 45 min.
4. Rinse thoroughly with distilled water, blot, allow to dry, and mount in synthetic neutral mountant.

A metaphase banded with the trypsin-Giemsa method is shown in Fig. 5 (See Note 4.4.).

3.2.2. R-Banding

R-banding produces a pattern along chromosomes of higher vertebrates that is essentially complementary to that produced by G-banding (i.e., dark R-bands are equivalent to pale G-bands, and vice versa). The method described here is slightly modified from that published by Sehested *(25)*.

In principle, R-banding can be used in the same situations as G-banding, but except in France, it is rarely used as the principal method for chromosome identification in higher vertebrates. There are, however, two situations in which R-banding is particularly useful. First, use of R-banding in combination with G-banding allows more precise delineation of chromosomal breakpoints *(26)*. G-banding is carried out first by incubating the 2-d-old slides, in the phosphate solution adjusted to pH 5.5 with sodium hydroxide, for 10 min at 67°C, followed by staining for 10 min in 5% Giemsa. After observation, the R-banding procedure described below is applied to the slides, but with the incubation time in the phosphate reduced to 5 min *(26)*.

Second, R-banding is valuable in situations where it is necessary to show the ends of chromosomes, which are normally very weakly stained with G-banding. This is useful in the study of various translocations and of terminal deletions of chromosomes.

Allow chromosome preparations to age for about 1 wk before use.

1. Incubate slides in $1M$ NaH_2PO_4 solution for 20 min at 88°C.
2. Rinse briefly with distilled water.
3. Stain with 5% Giemsa solution for 10 min.
4. Rinse with distilled water, blot, allow to dry thoroughly, and mount in a neutral synthetic mountant (e.g., DPX).

Human metaphase chromosomes stained using this technique are shown in Fig. 6 (*See* Note 4.5.).

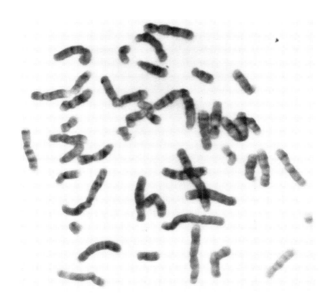

Fig. 5. A human metaphase chromosome spread G-banded using the trypsin method.

3.2.3. T-Banding (27)

This is really a variant of R-banding in which staining of most of the interstitial bands is largely suppressed, so that only the terminal segments of chromosomes, plus a few other regions, are strongly stained.

Use chromosome preparations that are a few days old.

1. Incubate slides in PBS or phosphate buffer, pH 5.1, for 20–60 min at 87°C.
2. Transfer directly to the Giemsa solution for 5–30 min at 87°C.
3. Rinse with distilled water, blot, allow to dry thoroughly, and mount in a neutral, synthetic mountant (e.g., DPX). A T-banded human metaphase is shown in Fig. 7 (*See* Note 4.6.).

3.3. Method for Nucleolar Organizers (NORs)

The sites of nucleolar organizers on chromosomes can be stained specifically with silver. Methods for doing this are referred to as Ag-NOR staining. The method given here was published by Howell and Black *(28)*.

Ag-NOR staining is used to locate NORs on chromosomes of both animals and plants, and is an essential part of the description of a species'

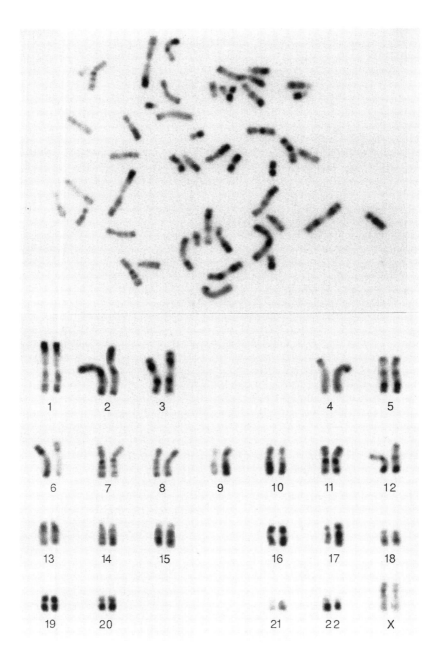

Fig. 6. An R-banded human metaphase chromosome spread and karyotype.

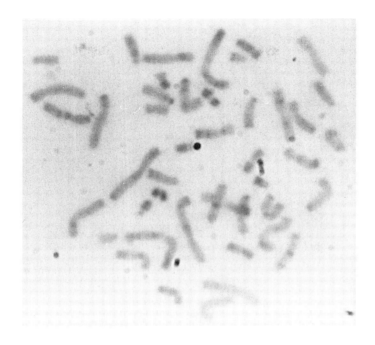

Fig. 7. A T-banded human metaphase chromosome spread.

karyotype. Ag-NOR staining actually reflects NOR activity, so that not all sites of genes for ribosomal RNA are necessarily stained *(2)*. Ag-NOR staining can therefore be used to study changes in ribosomal gene activity in embryonic development and during gametogenesis. Like C-bands, Ag-NOR bands show size heteromorphisms that are heritable, and are thus useful markers for gene mapping and studying the origin of extra chromosomes in trisomies or polyploids. Ag-NOR staining can also be used for studying the ultrastructural organization of the interphase nucleus *(29)*.

Slides are best used 2–3 d after the chromosomes have been spread.

1. Mix two drops of the colloidal developer and four drops of the silver nitrate solution in an Eppendorf tube. Pipet the mixture onto the slide, and cover with a coverslip.
2. Place on a hotplate preheated to approx 70°C. The slide should be removed when the solution turns golden yellow, after 1–2 min.

3. Remove the slide from the hotplate, and wash the coverslip off with a stream of distilled water. Wash thoroughly with distilled water.
4. Counterstain with Giemsa for about 5 min.
5. Rinse with distilled water, blot, allow to dry thoroughly, and mount with a synthetic neutral mountant (e.g., DPX) (*See* Note 4.7.).

Chromosomes showing Ag-NOR staining are illustrated in Fig. 8.

4. Notes
4.1. C-Banding

If the chromosomes are too darkly stained and differentiation is not obvious, it is unlikely to be because the slides have been overstained, but is likely to be because the earlier treatments have been inadequate. Similarly, very pale staining and swelling of the chromosomes are the result of overtreatment. To correct these faults adjust the barium hydroxide treatment: Increase the length of treatment if the chromosomes are too dark, and reduce it if the chromosomes are too pale. If a treatment with barium hydroxide as short as 1 min still seems excessive, reduce the temperature of the solution. Chandley and Fletcher *(30)* found that 37°C was a better temperature for meiotic chromosomes. If reducing the barium hydroxide treatment does not produce sufficient improvement, the treatment with hydrochloric acid may also be reduced, or even omitted completely.

Any other Romanowsky stain besides Giemsa (e.g., Leishman, Wright's, MacNeal's), as well as different formulations of Giemsa, can probably be used successfully instead of the Gurr's R66 specified above. However, it will probably be necessary to adjust the concentration and staining time for each new bottle of dye.

Glass Coplin jars have a distressing tendency to crack when heated, and for the barium hydroxide and 2X SSC solutions, plastic ones are to be preferred. Polypropylene jars remain rigid at the highest temperature used for chromosome banding and are therefore preferable to polythene ones, which may tend to soften. The type of jar without a broad foot is most convenient since it can be hung in the water bath through a metal plate with holes of the appropriate size cut in it.

4.2. G11 Banding

G11 staining is notoriously capricious, and it may be necessary to make minor adjustments in the proportions of the dyes in the staining solution and in the staining time to obtain optimal results. A low cell density on the slides is also required for good differentiation of G11 bands.

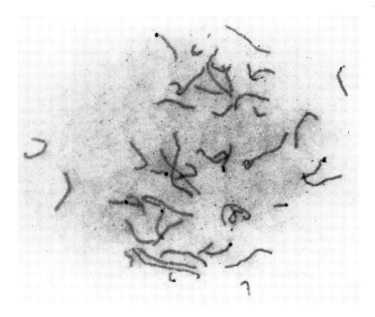

Fig. 8. Nucleolar organizers of human chromosomes stained with silver (Ag-NOR staining).

4.3. G-Banding: ASG Method

The most important factor in obtaining good banding with the ASG method is the use of good chromosome preparations. The chromosomes must be free of any surrounding cytoplasm. They must also not be too contracted, since the bands tend to fuse together as the chromosomes contract and detailed patterns cannot distinguished. If good banding is not obtained, there are few modifications that can be usefully made. Extending the incubation time, even to as much as 16 h, may help, but tends to result in poor chromosome morphology. If the staining is too dark, staining can be done for a shorter time or with a more dilute solution. If necessary, slides can be destained with alcohol (methanol or ethanol) and then restained.

4.4. G-Banding: Trypsin Method

As with the ASG method, good quality chromosome preparations are necessary to obtain satisfactory banding. The trypsin treatment will need to be adjusted, both in time and concentration, to produce optimal results on any particular batch of chromosome preparations. Trypsin, or indeed many other proteolytic enzymes, from a variety of sources may be substituted for the Difco product described above, although adjustments of time and concentration will be necessary.

Undertreated chromosomes will show dark staining and poor banding: Overtreatment produces pale chromosomes with ragged and distorted morphology. A small degree of swelling is required to obtain good banding, and this can be observed by phase-contrast microscopy.

Treatment of the chromosome preparations with hydrogen peroxide (50–60 vol, approx 15–18%) has been recommended for improving results with slides that are too fresh or too old *(31)*. The slides should be laid flat and the hydrogen peroxide poured onto them, left for 5–10 min, and washed off with PBS.

4.5. R-Banding

The original description of this method specified only 10-min incubation in the phosphate solution, and the time given above may therefore be reduced if it results in uniformly pale staining of the chromosomes. Temperature may also be adjusted by a degree or two either way to produce optimal results. R-banding originally suffered from excessively pale staining, and phase-contrast microscopy was recommended to make the bands more visible. However, this is rarely necessary with the method described here, which gives a greater intensity of staining.

4.6. T-Banding

T-band staining is generally rather weak. The times of incubation and of subsequent staining need to be adjusted to produce the best results.

4.7. NOR Staining

It is important to keep the silver staining time as short as necessary to show up NORs, since excessive staining produces a dirty background on the slides and may also result in other structures (e.g., kinetochores) staining. Silver is also deposited on any dirt on the slide, so it is necessary to keep the slides as clean as possible and use them before they have collected any dust.

The length of Giemsa staining should be adjusted so that the chromosome arms are clearly visible, but not so much as to obscure the black silver staining of the NORs. If the chromosomes are overstained, the dye may be extracted with methanol or ethanol, and then restained for a shorter time.

Note that the silver solutions should always be handled with care; otherwise everything they touch will be blackened. Good laboratory technique, plus the use of disposable gloves and a layer of protective paper on the bench, are useful precautions.

5. Microscopy and Photography

Practical details of how to set up a microscope for optimal results are given elsewhere *(32)* and will not be repeated here. Nevertheless, it must be emphasized that correct setting up is necessary to obtain the maximum resolution that is required to see the finest details of banding patterns. Many of these details are near the limit of resolution of light microscopy, and their study requires, therefore, a good microscope equipped with the highest quality objectives. A 10× objective is generally required to scan the slide to find metaphase plates, which are often scarce among a large number of nondividing nuclei. For detailed observation and photography, a 90× or 100× flat field oil immersion objective is used. Apochromatic correction of the objective is not necessary, since it is general practice to use a green filter, which provides maximum contrast and is most comfortable for the eye. Overstained chromosomes may be viewed with a red filter, but this is very tiring for the eye, and it is better to destain the slide and restain it less densely.

For certain purposes, it is useful to prepare banding profiles, that is, scans of the density variation along the banded chromosome. This procedure can bring out details not immediately apparent to the eye, and can be used to make objective comparisons, as for example, between homologs in the same cell or between similar chromosomes in the same or different species. The chromosomes can be scanned directly under a microscope equipped with appropriate photometric facilities, or photographs can be measured using a scanning densitometer. For an example of the results of this procedure, *see* Fig. 9.

General principles of photomicrography have been described by Thomson and Bradbury *(33)*, and Davidson *(34)* has described special requirements for photographing banded chromosomes. Absorption banding generally does not impose especially strict requirements on the photomicrographic system. It is, nevertheless, a good idea to take

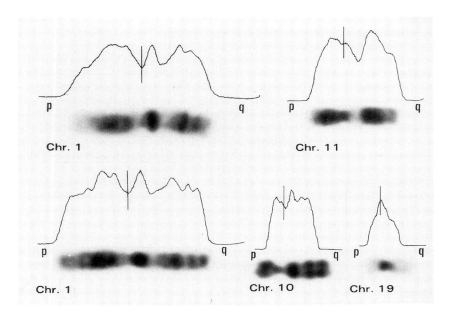

Fig. 9. Optical density profiles of selected G-banded human chromosomes (ASG method). The vertical lines on the profiles mark the position of the centromeres. Reproduced from Sumner (1989) *(37)* by permission of Oxford University Press.

a test strip to determine the optimal conditions for any combination of camera, film, developer, and banding technique. Different exposures can be made by adjusting the exposure time (on a manual camera system) or by altering the film speed setting (on an automatic system). The conditions (i.e., lamp voltages, filters, film type, development conditions, and so forth) must of course be recorded for future reference. A fine grain film is best (e.g., Kodak Technical Pan; Ilford Pan F), and for absorption staining, the relatively slow speed of such films is not a problem. For weakly stained subjects with low contrast, such as R- or T-banding in many cases, it may be desirable to use special developing conditions to produce the greatest contrast on the film. Refer to the manufacturer's literature for information on this point.

6. Karyotyping

One of the main aims of a cytogenetic analysis, particularly when studying banded chromosomes, is to prepare a *karyotype,* in which the chromosomes are arranged in homologous pairs, usually in order of decreasing size, often subdivided according to centromere position (*see* Figs. 4 and 6). Karyotyping necessarily involves taking photographs, and the individual chromosomes are cut out and arranged on a sheet of card or stiff paper. (However, machines are now becoming available for human karyotyping that can perform this process semiautomatically, *see* Chapter 11). For technical reasons, not every metaphase spread will be complete, and ideally, the metaphase should not contain any overlapping chromosomes. If overlaps cannot be avoided, more than one print of the metaphase will be needed to prepare the karyotype. Standard karyotypes have now been published for many mammalian species (*see* Table 2.4 in ref. *2*) in particular for humans *(35)* and mouse *(36).* The system used for numbering chromosome bands devised for human chromosomes *(35)* has been adopted for most other mammalian species, although the system for mouse chromosomes is slightly different *(36).* Such detailed systems for denoting individual bands are, however, less appropriate for species in which euchromatic bands (i.e., G- or R-bands) cannot be obtained.

Once karyotypes have been prepared, a diagrammatic representation of the chromosomes, or *idiogram,* can be prepared. This is based on average measurements of the relative sizes of the chromosomes from a number of different metaphases, and shows the relative positions and sizes of the bands. An idiogram is generally the most satisfactory way of describing the chromosome complement of a species, since it is rare to find a perfectly banded, complete, and undistorted metaphase that can be used to illustrate all the relevant features.

References

1. Sumner, A. T. (1982) The nature and mechanisms of chromosome banding. *Cancer Genet. Cytogenet.* **6,** 59–87.
2. Sumner, A. T. (1990) *Chromosome Banding.* Unwin Hyman, London.
3. Bickmore, W. and Sumner, A. T. (1989) Mammalian chromosome banding— an expression of genome organization. *Trends Genet.* **5,** 144–148.
4. Kanda, N. (1973) A new differential technique for staining the heteropycnotic X-chromosome in female mice. *Exp. Cell Res.* **80,** 463–467.
5. Holmquist, G. P. (1989) Evolution of chromosome bands: molecular ecology of noncoding DNA. *J. Mol. Evol.* **28,** 469–486.
6. Sumner, A. T. (1972) A simple technique for demonstrating centromeric heterochromatin. *Exp. Cell Res.* **75,** 304–306.
7. Macgregor, H. C. and Varley, J. M. (1988) *Working with Animal Chromosomes,* 2nd ed. Wiley, Chichester.

8. Hsu, T. C., Cooper, J. E. K., Mace, M. L., and Brinkley, B. R. (1971) Arrangement of centromeres in mouse cells. *Chromosoma* **34,** 73–87.

9. Fussell, C. P. (1975) The position of interphase chromosomes and late replicating DNA in centromere and telomere regions of *Allium cepa* L. *Chromosoma* **50,** 201–210.

10. Davisson, M. T. (1989) Centromeric heterochromatin variants, in *Genetic Variants and Strains of the Laboratory Mouse* (Lyon, M. F. and Searle, A. G., eds.) Oxford University Press, Oxford, UK, pp. 617–618.

11. Webb, G. C., White M. J. D., Contreras, N., and Cheney, J. (1978) Cytogenetics of the parthenogenetic grasshopper *Warramaba* (formerly *Maraba*) *virgo* and its bisexual relatives. IV Chromosome banding studies. *Chromosoma* **67,** 309–339.

12. Hsu, L. Y. F., Benn, P. A., Tannenbaum, H. L., Perlis, T. E., and Carlson, A. D. (1987) Chromosomal polymorphisms of 1, 9, 16 and Y in 4 major ethnic groups: a large prenatal study. *Amer. J. Med. Genet.* **26,** 95–101.

13. Atkin, N. B. and Brito-Babapulle, V. (1981) Heterochromatin polymorphism and human cancer. *Cancer Genet. Cytogenet.* **3,** 261–272.

14. Hassold, T, Jacobs, P. A., Leppert, M., and Sheldon, M. (1987) Cytogenetic and molecular studies of trisomy 13. *J. Med. Genet.* **24,** 725–732.

15. Khokhar, M. T., Lawler, S. D., Powles, R. L., and Millar, J. L. (1987) Cytogenetic studies using Q-band polymorphisms in patients with AML receiving marrow from like-sex donors. *Human Genet.* **76,** 176–180.

16. Magenis, R. E., Donlon, T. A., and Wyandt, H. E. (1978) Giemsa-11 staining of chromosome 1: a newly described heteromorphism. *Science* **202,** 64–65.

17. Buhler, E. M. (1984) Formal analysis of the Y chromosome in *Aspects of Human Genetics.* (San Roman Cos-Gayon, C. and McDermott, A., eds.) Karger, Basel, pp. 106–118.

18. Donlon, T. A. and Magenis, R. E. (1981) Structural organization of the heterochromatic region of human chromosome 9. *Chromosoma* **84,** 353–363.

19. Buys, C. H. C. M., Aanstoot, G. H., and Nienhaus, A. J. (1984) The Giemsa-11 technique for species-specific chromosome differentiation. *Histochemistry* **81,** 465–468.

20. Bobrow, M. and Cross, J. (1974) Differential staining of human and mouse chromosomes in interspecific cell hybrids. *Nature* **251,** 77–79.

21. Bobrow, M., Madan, K., and Pearson, P. L. (1972) Staining of some specific regions of human chromosomes, particularly the secondary constriction of no 9. *Nature New Biol.* **238,** 122–124.

22. Gagne, R. and Laberge, C. (1972) Specific cytological recognition of the heterochromatic segment of number 9 chromosome in man. *Exp. Cell Res.* **73,** 239–242.

23. Sumner, A. T., Evans, H. J., and Buckland, R. A. (1971) New technique for distinguishing between human chromosomes. *Nature New Biol.* **232,** 31–32.

24. Seabright, M. (1971) A rapid banding technique for human chromosomes. *Lancet* **2,** 971–972.

25. Sehested, J. (1974) A simple method for R-banding of human chromosomes, showing a pH-dependent connection between R and G bands. *Humangenetik* **21,** 55–58.
26. Buckton, K. E. (1976) Identification with G and R banding of the position of breakage points induced in human chromosomes by *in vitro* X-irradiation. *Int. J. Radiat. Biol.* **29,** 475–488.
27. Dutrillaux, B. (1973) Nouveau systeme de marquage chromosomique: les bandes T. *Chromosoma* **41,** 395–402.
28. Howell, W. M. and Black, D. A. (1980) Controlled silver staining of nucleolus organizer regions with a protective colloidal developer: a 1-step method. *Experientia* **36,** 1014–1015.
29. Hernandez-Verdun, D., Hubert, J, Bourgeois, C. A., and Bouteille, M. (1980) Ultrastructural localization of Ag-NOR stained proteins in the nucleolus during the cell cycle and in other nucleolar structures. *Chromosoma* **79,** 349–362.
30. Chandley, A. C. and Fletcher, J. M. (1973) Centromere staining at meiosis in man. *Humangenetik* **18,** 247–252.
31. Seabright, M. (1973) Improvement of trypsin method for banding chromosomes. *Lancet* **1,** 1249,1250.
32. Bradbury, S. (1989) *An Introduction to the Optical Microscope* (rev. ed.), Oxford University Press, Oxford, UK.
33. Thomson, D. J. and Bradbury, S. (1987) *An Introduction to Photomicrography.* Oxford University Press, Oxford, UK.
34. Davidson, N. R. (1973) Photographic techniques for recording chromosome banding patterns. *J. Med. Genet.* **10,** 122–126.
35. ISCN (1985) *An International System for Human Cytogenetic Nomenclature.* (Harnden, D. G. and Klinger, H. P., eds.) Karger, Basel, Switzerland.
36. Evans, E. P. (1989) Standard normal chromosomes (Lyon, M. F. and Searle, A. G., eds.) Oxford University Press, Oxford, UK, pp. 576–581.
37. Sumner, A. T. (1989) Chromosome banding, in *Light Microscopy in Biology* (Lacey, A. J., ed.) IRL, Oxford, UK, pp. 279–314.

CHAPTER 7

Chromosome Banding and Identification

Fluorescence

Adrian T. Sumner

1. Introduction

General characteristics of chromosome banding and banding techniques have been described in the previous chapter (Chapter 6). In general, fluorescence banding provides much the same information as banding using absorption staining, but fluorescence staining methods are generally simpler than banding methods using absorption staining and, in many respects, are more reliable. On the other hand, fluorescent preparations are not permanent and have to be examined using a fluorescence microscope. As well as providing the same general information as banding with absorption staining, most fluorescence banding methods also provide specific types of information (for example, on heteromorphisms of heterochromatin) that are not shown by other methods. Details of these applications will be given under the specific methods.

2. Solutions
2.1. Q-Banding with Quinacrine

1. Aqueous solution of quinacrine (0.5%): Although this dye is generally sold as quinacrine or quinacrine dihydrochloride, note that it is also known as atabrine, atebrin, or mepacrine. This solution is stable, but should be kept in the dark.

From: *Methods in Molecular Biology, Vol. 29: Chromosome Analysis Protocols*
Edited by: J. R. Gosden Copyright ©1994 Humana Press Inc., Totowa, NJ

2.2. *Q-Banding with (CMA)$_2$S*

1. Phosphate buffer, pH 6.5: 10 mM disodium hydrogen phosphate (Na$_2$ HPO$_4$ 2H$_2$O; 1.78 g/L), adjusted to pH 6.5 with 0.2M hydrochloric acid (17.2 mL of concentrated acid/L).
2. Spermine *bis*-acridine, (CMA)$_2$S: Dissolve 5 mg of (CMA)$_2$S in 2 mL of methanol, and make up to 100 mL with phosphate buffer, pH 6.5.

It was formerly necessary to synthesize this compound in the laboratory (*see* ref. *1* and Chapter 18 for a description of the synthesis), but this involves some rather dangerous procedures that should not be attempted by anyone without good practical experience of chemical procedure. Fortunately, (CMA)$_2$S is now available commercially (*bis*-[6-chloro-2 methoxy-9-acridinyl] spermine, Molecular Probes, Inc., 4849 Pitchford Avenue, Eugene, OR 97402. UK agents: Cambridge Bio Science, 25 Signet Court, Newmarket Road, Cambridge CB5 8LA.

2.3. *Hoechst 33258 Banding*

1. Phosphate buffered saline (PBS): Use PBS tablets (Dulbecco "A"; Oxoid Ltd., Basingstoke, UK), and dissolve according to manufacturer's instructions.
2. Stock solution: Dissolve Hoechst 33258 at a concentration of 50 µg/mL in PBS. This solution may be stored indefinitely in the refrigerator.
3. Working solution: Dilute the stock solution 100-fold with PBS to make the staining solution.
4. Mountant: PBS containing 1% sodium dithionite.

2.4. *Chromomycin Staining*

1. Stock buffer: McIlvaine's phosphate-citrate, pH 7. Mix 17.65 mL of 0.1M citric acid (monohydrate, 21.01 g/L) and 82.35 mL of 0.2M disodium hydrogen phosphate (Na$_2$HPO$_4$, 2H$_2$O; 35.60 g/L). Add magnesium chloride to make a concentration of 5 mM (MgCl$_2$ · 6H$_2$O, 0.1017 g/100 mL buffer).
2. Staining solution: Dilute the stock buffer 1:1 with distilled water, dissolve 0.5 mg/mL of chromomycin A$_3$ in the buffer, and add paraformaldehyde to 4%. A stock solution of paraformaldehyde is made by adding 4 g paraformaldehyde to 6 mL of distilled water containing two drops of 5M sodium hydroxide (20%). This mixture is heated until it just boils, allowed to cool, and 1 mL methanol added. After filtering, the solution can be stored at room temperature in the dark. Old staining solutions give better, more stable fluorescence than freshly made ones.

3. Washing buffer: stock buffer diluted 1:1 with distilled water.
4. Mountant: stock buffer diluted 1:1 with glycerol.

2.5. Acridine Orange R-Banding

1. Phosphate buffer, pH 6.5. This consists of 32 mL of 0.07M disodium hydrogen phosphate (12.46 g $Na_2 \cdot HPO_4 \cdot 2H_2O$/L) plus 68 mL of 0.07$M$ potassium dihydrogen phosphate (9.532 g KH_2PO_4/L).
2. Acridine orange, 0.05% in the phosphate buffer, pH 6.5.

3. Methods
3.1. Q-Banding

Q-banding was the first banding technique to come into general use and originally employed the compound quinacrine mustard *(2,3)*, but quinacrine, which is rather safer to handle, is now generally used. An alternative dye, a dimeric analog of quinacrine, gives brighter and more stable fluorescence *(4):* Methods using both dyes are given here.

Q-banding is not particularly sensitive to the method of chromosome preparation. As well as methanol–acetic acid fixed, air-dried preparations (Chapters 1, 2, and 5), squash preparations of material from plants, invertebrates, and lower vertebrates *(5,6)* can be banded successfully with quinacrine.

In higher vertebrates (reptiles, birds, and particularly mammals), Q-banding can be used as an alternative to G-banding for identification of chromosomes. Although less used than formerly for this purpose, its greater reliability makes it valuable where material is scarce or difficult to band, as for example in cancer cells *(7),* in studies of sperm chromosomes made visible by in vitro fertilization of hamster eggs *(8),* and for identification of human pachytene bivalents *(9).* Q-banding can also be combined successfully with procedures for *in situ* hybridization.

Q-banding also stains many, but by no means all, heterochromatic bands. It is, therefore, valuable for identifying chromosomes in lower organisms that lack euchromatic bands (*see* Fig. 1). Quinacrine positive heterochromatic bands, like other blocks of heterochromatin, show size heteromorphisms; in addition, various segments on human chromosomes are heteromorphic for quinacrine brightness (Fig. 2) *(11).* These heteromorphisms provide valuable markers for determining the origin of extra chromosomes in human trisomies *(12,13)* and

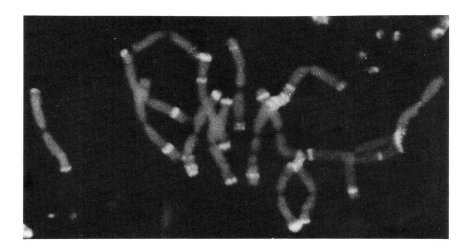

Fig. 1. Q-banded metaphase chromosomes from the plant, *Allium carinatum.* Note that only blocks of heterochromatin stain distinctively. Reproduced from ref. *10* by permission of the author and Springer-Verlag.

triploidies *(13),* as well as distinguishing between donor and recipient cells in bone marrow transplants *(14).*

3.1.1. Q-Banding with Quinacrine

1. Stain the preparations for 6–10 min in the quinacrine solution.
2. Wash in running tap water for 3 min.
3. Rinse and mount in distilled water. Carefully press down on the coverslip with filter paper to remove surplus water, and seal the edges with rubber solution. A fairly runny solution, such as "Pang Supersolution" (Fritz Hesselbein Chemische Fabrik, 2000 Norderstedt, Germany; Pang [UK] Ltd., Newmarket, Suffolk CB8 7A4; Dunfermline, Fife, Scotland) is suitable.

Mounted preparations may be stored overnight for a day or two in the refrigerator, but the quality tends to deteriorate with time. A Q-banded karyotype is illustrated in Fig. 3.

*3.1.2. Q-Banding with Spermine-*Bis*-Acridine ([CMA]$_2$S)*

1. Stain the chromosome preparations for 10 min in the dye solution.
2. Wash with running tap water for 2–3 min.
3. Mount in deionized water, or phosphate buffer, pH 6.5. Blot off surplus mountant, and seal with rubber solution, as for quinacrine staining (Section 3.1.1.).

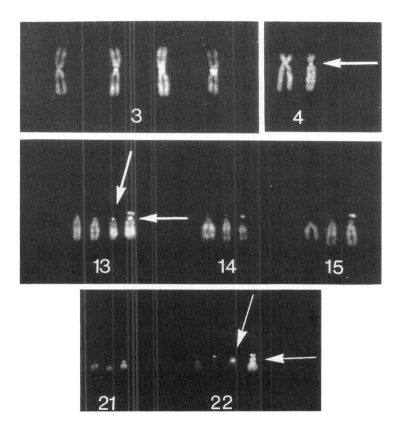

Fig. 2. Quinacrine fluorescence heteromorphisms of human chromosomes. Reproduced from ref. *11,* by permission of Springer-Verlag.

Results are identical with those obtained with quinacrine (*see* Fig. 1), but the fluorescence is brighter and more stable. This is a very reliable method, claimed to give excellent definition of bands even on old chromosome preparations.

3.2. Banding with Hoechst 33258

Hoechst 33258, like quinacrine, produces a pattern on chromosomes of higher vertebrates that resembles G-banding. In the case of Hoechst 33258, however, this pattern is relatively weak, and the dye is more commonly used to distinguish blocks of heterochromatin that contain A + T-rich DNA *(16)*.

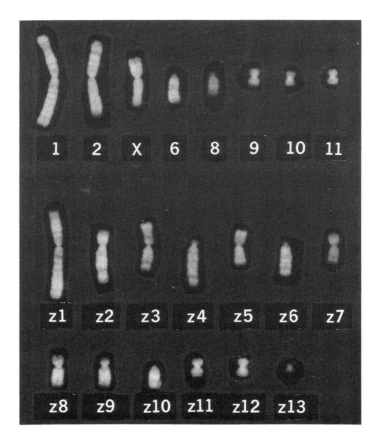

Fig. 3. Karyotype of Q-banded chromosomes from the Chinese hamster ovary (CHO) cell line. The prefix "z" denotes chromosomes that have been modified since they were derived from the animal. Reproduced from ref. *15* by permission of Springer-Verlag.

1. Stain for up to 40 min in the working solution.
2. Rinse with PBS.
3. Mount in PBS solution containing 1% sodium dithionite. Blot off surplus liquid, and seal with rubber solution (*see* Section 3.1.1.).

Mouse chromosomes stained by this procedure are illustrated in Fig. 4. Note the brighter fluorescence of the centromeres of the acrocentric chromosomes, which contain A + T-rich satellite DNA.

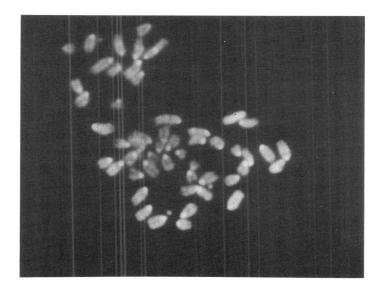

Fig. 4. Chromosomes from a mouse cell line stained with Hoechst 33258, showing brighter fluorescence of the centromeric heterochromatin.

3.3. Banding with Chromomycin and Related Compounds

Chromomycin, and the closely related antibodies mithramycin and olivomycin, bind preferentially to G + C-rich DNA. When used to stain mammalian chromosomes, they produce a fluorescent pattern resembling R-banding. In addition, they produce strong fluorescence with blocks of G + C-rich heterochromatin, including the heterochromatin associated with nucleolar organizers in many species *(17–19)*.

The method described here is based on that published by Schweizer *(20),* with modifications recommended by P. F. Ambros (personal communication).

1. Stain with chromomycin solution for 30–45 min.
2. Rinse briefly with the washing buffer.
3. Mount in the buffer–glycerol mixture. Blot off surplus mountant seal with rubber solution.
4. Age the mounted slides in the dark at 37°C for 3 d before examination.

A metaphase stained with chromomycin is shown in Fig. 5.

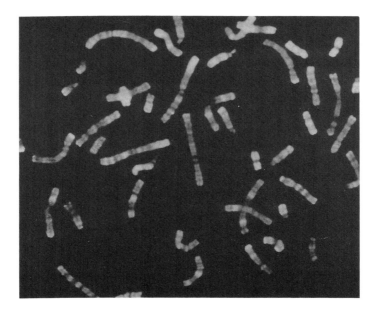

Fig. 5. Human metaphase chromosomes stained with chromomycin A_3. Micrograph kindly provided by P. F. Ambros, and reproduced from ref. *14*.

3.4. Acridine Orange R-Banding

As an alternative to R-banding with Giemsa (Chapter 6), fluorescent R-banding can be obtained using acridine orange. Unlike the other methods described in this chapter, a pretreatment of the chromosome preparations before staining is required. Compared with Giemsa R-banding, acridine orange R-banding generally gives better contrasted and sharper bands. In addition, the short arms of the human acrocentric chromosomes show a fluorescence color polymorphism *(21)*. The method described here is modified from that of Verma and Lubs *(22)*.

Use chromosome preparations approx 1 wk old.

1. Incubate slides for 25 min in phosphate buffer, pH 6.5, preheated to 88°C. Put the solution in a polypropylene slide jar suspended over a water bath.
2. Transfer the slides directly (without rinsing) to the acridine orange solution, and stain for 5 min.

3. Rinse in the phosphate buffer.
4. Mount in the phosphate buffer, blot off surplus buffer, and seal with rubber solution.

A human metaphase spread and karyotype stained by this method is illustrated in Fig. 6. Positive R-bands show yellow-green fluorescence, whereas negative R-bands fluoresce orange-red.

4. Notes

4.1. Q-Banding

Q-banding is a robust technique and normally produces recognizable banding patterns. As with all banding techniques, chromosomes that are reasonably well extended and well spread give the best results.

4.2. Banding with Hoechst 33258

Successful differentiation of A + T-rich heterochromatin is highly dependent on the degree of staining with Hoechst 33258. Overstained chromosomes will tend to show uniform fluorescence. If this happens, both the concentration of the dye and the staining time can be reduced. The concentration of the staining solution may be reduced to as little as 0.05 μg/mL, and the staining time to 10 min. Somewhere between these figures and those given in Section 3.2. for the standard staining method, should give acceptable results. It is helpful to experiment on chromosomes known to contain A + T-rich DNA (e.g., those of the laboratory mouse), although finding a successful combination of dye concentration and staining time for this material does not guarantee success with chromosomes from a different species that may have been prepared in a totally different way. Chromosomes stained with Hoechst 33258 often fade rather rapidly when examined with a fluorescence microscope, but the addition of sodium dithionite to the mounting medium reduces the rate of fading.

4.3. Chromomycin Banding

The main problem with chromomycin is the severe fading of fluorescence that occurs when illuminated. This is greatly reduced, first, by using old dye solutions, and second, by aging the slides for 3 d after they have been stained.

If satisfactory staining is not obtained under the conditions described in Section 3.3., it may help to increase the staining time, even up to

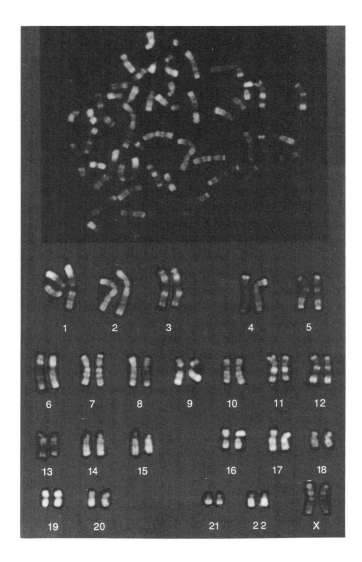

Fig. 6. Acridine orange R-banding of a human metaphase chromosome spread, plus karyotype.

several hours. The inclusion of paraformaldehyde in the solution prevents swelling of the chromosomes during staining. If necessary, the concentration of the stain can also be adjusted.

4.4. Acridine Orange R-Banding

Acridine orange R-banded preparations may range in color from wholly green to wholly red fluorescence. This variation may result from two different factors. Insufficient incubation in the buffer will result in uniform green fluorescence; this can be corrected by using a longer incubation or higher temperature. Excessive incubation results in uniform red fluorescence; this fault can only be cured by incubating another slide for a shorter time or at a lower temperature (the original method prescribed 85°C).

The same effects can be produced by insufficient staining (uniform green fluorescence, which can be corrected by longer staining or a higher dye concentration) or by excessive staining (uniform orange-red fluorescence, which can be corrected by additional rinsing or, for subsequent slides, a shorter staining time or a lower dye concentration—the original method recommended 0.01% acridine orange).

4.5. Microscopy and Photography of Fluorescent-Banded Chromosome Preparations

Fluorescent-banded chromosomes generally produce a low level of fluorescence and tend to fade. Therefore a fluorescence microscope system of the highest efficiency is necessary to obtain satisfactory results. Characteristics of such systems are described in detail elsewhere *(23,24)*. The most important features are the maximum efficiency of illumination and light collection, which are achieved using epi-illumination (incident illumination through the objective) and special objectives for fluorescence work with high light transmission. Such objectives are available from the major microscope manufacturers. It is important to use flat field objectives, especially for photography, but apochromatic correction of the objectives is undesirable, since the large number of lenses in such objectives reduces the light transmission substantially. A low-power oil immersion objective is particularly useful for scanning the slide.

To obtain separation of the incident, exciting radiation, and the fluorescent light, a system of exciter and barrier filters is required. Normally, these are incorporated in a single module with a dichroic mirror to produce the epi-illumination. It is very important for obtaining satisfactory results that the correct filter module is used to match the characteristics of the fluorescent dye being used. Unfortunately there is no universal system of nomenclature for these filter modules, but the different microscope manufacturers should be able to advise on the appropriate filter modules to use with different fluorochromes.

Because fluorescently banded chromosome preparations fade under illumination and are not permanent, it is always necessary to photograph chromosome spreads for analysis. General principles of photomicrography are described in references *(25)* and *(26),* and principles for the photography of banded chromosomes have been described by Davidson *(27).* It is fundamentally important that the microscope be correctly set up and also that, whether an automatic or a manual camera is used, a test strip of the chosen film be exposed with a range of exposure times to establish the optimal conditions. Because of the specialized conditions under which the film is used, the manufacturer's recommended film speed setting is often inappropriate. All relevant details, such as filters and exposure time, as well as the type of film and method of development must, of course, be recorded for future reference.

Because the fluorescence is relatively weak and tends to fade, it would be desirable to use as fast a film as possible. Formerly, this necessitated a compromise, since fast films had a relatively coarse grain that produced a noisy image. Now, however, fast films with a finer grain are available (e.g., Kodak T-max 100 and T-max 400, and Ilford HP5 Plus), and such films are strongly recommended for photographing fluorescently banded chromosomes.

Color transparencies of fluorescent chromosomes are often particularly useful for lectures. Daylight reversal films are generally best, since these reproduce the colors most accurately. Color negative film is generally unsuitable, since the colors often become distorted during the making of prints. As with black-and-white film, the fastest emulsion that will give acceptable results should be used, and correct exposure judged by exposing a test strip.

References

1. Sumner, A. T. (1989) Chromosome banding, in *Light Microscopy in Biology* (Lacey, A. J., ed.) IRL, Oxford, UK, pp. 279–314.
2. Caspersson, T., Farber, S., Foley, G. E., Kudynowski, J., Modest, E. J., Simonsson, E., Wagh, U., and Zech, L. (1968) Chemical differentiation along metaphase chromosomes. *Exp. Cell Res.* **49,** 219–222.

3. Caspersson, T., Zech, L., Modest, E. J., Foley, G. E., Wagh, U., and Simonsson, E. (1969) Chemical differentiation with fluorescent alkylating agents in *Vicia faba* metaphase chromosomes. *Exp. Cell Res.* **58,** 128–140.
4. van de Sande, J. H., Lin, C. C., and Deugan, K. V. (1979) Clearly differentiated and stable chromosome bands produced by a spermine bis-acridine, a bifunctional intercalating analogue of quinacrine. *Exp. Cell Res.* **120,** 439–444.
5. Macgregor, H. and Varley, J. (1988) *Working with Animal Chromosomes,* 2nd ed, Wiley, Chichester, UK.
6. Schwarzacher, T., Ambros, P., and Schweizer, D. (1980) Application of Giemsa banding to orchid karyotype analysis. *Plant Syst. Evol.* **134,** 293–297.
7. Oshimura, M. and Barrett, J. C. (1985) Double nondisjunction during karyotypic progression of chemically induced Syrian hamster cell lines. *Cancer Genet. Cytogenet.* **18,** 131–139.
8. Martin, R. H., Balkan, W., Burns, K., Rademaker, A. W., Lin, C. C., and Rudd, N. L. (1983) The chromosome constitution of 1000 human spermatozoa. *Human Genet.* **63,** 305–309.
9. de Torres, M. L. and Abrisqueta, J. A. (1978) Study of human male meiosis. II. Q-banding in pachytene bivalents. *Human Genet.* **42,** 283–289.
10. Vosa, C. G. (1971) The quinacrine-fluorescence patterns of the chromosomes of *Allium carinatum. Chromosoma* **33,** 382–385.
11. Evans, H. J., Buckton, K. E., and Sumner, A. T. (1971) Cytological mapping or human chromosomes: results obtained with quinacrine fluorescence and the acetic-saline-Giemsa techniques. *Chromosoma,* **35,** 310–325.
12. Hassold, T., Kumlin, E., Takaesu, N., and Leppert, M. (1985) The use of restriction fragment length polymorphisms to study the origin of human aneuploidy. *Ann. NY Acad. Sci.* **450,** 179–189.
13. Meulenbroek, G. H. M. and Geraedts, J. P. M. (1982) Parental origin of chromosome abnormalities in spontaneous abortions. *Human Genet.* **62,** 129–133.
14. Khokhar, M. T., Lawler, S. D., Powles, R. L., and Millar, J. L. (1987) Cytogenetic studies using Q-band polymorphisms in patients with AML receiving marrow from like-sex donors. *Human Genet.* **76,** 176–180.
15. Sumner, A. T. (1981) The distribution of quinacrine on chromosomes as determined by X-ray microanalysis. I. Q-bands on CHO chromosomes. *Chromosoma* **82,** 717–734.
16. Sumner, A. T. (1990) *Chromosome Banding.* Unwin Hyman, London, UK.
17. Schweizer, D. (1976) Reverse fluorescent chromosome banding with chromomycin and DAPI. *Chromosoma* **58,** 307–324.
18. Schmid, M. (1980) Chromosome banding in amphibia IV. Differentiation of GC- and AT-rich chromosome regions in Anura. *Chromosoma* **77,** 83–103.
19. Schweizer, D., Mendelak, M., White, M. J. D., and Contreras, N. (1983) Cytogenetics of the parthenogenetic grasshopper *Warramaba virgo* and its bisexual relatives. X. Patterns of fluorescent banding. *Chromosoma* **88,** 227–236.
20. Schweizer, D. (1980) Simultaneous fluorescent staining of R bands, and specific heterochromatic regions (DA-DAPI bands) in human chromosomes. *Cytogenet. Cell Genet.* **27,** 190–193.

21. Verma, R. S. and Lubs, H. A. (1976) Inheritance of acridine orange R variants in human acrocentric chromosomes. *Human Hered.* **26,** 315–318.
22. Verma, R. S. and Lubs, H. A. (1975) A simple R-banding technic. *Am. J. Hum. Genet.* **27,** 110–117.
23. Ploem, J. S. and Tanke, H. J. (1987) *Introduction to Fluorescence Microscopy.* Oxford University Press, Oxford, UK.
24. Ploem, J. S. (1989) Fluorescence microscopy, in *Light Microscopy in Biology: A Practical Approach* (Lacey, A. J., ed.) IRL, Oxford, UK.
25. Thomson, D. J. and Bradbury, S. (1987) *An Introduction to Photomicrography.* Oxford University Press, Oxford, UK.
26. Evennett, P. J. (1989) Image recording, in *Light Microscopy in Biology: A Practical Approach* (Lacey, A. J., ed.) IRL, Oxford, UK.
27. Davidson, N. R. (1973) Photographic techniques for recording chromosome banding patterns. *J. Med. Genet.* **10,** 122–126.

CHAPTER 8

Chromosome Banding

Stain Combinations for Specific Regions

Dieter Schweizer and Peter F. Ambros

1. Introduction

The chromosome banding patterns produced by certain DNA binding *fluorescent* dyes (*primary stain*) can be enhanced or modified by an appropriately chosen DNA binding *counterstain* (Fig. 1). The latter ligand is usually nonfluorescent or may be fluorescent, but not in the wavelength range of the primary stain (reviewed in *1,2*). Two such methods have proved indispensable in routine human cytogenetic diagnosis, namely, DA-DAPI banding *(3,4)* and chromomycin R-banding *(5)*. The mechanisms of fluorescence contrast enhancement on counterstaining have been studied in some detail *(1,2,6–11)*.

Counterstain-enhanced fluorescent chromosome banding is technically simple and usually more reliable than the corresponding cytochemical technique using absorption staining. The staining is usually carried out at room temperature and consists of consecutive incubations of the chromosome preparation with buffered solutions of selected ligands interrupted by brief rinses with demineralized water. The critical variables are the ligand concentration, the composition of the dye-buffer, and last but not least, the composition of the mounting buffer. The fluorescent techniques described in the following can be applied sequentially with other chromosome banding techniques, including nonradioactive *in situ* hybridization *(12–14)* (*see* Notes 1 and 7).

From: *Methods in Molecular Biology, Vol. 29: Chromosome Analysis Protocols*
Edited by: J. R. Gosden Copyright ©1994 Humana Press Inc., Totowa, NJ

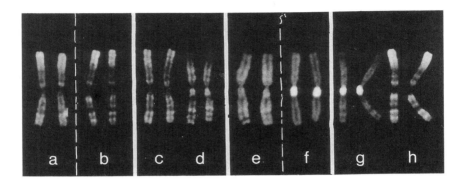

Fig. 1. Effect of counterstaining with one or two DNA ligands on DAPI fluorescence and on chromomycin fluorescence, respectively, of human chromosome no. 1: **a.** chromomycin in the absence of any counterstain; **b.** chromomycin R-banding, counterstain: distamycin A; **c.** chromomycin R-banding, counterstain: DAPI; **d.** same chromosome as in **c,** DAPI fluorescence, counterstain: chromomycin; **e.** DAPI in the absence of any counterstain; **f.** DAPI fluorescence, counterstain: distamycin A; **g.** DAPI fluorescence, counterstains: distamycin A and chromomycin; **h.** same chromosome as in **g** chromomycin R-banding, counterstains distamycin A and DAPI.

2. Materials
2.1. Solutions for DA/DAPI Staining

1. McIlvaine's citric acid-Na_2HPO_4 buffer, pH 7.0: Prepare solution A, $0.1M$ citric acid, and solution B, $0.2M$ disodium hydrogenphosphate. For pH 7, mix 82 mL of B plus 18 mL of A.
2. DAPI (4'-6-diamidino-2-phenylindole-2HCl): Prepare stock solution of 2 mg/mL in distilled water. DAPI stock solution is stored frozen at –20°C.
3. DAPI staining solution: 0.2–2 μg/mL in McIlvaine's buffer, pH 7.
4. Distamycin (SERVA) staining solution: 0.1–0.2 mg/mL of McIlvaine's pH 7 buffer. Note: Distamycin A (DA) tends to lack stability in aqueous solution, and it is not advisable to store it in solution at room temperature or in the refrigerator at 1–4°C. It is recommended to store aliquots of the DA staining solution at –20°C.
5. Mounting solution for DA/DAPI: glycerol (Merck [Rahway, NJ] "for fluorescence microscopy") and pH 7-McIlvaine's buffer mixed 1:1 (or 1:2).

2.2. Solutions for Chromomycin/ Distamycin/DAPI (CDD) Staining

1. McIlvaine's citric acid-Na_2HPO_4 buffer, pH 7 (*see* Section 2.1.), diluted 1:1 with distilled water; add $MgCl_2$ from stock solution ($1M$) to give 5 mM final concentration.

2. Chromomycin A_3 (CMA) (USB, Cleveland, OH; SERVA, Heidelberg, Germany) staining solution: 0.5 mg CMA/mL of pH 7 buffer containing 5 mM MgCl$_2$ (*see* Section 2.2., point 1). Note: Add sterile buffer slowly to the chromomycin A_3 powder without stirring, and dissolve the antibiotic slowly by leaving in the refrigerator at about 4°C overnight. The chromomycin solution may be kept in the refrigerator for some months if microbial contamination is avoided. It appeared that "aged" chromomycin solutions gave even better staining than new ones. To avoid swelling of the chromosomes, it proved useful or necessary to introduce a paraformaldehyde fixation step. A 4% paraformaldehyde (*see* Section 2.2., point 3) fixation can be done before the CMA incubation step or can be achieved by the addition of paraformaldehyde (immediately before use) to the CMA staining solution to give a final concentration of 4%.
3. Paraformaldehyde stock solution: It is made by adding 4 g paraformaldehyde to 6 mL of distilled water containing two drops of 5M sodium hydroxide (20%). This mixture is heated until it just boils, allowed to cool, 1 mL methanol added, and filled up with distilled water to give a final vol of 10 mL. After filtering, the solution can be stored at room temperature in the dark for 2–6 wk.
4. Distamycin (SERVA) staining solution: 0.1–0.2 mg/mL of McIlvaine's buffer, pH 7 (*see also* note on DA stability in Section 2.1., point 4).
5. DAPI stock solution: 2 mg/mL in distilled water (*see* Section 2.1., point 2).
6. DAPI staining solution: 0.2 µg/mL of McIlvaine's buffer, pH 7.
7. Mounting solution for CMA/DA/DAPI tristaining: glycerol (Merck, "for fluorescence microscopy") is mixed (1:1) with McIlvaine's pH 7 buffer (the latter containing 5 mM MgCl$_2$ to give a final magnesium concentration in the mixture of 2.5 mM).

2.3. Solutions for Chromomycin/Methyl Green

1. Chromomycin A_3 (CMA) staining solution: 0.5 mg CMA/mL of pH 7 buffer. For details of the CMA staining solution as well as the paraformaldehyde fixation step, *see* Section 2.2., point 2.
2. Methyl green (SERVA) stock solution: 5 mg/mL in 0.01M Tris HCl, pH 4. Note that this solution is stable only for some days; it is recommended to prepare a new stock solution as well as a new working solution if intervals between experiments are longer.
3. Methyl green staining solution: 1–5 µg/mL in 0.1M Tris-HCl, pH 7.
4. Mounting medium for methyl green: glycerol (Merck, "for fluorescence microscopy").

2.4. Solutions for DAPI/Actinomycin D

1. McIlvaine's citric acid-Na$_2$HPO$_4$ buffer, pH 7 (*see* Section 2.1., point 1).
2. DAPI stock solution 0.2 mg/mL in distilled water.
3. DAPI staining solution 0.2–0.4 µg/mL in McIlvaine's buffer, pH 7.
4. Actinomycin D (AMD) staining solution: 0.2–0.3 mg/mL in 10 mM sodium phosphate buffer (pH 7.0) containing 1 mM EDTA. (AMD is first dissolved in one to two drops of methanol, and then buffer is added). This solution may be kept in the refrigerator for several months. AMD is highly toxic; therefore, rubber gloves should be used when handling it.
5. Mounting medium for actinomycin D: Glycerol is mixed (1:2) with McIlvaine's pH 7 buffer.

2.5. Solutions for the DAPI-Derived Stains D 288/45 and D 287/170

1. D 287/170 and D 288/45 stock solutions: 1 mg dye/mL of distilled water. The dyes are not available commercially. Samples of DAPI derivatives can be obtained by O. Dann, Louis-Störzbach-Straße 5, D-6930 Eberbach am Neckar, Germany, or from D. Schweizer, Department of Cytology and Genetics, Institute of Botany, University of Vienna, Rennweg 14, A-1030 Vienna, Austria.
2. D 287/170 (or D 288/45) staining solution (should be made *immediately* before use): The final concentration of D 287/170 is 0.01–0.05 mg/mL of sodium phosphate buffer containing 10% DMSO. The latter staining buffer is made by mixing nine parts of pH 7 McIlvaine's buffer with nine parts of distilled water and two parts of dimethylsulfoxid (DMSO). D 288/45 staining solution: 0.5–1 µg/mL DMSO pH 7 buffer.
3. Mounting medium for D 287/170: 1:1 mixture of glycerol and 0.2M Na$_2$HPO$_4$.
4. Mounting medium for D 288/45: 1:2 mixture of glycerol and pH 7.0 McIlvaine's buffer.

3. Methods

3.1. Distamycin A plus DAPI (DA/DAPI) Heterochromatin Staining

The DA/DAPI method of Schweizer et al. *(3,4)* and Schweizer *(9)* consists of a preincubation of the chromosome preparation with the AT-specific nonfluorescent DNA-binding peptide antibiotic distamycin A (DA), followed by incubation with a likewise AT-specific fluorescent DNA ligand 4'-6-diamidino-2-phenylindole (DAPI). Differential DAPI fluorescence of C-bands results from competition binding effects of the DNA groove binders DAPI and distamycin A *(1,6,9)* (*see* Note 1). In humans, the paracentromeric heterochromatin blocks of chromosomes 1, 9, 16 and the heterochromatin of the long arm of the Y chromosome, together with a C-band in the short arm of chromosome 15, exhibit bright fluorescence after DA/DAPI staining (Figs. 2c,3b). DA/DAPI bands have been reported for a variety of animal species, both invertebrates and vertebrates, but so far not in plants.

1. Flood the slide with DA solution, cover with a coverslip, and incubate at room temperature for about 10 min.
2. Remove the coverslip, and rinse briefly with demineralized water.
3. Flood with DAPI solution, cover with coverslip, and incubate at room temperature for about 10 min in the dark.
4. Rinse briefly with demineralized water.
5. Mount in buffer, pH 7.0 (or in a 1:1 mixture of glycerol and pH 7.0 buffer; *see* Note 1); remove excess buffer by blotting over coverslip. Seal with rubber solution (*see* Note 1).
6. Chromosomal DAPI fluorescence is observed under short-wavelength blue light excitation (360 nm). The DAPI fluorescence emission spectrum has a maximum around 460 nm.

3.2. Chromomycin/Distamycin/DAPI (CDD) Staining for Simultaneous Production of Reverse (R) and DA-DAPI Bands

The method provides from the same metaphase spread a distinct fluorescent R-banding pattern, as well as DA-DAPI bands depending on the excitation light used *(5)* (*see* Note 6). Using appropriate combinations of excitation and barrier filters, chromomycin R-banding appears yellow-red, whereas DA-DAPI banding is light-blue *(1)* (*see* Note 2). CDD staining is the only simple and reliable method known that simultaneously provides a general (R) as well as regional (C) chromosome banding pattern (Figs. 1g and h; 2a and c; 3a and b; 4b). CDD staining has recently proven most useful in conjunction with nonisotopic *in situ* hybridization *(12,13)* (*see* Note 7).

1. Flood slide with chromomycin A_3 (CMA) staining solution (if necessary, containing 4% paraformaldehyde), cover with coverslip, and incubate at room temperature in the dark overnight. The duration of staining may be extended but care should be taken to avoid drying out the slide.
2. Remove coverslip, and rinse briefly with demineralized water. Then shake off water droplets, and blow the slide dry by means of a medical rubber bulb.

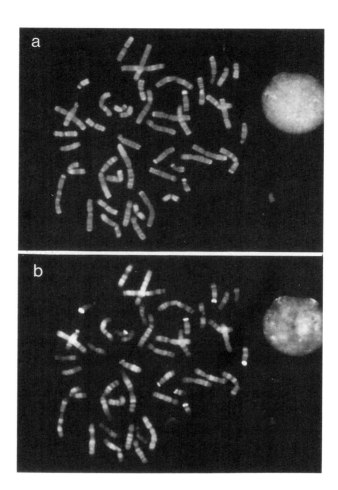

Fig. 2. CDD tristaining followed by DAPI/AMD and Giemsa C-banding of the same metaphase chromosome spread of a male chimpanzee (*Pan troglodytes*). Note differential staining response of centric and terminal C-bands and NOR-satellites. **a.** Chromomycin R-banding (counterstains: distamycin and DAPI). **b.** DAPI counterstained with actinomycin D.

3. Flood slide with distamycin A solution, cover with coverslip, and stain at room temperature in the dark for about 10 min.
4. Float off coverslip, and rinse briefly with demineralized water. Then shake water droplets off and blow dry.
5. Flood slide with DAPI solution, cover with coverslip, and stain in the dark at room temperature for 15 min.

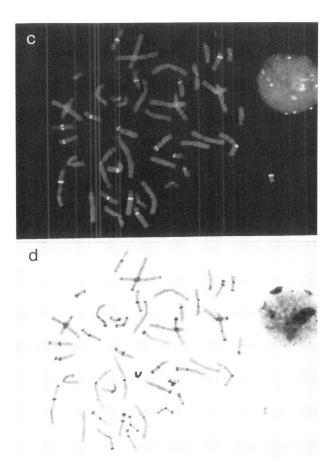

c. Banding pattern of chimpanzee chromosomes as obtained by distamycin/DAPI.
d. Giemsa C-band pattern of the same metaphase shown in a–c.

6. Remove coverslip, and rinse briefly with demineralized water followed
   by brief air-drying.
7. Mount in a 1:1 mixture of glycerol/pH 7 McIlvaine's buffer (plus
   2.5 mM MgCl$_2$). Remove excess buffer by pressing gently between
   filter paper and blotting repeatedly over coverslip. Seal with rubber
   solution.
8. Age the slide prior to examination by storing it in the dark at 30–37°C
   for a minimum of 1 d (preferably 2–3 d; ref. *17*), or at room temperature for 3–6 d (*see* Note 2).

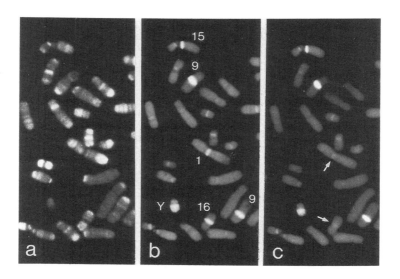

Fig. 3. Part of human metaphase of a male individual with inv(9)(qh) first CDD stained, then destained, and restained with D 287/170. **a.** Chromomycin R-banding; **b.** DA/DAPI banding pattern; **c.** D 287/170 banding; note that D 287/170 preferentially stains 9qh, 15p, and part of the long arm of the Y, but not the heterochromatins of chromosomes 1 and 16 (arrows).

9. Fluorescence microscopy: The specific band patterns, either DA/DAPI or reverse bands, can be viewed and photographed from the same cell by choosing the appropriate filters. For DA/DAPI bands, use excitation light in the wavelength range of 360–370 nm. Selective excitation of chromomycin A_3 fluorescence is achieved by using a narrow filter (435 nm ± 10 nm; e.g., Leitz filter E_3) (*see* Note 6).

3.3. R-Banding by Chromomycin/Methyl Green

This is a simple method for fluorescent R-banding of chromosomes. It was originally introduced by Schweizer in 1976 for demonstrating GC-rich nucleolar organizers and C-bands in plants *(15)*, and subsequently adopted by other laboratories for staining mammalian chromosomes (e.g., ref. *8*). Original work on methyl green DNA binding studies in solution was done by Müller and Gautier *(16)*. The method described here is based on that published by Schweizer *(15)*, with modifications worked out by P. F. Ambros, D. Schweizer, and P. M. Kroisel

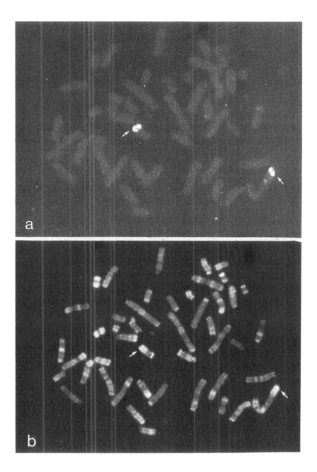

Fig. 4. Example of a TRITC-based *in situ* hybridization of a 1p36.3-specific human VNTR-sequence (DZ2) on a Ewing tumor cell (kindly provided by Sabine Strehl, Vienna): **a.** Beside the normal chromosome 1 (bottom right), a transloca-tion of the tip of chromosome 1 onto another chromosome can be noted (arrows). **b.** Chromomycin R-band pattern by CDD staining of the same metaphase spread as in a. Also a DA/DAPI banding can be induced from the same cell by excitation around 360 nm (not shown).

(unpublished observations and ref. *17*). Methyl green can be replaced in this method by distamycin A (*see* steps 1–3 of Section 3.2.).

1. Stain with chromomycin solution for 1 h or longer.
2. Rinse briefly with demineralized water.

3. Counterstain for 10–20 min with methyl green solution (*see* Note 3).
4. Rinse briefly with demineralized water.
5. Mount in glycerol. Blot off surplus glycerol, and seal with rubber solution. Store preparations for 1 d at 37°C prior to analysis by epifluorescent microscopy (excitation wavelength range 430–450 nm) (*see* Note 3).

3.4. Counterstaining of DAPI with Actinomycin D

This was the first example of counterstain-enhanced chromosome banding making use of an appropriately chosen combination of DNA binding dyes, fluorescent and nonfluorescent, and with complementary base pair binding specificity, AT-specific and GC-specific (*15;* for earlier references, *see* ref. *12*).

The reliable method provides a distinct bright and stable Q-banding differentiation of metaphase chromosomes. In addition, some AT-rich C-bands are enhanced (1qh, 3cen, 16qh, distal Y, and certain satellites of D- and G-group chromosomes of the human).

TActinomycinD(AMD) counterstaining is also recommended for the DAPI-derived dye D 288/45 (*see* Section 3.5. and ref. *6*). With this dye combination, in some species, a slightly different set of C-bands is enhanced than with DAPI/AMD *(6)*.

The method may also be applied sequentially in conjunction with other banding techniques (e.g., subsequent to tristaining with chromomycin/distamycin/DAPI). As an example, sequential CDD and DAPI/ AMD and Giemsa C-banding are shown for a metaphase cell of the chimpanzee (Fig. 2a–d).

1. Flood the slide with DAPI staining solution, cover with coverslip, and, incubate at room temperature for 20–30 min.
2. Remove coverslip and rinse briefly with deionized water. Shake and blow dry (e.g., by means of a medical rubber bulb).
3. Flood slide with actinomycin D staining solution, cover with coverslip and stain in the dark at room temperature for 15–20 min. (*see* Note 4).
4. Rinse briefly with demineralized water, then blow dry (*see* Note 4).
5. Mount in pH 7.0–7.5-McIlvaine's buffer, remove excess buffer by blotting over coverslip. Seal with rubber solution. Alternatively, the slides may be mounted in a 1:2 mixture of glycerol and pH 7.5 McIlvaine's buffer. Addition of glycerol stabilizes DAPI fluorescence and prevents the slides from drying out. The DAPI fluorescence is, however, slightly less intense than with buffer alone.

6. Chromosomal DAPI fluorescence is observed under short wavelength blue light excitation (360 nm).

3.5. DAPI-Derived Stains
for Specific Regions: D 288/45 and D 287/170

D 288/45 is a DAPI derivative that exhibits similar, but not identical, binding and fluorescence properties as DAPI *(6)*. Certain types of C-bands can be differentially stained by this dye. D 288/45 is employed alone or in conjunction with counterstains, such as distamycin or actinomycin D (*see* Section 3.1. and 3.4.) (*see* Note 5).

Direct staining of human chromosomes with D 287/170 results in brilliant fluorescence of the paracentromeric C-band of chromosome 9, of a proximal short-arm segment of chromosome 15, and of certain heterochromatic regions in the Y *(18)*. Bright, but less conspicuous fluorescence is occasionally seen at the centromeres of other chromosomes (Fig. 3c). The staining differentiation obtained by D 287/170 (which is similar, but not identical to DA/DAPI) is very distinct, and the intensity of the fluorescent light is unusually high. The fluorochrome has proven useful for rapid detection of human chromosome 9 heterochromatin at various stages of the cell cycle.

1. Flood slide with D 287/170 staining solution (or with D 288/45 staining solution), cover with coverslip, and incubate at room temperature in the dark for 15–30 min (*see* Note 5).
2. Remove coverslip, and rinse thoroughly with deionized water.
3. Mount preparations stained with D 287/170 in a 1:1 mixture of glycerol and $0.2M$ Na_2HPO_4. Preparations stained with D 288/45 are mounted in a 1:2 mixture of glycerol and McIlvaine's pH 7.0 buffer. Remove excess mounting medium by pressing gently between filter paper and blotting repeatedly over coverslip. Seal with rubber solution. "Age" the slides by storing in the dark for a minimum of 1 d prior to examination (*see* Note 5).
4. Fluorescence microscopy: Use same filter combination as recommended for quinacrine (*see* Chapter 7).

4. Notes

1. The specific DA/DAPI chromosomal banding pattern can also be obtained with related compounds; e.g., Hoechst 33258 can be substituted for DAPI and netropsin can be used instead of distamycin A *(1,2,19)*. The sequence of the staining can be reversed, i.e., DAPI first followed by DA.

The stained preparations may fade rapidly when first examined, but usually stabilize after a day or so stored at 4°C. A stabilizing influence of glycerol was observed for DA/DAPI banding *(1,2,5)*; however, the overall DAPI fluorescence was quenched, as established by cytofluorometry. If preparations stained with distamycin plus DAPI were mounted in glycerol, the DAPI fluorescence of metaphases was less than half the value of controls (which were mounted in pH 7.0 McIlvaine's buffer). A 1:1 mixture of glycerol and pH 7.0 McIlvaine's buffer proved to be a suitable compromise, because the fluorescence pattern was still stabilized whereas DAPI was quenched by only 17% *(5)*.

DA/DAPI staining can profitably be combined in a tristaining procedure with chromomycin R-banding (*see* Section 3.2.). DA/DAPI can be followed by any banding both fluorescent or absorption stain (*see* Chapters 6 and 7). Destaining of fluorescent slides is done as follows: Remove rubber seal and float off coverslip by rinsing with pH 7 buffer, and then blow the slide dry. Incubate the preparation overnight in methanol/acetic acid glacial (3:1), and then blow dry; another banding procedure can follow.

2. In the CDD procedure, one or the other of the stains may be replaced by a closely related dye, e.g., chromomycin by olivomycin or mithramycin, distamycin by netropsin, DAPI by Hoechst 33258 *(1,2)*. Using BrdU-substituted chromosomes, the dye triplet chromomycin/methyl green/DAPI has proven useful for the simultaneous production of R-bands, and either replication patterns or sister chromatid differentiation *(17)*. Air-dried chromosome spreads, a few days up to several weeks old, give the best results. Too fresh or very old slides may exhibit swelling of nuclei and chromosomes. Flame-dried and/or old preparations usually stain less intensely with chromomycin A_3. The inclusion of paraformaldehyde (4%) in the chromomycin staining solution greatly helps to prevent swelling of the chromosomes during staining *(12,14)*.

CDD-stained preparations may exhibit rapid fading of chromomycin (R-band) fluorescence when first examined, but usually stabilize when "aged" for 2–3 d or longer in the dark at 30–37°C *(12,17)*. CDD-tristained slides may be kept at 4°C for up to 1 yr or longer without loss of quality of the fluorescence patterns.

The CDD staining technique can be followed by any other banding method (*see* as an example Fig. 2a–d of a sequentially banded *Pan troglodytes* metaphase). Triple CDD staining is the method of choice for R-banding after flourescent *in situ* hybridization (FISH) procedures. It allows unambiguous chromosome identification and the assignment of the FISH signals to specific chromosome bands (*see* Fig. 4a,b).

3. Immediately after counterstaining with methyl green, no detectable R-banding can be seen. R-banding differentiation appears after 24 h of aging in the dark at room temperature or at 37°C. A longer aging of the slides will help to stabilize and brighten the R-banding pattern. Using the CMA filter block (e.g., Leitz filter block E$_3$), the R-band positive material has a yellow fluorescence, whereas the non-R-band material should appear orange in color. If necessary, several methyl green concentrations should be tested in a preliminary experiment to avoid overstaining. Methyl green staining can be monitored by a TRITC excitation filter (e.g., Leitz N$_2$), where it results in a rather uniform faint magenta fluorescence. By absorption microscopy, the hue of the chromosomes and nuclei should appear slightly greenish.

4. The method is simple and reliable, and can be applied prior or subsequent to other fluorescent banding techniques. In Section 3.4., DAPI can be replaced by Hoechst 33258 or by D 288/45 *(1,2,6)*. The sequence of the staining can be reversed, i.e., AMD first followed by DAPI. **Note:** To the washing buffers containing the toxic AMD prior to disposal 1N HCl (10 parts of vol) is added.

5. The application of the DAPI derivative D 288/45 follows in principle the protocols worked out for DAPI (e.g., 3.1. DA/DAPI banding, 3.4. DAPI/actinomycin D banding). The solubility in phosphate-containing buffer of D 288/45 (and also of D 287/170) is much lower than that of DAPI. This can be overcome by the addition of dimethylsulfoxid (DMSO) to the staining solution. It was found that the staining of cell nuclei with a freshly prepared pH 7-buffered dye solution (*see* Section 2.5.) was superior to that obtained with this type of dye dissolved in water only.

    The fluorescence pattern of D 287/170-stained chromosomes was influenced by the concentration of the dye. Preferential fluorescent staining of human chromosome 9 C-band material was usually seen in a concentration range 10X higher than that routinely employed for DAPI. Too low a dye concentration results in a typical QFH-type banding pattern; too high a concentration of D 287/170 results in uniform overstaining. Air-dried chromosome spreads not older than a month appeared to give the best results. Sometimes with new or very old preparations, the chromosomes may become swollen and artificially distorted during staining. In such cases, it is advisable to pretreat the chromosome preparations with a 4% solution of paraformaldehyde (buffered at about pH 7–8) for 30 min to 1 h (*see* Section 2.2., point 3).

6. Fluorescence microscopy and photography: Chromosomal fluorescence is excited with light from a high-pressure mercury lamp in conjunction with an incident ("epi") illumination system. For chromomycin/

distamycin/DAPI banding, special filter systems should be employed
that limit the spectrum of the excitation light to rather narrow wavelength ranges: i.e., for DA/DAPI bands, use excitation light around 360–
370 nm (e.g., Leitz Ploem-Opak filter block A); for chromomycin
R-bands, use excitation wavelength range 435–445 nm (e.g., Leitz filter block E$_3$). Using human chromosomes as a test system, it should be
checked that neither of the two filter blocks produces a mixed fluorescence (e.g., region 1qh, when examined with filters for chromomycin
R-banding, should be negative). Because chromomycin fluorescence is
comparatively weak (<10% of DAPI fluorescence intensity, ref. *2*), it is
necessary to employ a high-speed film, or a CCD or low light camera
capable of capturing fluorescence images (e.g., Genevision Applied
Imaging, Santa Clara, CA).

7. *In situ* hybridization and chromosome banding: Chromosome identification and the assignment of hybridization signals after nonisotopic *in
situ* hybridization (ISH) very often are hampered by the deteriorated
morphology of chromosomal band patterns. Chromosomal erosion seems
to be more pronounced in G-(Q-)band material rather than in R-bands.
The exact chromosome identification and the unambiguous assignment
of ISH signals to specific bands or even subbands can be achieved by
the chromomycin R-banding techniques (*see* Sections 3.2. and 3.3.).
These techniques allow an exact mapping of viral DNA in the human
complement *(12)* or the exact localization of single copy genes *(13)*
after peroxidase-based ISH.

A simultaneous visualization of the fluorescence *in situ* hybridization
(FISH) signals and R as well as DA/DAPI bands can be achieved by simply changing the appropriate filters *(14)* when making use of the fluorochromes rhodamine (TRITC), chromomycin (CMA), and DAPI,
respectively. Figure 4 shows a FISH with TRITC-labeled antibodies recognizing human VNTR sequences on 1p36.3. This technique is especially
useful in identifying somatic cell hybrids, analyzing translocations or
marker chromosomes, and for the assignment of single-copy genes, VNTR
sequences, cosmids, or YAC clones to specific chromosomal bands.

References

1. Schweizer, D. (1981) Counterstain-enhanced chromosome banding. *Hum.
   Genet.* **57,** 1–14.
2. Schweizer, D. (1980) Fluorescent chromosome banding in plants: applications,
   mechanisms, and implications for chromosome structure, in *The Plant Genome,
   Proceedings of the Fourth John Innes Symposium* (Davies, D. R. and Hopwood,
   D. A., eds.) John Innes Charity, Norwich, UK, pp. 61–72.

3. Schweizer, D., Ambros, P. F., and Andrle, M. (1978) Modification of DAPI banding on human chromosomes by prestaining with a DNA-binding oligopeptide antibiotic, distamycin A. *Exp. Cell Res.* **111,** 327–332.
4. Schweizer, D., Ambros, P., Andrle, M., Rett, A., and Fiedler, W. (1979) Demonstration of specific heterochromatic segments in the orangutan (*Pongo pygmaeus*) by a distamycin/DAPI double staining technique. *Cytogenet. Cell Genet.* **24,** 7–14.
5. Schweizer, D. (1980) Simultaneous fluorescent staining of R bands and specific heterochromatic regions (DA-DAPI bands) in human chromosomes. *Cytogenet. Cell Genet.* **27,** 190–193.
6. Burckhardt, G., Votavova, H., Jantsch, M., Zimmer, C., Lown, J. W., and Schweizer, D. (1993) Mechanisms of distamycin/DAPI chromosome staining I. Competition binding effects of non-intercalative DNA groove binding drugs in situ and in vitro. *Cytogenet. Cell Genet.* **62,** 19–25.
7. Jorgenson, K. F., van de Sande, J. H., and Lin, C. C. (1978) The use of base pair specific DNA binding agents as affinity labels for the study of mammalian chromosomes. *Chromosoma* **68,** 287–302.
8. Sahar, E. and Latt, S. A. (1980) Energy transfer and binding competition between dyes used to enhance staining differentiation in metaphase chromosomes. *Chromosoma* **79,** 1–28.
9. Schweizer, D. (1983) Distamycin-DAPI bands: properties and occurrence in species, in *Kew Chromosome Conference II* (Brandham, P. E. and Bennett, M. D., eds.) George Allen and Unwin, London, pp. 43–51.
10. Schweizer, D., Loidl, J., and Hamilton, B. (1987) Heterochromatin and the phenomenon of chromosome banding, in *Results and Problems in Cell Differentiation 14* (Hennig, W., ed.) Springer-Verlag, Berlin, pp. 235–254.
11. Zimmer, Ch. and Wähnert, U. (1986) Nonintercalating DNA-binding ligands: Specificity of the interaction and their use as tools in biophysical, biochemical and biological investigations of the genetic material. *Prog. Biophys. Molec. Biol.* **47,** 31–112.
12. Ambros, P. F. and Karlic, H. I. (1987) Chromosomal insertion of human papillomavirus 18 sequences in HeLa cells detected by nonisotopic in situ hybridization and reflection contrast microscopy. *Hum. Genet.* **77,** 251–254.
13. Ambros, P. F., Bartram, C. R., Haas, O. A., Karlic, H. I., and Gadner, H. (1987) Nonisotopic in situ hybridization for mapping oncogenic sequences, in *Modern Trends in Human Leukemia VII* (Neth, R., Gallo, R. C., Greaves, M. F., and Kabisch, H., eds.) Springer-Verlag, Berlin, pp. 141–144.
14. Dworzak, M., Stock, C., Strehl, S., Gadner, H., and Ambros, P. F. (1992) Ewing's tumor x mouse hybrids expressing the MIC2 antigen: analysis using fluorescence CDD-banding and non-isotopic ISH. *Hum. Genet.* **88,** 273–278.
15. Schweizer, D. (1976) Reverse fluorescent chromosome banding with chromomycin and DAPI. *Chromosoma* **58,** 307–324.
16. Müller, W. and Gautier, F. (1975) Interactions of heteroaromatic compounds with nucleic acids. A-T-specific non-intercalating DNA ligands. *Eur. J. Biochem.* **54,** 385–394.

17. Kroisel, P. M., Rosenkranz, W., and Schweizer, D. (1985) Simultaneous production of R-bands and either replication patterns or sister chromatid differentiation. *Hum. Genet.* **71,** 333–341.
18. Schnedl, W., Abraham, R., Dann, O., Geber, G., and Schweizer, D. (1981) Preferential fluorescent staining of heterochromatic regions in human chromosomes 9, 15, and the Y by D 287/170. *Hum. Genet.* **59,** 10–13.
19. Schnedl, W., Dann, O., and Schweizer, D. (1980) Effects of counterstaining with DNA binding drugs on fluorescent banding patterns of human and mammalian chromosomes. *Europ. J. Cell Biol.* **20,** 290–296.

CHAPTER 9

Inhibition
of Chromosome Condensation

Adrian T. Sumner and Arthur R. Mitchell

1. Introduction

In the fully contracted metaphase chromosome, the length of DNA is compacted at least 10,000 times, and many details of chromosome organization cannot be distinguished. Study of the more elongated prophase chromosomes permits the observation of finer details; for example, the number of bands in a human haploid chromosome set increases from about 300 in metaphase *(1)* to as many as 2000 in prophase *(2)*. However, the number of naturally occurring prophases in normal mitotic chromosome preparations is usually very small, and artificial means are required to increase the number of elongated prophase chromosomes to an acceptable level for high-resolution analysis. One method used for high-resolution banding (Chapter 1) is the synchronization of cells in interphase, followed by release of the block and harvesting of the cells an appropriate time later when the cells have progressed through to prophase. An alternative approach, which will be described here, is to add to the cultured cells some substance that will either be incorporated in the chromosomal DNA or, more usually, bind to the chromosomal DNA, and thereby inhibit condensation of the chromosomes. Such substances may either inhibit the condensation of whole chromosomes or of specific parts, normally heterochromatin.

Cultures treated in the various ways described in this chapter may be fixed by the conventional method using methanol-acetic acid (Chapter 1) or spread unfixed using a cytocentrifuge (Chapter 15).

From: *Methods in Molecular Biology, Vol. 29: Chromosome Analysis Protocols*
Edited by: J. R. Gosden Copyright ©1994 Humana Press Inc., Totowa, NJ

2. Materials (*see* Note 1)

1. Ethidium bromide: 4 mg/10 mL distilled water (1 m*M*). This solution is stable indefinitely if kept in the dark in the refrigerator.
2. FdU (deoxy-5-fluorouridine): 0.025 mg/mL in sterile distilled water (0.1 m*M*). The solution is stable for many months if kept in the dark in the refrigerator.
3. Uridine: 0.244 mg/mL (1 m*M*) in sterile distilled water. The solution is stable for many months if kept in the dark in the refrigerator.
4. 5'-Azacytidine: 0.73 mg/mL ($3.7 \times 10^{-5}M$) in sterile distilled water. Store at –20°C.
5. 5'-Azadeoxycytidine: 0.227 mg/mL ($10^{-3}M$) in sterile distilled water. Store at –20°C.
6. Thymidine: 2.43 mg/mL (10 m*M*) in sterile distilled water. This is stable for many months at 4°C.
7. DAPI (4'-6-diamidino-2-phenylindole): 10 mg/mL in sterile distilled water. Store at 4°C protected from light.
8. Berenil (diminazene aceturate): 50 mg/mL in sterile distilled water. This compound can be obtained from Sigma (Poole UK; St. Louis, MO).
9. Hoechst 33258: 40 mg/mL in sterile distilled water. Store at 4°C protected from light.
10. Colcemid: 0.1 mg/mL in sterile distilled water. Store at 4°C.

3. Methods

3.1. Inhibition of Condensation of Whole Chromosomes

*3.1.1. Ethidium (*See *Note 2)*

The fluorescent dye ethidium bromide, when added to human lymphocyte cultures, inhibits condensation throughout the length of the chromosomes *(3)*. This is a useful pretreatment for high-resolution banding *(3,4)* (*see* Chapter 1).

At the same time that colchicine is added to the culture to arrest cells in metaphase (*see* Chapter 1), add 10–25 µL of the ethidium bromide solution/1 mL of culture medium. After continuing the culture for an appropriate length of time to accumulate enough dividing cells, treat with hypotonic solution and fix in the usual way (*see* Chapter 1).

A dividing human lymphocyte from a culture treated in this way is illustrated in Fig. 1. Note the relatively elongated chromosomes.

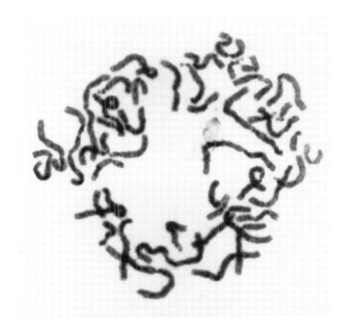

Fig. 1. Metaphase chromosome spread from a human lymphocyte culture treated with ethidium bromide. Note the uniform elongation of the chromosomes—Methanol-acetic acid fixation.

3.1.2. Decondensation Using
an FdU / Uridine Block (see Note 3)

This procedure appears to prevent the condensation of the G-positive bands in the chromosome arms. The result is the production of extended chromosomes that can, in some instances, be of a considerable length. The applications of this technique can therefore be used in studies of both centromeric domains and G-positive bands. A disadvantage is the relatively small number of mitoses produced.

Both FdU and uridine are added to the cell culture to the concentrations specified above (i.e., 1 μL for every 1 mL of culture medium). This should be carried out 18 h prior to harvesting the cells. Five hours before harvesting, the FdU/uridine block is removed by the addition of thymidine to a final concentration of 10 μM (i.e., 1 μL/mL

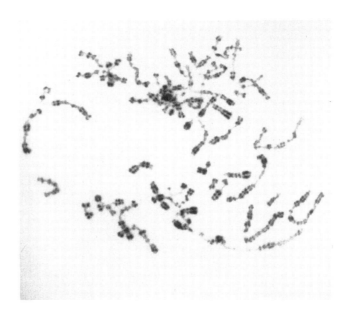

Fig. 2. Human metaphase chromosomes showing preferential inhibition of condensation of G-positive bands after culture in the presence of FdU/uridine—Methanol-acetic acid fixation.

of culture). At this time, 5'-azacytidine should also be added as described in Section 3.2.1. A human metaphase treated in this way is shown in Fig. 2.

3.2. Inhibition of Condensation
of Heterochromatin

The techniques described here concern chromosomes that contain heterochromatic domains, which under normal cellular conditions remain compact and can be C-banded *(5)*. This type of chromatin is generally referred to as constitutive heterochromatin to distinguish it from the facultative heterochromatin of, for example, the inactive X chromosome in female mammals *(6)*. In humans, the chromosomes affected by this procedure are: chromosomes 1, 9, 13, 14, 15, 16, 21, 22, and the Y chromosome. In mouse (i.e., *Mus* species), all of the chromosomes with the exception of the Y chromosome are affected.

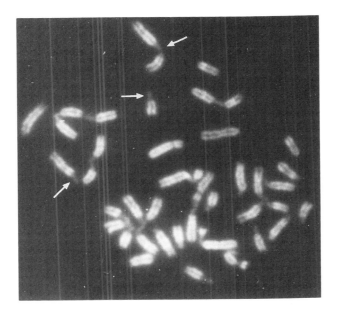

Fig. 3. Human metaphase chromosomes from a culture treated with 5'-azacytidine, showing decondensation of heterochromatin on chromosome 9 (arrowed)—Cytocentrifuge preparation.

3.2.1. Decondensation Using 5'-Azacytidine

The cytosine analog (5'-azacytidine) inhibits the condensation of centromeric constitutive heterochromatin in both human and mouse chromosomes (with the exception of the Y chromosome in both species) *(7)*. 5'-Azacytidine is added to the cell culture 5 h before harvesting to a final concentration of 0.37 μM (i.e., 10 μL of the 5'-azacytidine solution is added for every 1 mL of culture). One hour before harvesting, colcemid (to a final concentration of 0.1 μg/mL again, 1 μL of stock solution for every 1 mL culture) is added. (*see* Note 4). A human metaphase treated in this way is shown in Fig. 3.

5'-Aza-deoxycytidine can be used to produce the same effect as 5'-azacytidine *(8)*. One possible advantage of using the latter is the ability to grow cells in the presence of this analog for up to three generations. Both analogs of cytosine are thought to become incorporated into the

DNA molecule and to prevent methylation of this base from occurring. However, this is by no means certain; evidence *(8)* to the contrary has been presented, and the possibility exists that the absence of a specific protein may give rise to this phenomenon.

3.2.2. Decondensation of the Constitutive Heterochromatin Present on the X Chromosome of Microtus agrestis

A substantial proportion of the chromatin of the X chromosome of the vole *Microtus agrestis* comprises C-banded heterochromatin. This can be decondensed specifically by growing cells in 5'-azadeoxycytidine *(8)*.

5'-Aza-deoxycytidine is added to the growing cells 2 h before harvesting to a final concentration of $10^{-5}M$ (10 μL/mL culture) (*see* Note 4). Colcemid to a final concentration of 0.1 μg/mL is added 1 h before harvesting. The colcemid is prepared and stored as described in Section 2.

3.2.3. Decondensation Using DAPI

The procedure described here once again applies to human lymphocyte blood cultures and may have to be adapted for other cell lines. DAPI is 4'-6-diamidino-2-phenylindole. It binds primarily to A + T rich DNA molecules, and this has to be remembered when using this compound to extend heterochromatin at the centromeres of chromosomes. In humans and in the mouse, its effect is the same as that seen with the cytosine analogs. That is, the chromosomes containing constitutive heterochromatin show decondensation of this chromatin.

DAPI is added to a final concentration of 100 μg/mL to the growing cells 16–18 h before harvesting (*see* Note 5). Colcemid is again added to the culture to arrest the cells in metaphase as described above (Section 3.2.2.). Chromosomes from cultures treated in this way have an appearance similar to those from cultures treated with 5'-azacytidine.

3.2.4. Decondensation of the Human Y Chromosome

The procedures described above are not usually successful when applied to the human Y chromosome. To obtain decondensation of the constitutive heterochromatin of the human Y chromosome reliably, it is necessary to use the ligand Berenil. This ligand binds specifically to the A + T rich DNA sequences of the human Y chromosome *(9)*.

Berenil is added to a final concentration of 150 µg/mL (3 µL/1 mL culture) 24 h before harvesting the cells (*see* Note 6). Colcemid is not added to the culture medium in this instance.

3.2.5. Decondensation
of the Centromeric Constitutive Heterochromatin
of Mouse L-Cells

The benzimidazole derivative "33258 Hoechst" (2,2[4-hydroxy-phenyl]-6-benzimidazolyl-6-[1-methyl-4-piperazyl]-benzimidazol-trihydrochloride) binds preferentially to A + T rich DNA molecules. It does also bind to G + G rich DNAs, but to a lesser degree. Growing L-cells in the presence of the benzimidazole "33258 Hoechst" will decondense the constitutive heterochromatin of the centromeres *(10)*. Human cells seem to be relatively insensitive to this drug.

Hoechst 33258 is added to the cell culture to a final concentration of 40 µg/mL (1 µL/mL culture) 30 h before harvesting. Colcemid to 1 µg/mL is added for the last 3 h before the cells are harvested. A mouse metaphase treated by this procedure is shown in Fig. 4.

4. Notes

1. It should be borne in mind that most the compounds described in this chapter are hazardous, and care should be exercised in their usage. Gloves should be used at all times when these compounds are used. Care should be taken when weighing out these chemicals. At all times, avoid inhalation of the powdered compounds during weighing them on balances. (For disposal methods for ethidium bromide, *see* refs. *11–13*).
2. The method described applies essentially to human lymphocyte cultures, and other types of cells may require higher or lower concentrations of ethidium. However, too high a concentration of ethidium may prove damaging to the cells and reduce the mitotic index. Prolonged treatment with colchicine to accumulate a large number or metaphase cells also results in excessive contraction of the chromosomes, which cannot be entirely counteracted by the use of ethidium; for best results, therefore, the time of treatment with colchicine should be kept short (preferably <3 h).
3. It is important to note that no colcemid is added in this procedure. This is one of the reasons for the relatively poor yield of mitoses using this technique. Addition of colcemid will result in a good mitotic index with few if any chromosomes showing chromatin decondensation of any sort.

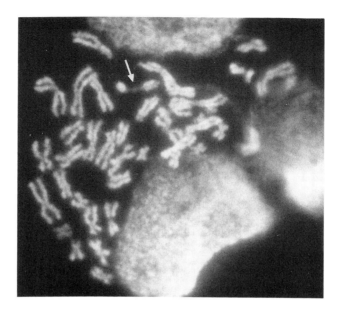

Fig. 4. A mouse metaphase spread from a culture treated with Hoechst 33258, showing decondensation of centromeric heterochromatin (arrowed). Fixed with methanol-acetic acid and stained with Hoechst 33258.

4. The conditions described apply to the culturing of human lymphocytes. Other cell lines appear to vary somewhat in their tolerance to both kinds of cytosine analog. A poor mitotic yield indicates that the concentration should be reduced somewhat (a factor of 10 is usually sufficient). On the other hand, the production of too many mitoses indicates that the concentration of the analog should be increased (again a factor of 10 should be tried).
5. As stated for 5'-azacytidine, different cell lines may have different sensitivities to DAPI. It may be necessary to adjust the concentrations of the DAPI accordingly.
6. Berenil becomes toxic to cells above 200 µg/mL in concentration. Care should therefore be taken to ensure that the concentrations used do not exceed 150 µg/mL.

References

1. ISCN (1985) *An International System for Human Cytogenetic Nomenclature* (Harnden, D. G. and Klinger, H. P., eds.) S. Karger, Basel.
2. Yunis, J. J. (1981) Mid-prophase human chromosomes. The attainment of 2000 bands. *Hum. Genet.* **56,** 293–298.

3. Ikeuchi, T. (1984) Inhibitory effect of ethidium bromide on mitotic chromosome condensation and its application to high-resolution chromosome banding. *Cytogenet. Cell. Genet.* **38**, 56–61.
4. Rønne, M. (1985) Double synchronization of human lymphocyte cultures: selection for high-resolution banded metaphases in the first and second division. *Cytogenet. Cell Genet.* **39**, 292–295.
5. Sumner, A. T. (1990) *Chromosome Banding.* Unwin Hyman, London, UK.
6. Brown, S. W. (1966) Heterochromatin. *Science* **151**, 417–425.
7. Schmid, M., Grunert, D., Haaf, T., and Engel, W. (1983) A direct demonstration of somatically paired heterochromatin of human chromosomes. *Cytogenet. Cell. Genet.* **36**, 554–561.
8. Haaf, T. and Schmid, M. (1989) 5-Azadeoxycytidine induced undercondensation in the giant X chromosome of *Microtus agrestis. Chromosoma* **98**, 93–98.
9. Haaf, T., Feichtinger, W., Guttenbach, M., Sanchez, L., Muller, C. R., and Schmid, M. (1989) Berenil-induced undercondensation in human heterochromatin. *Cytogenet. Cell Genet.* **50**, 27–33.
10. Hilwig, I. and Gropp, A. (1973) Decondensation of constitutive heterochromatin in L cell chromosomes by a benzimidazole compound ("33258 Hoechst"). *Exp. Cell Res.* **81**, 474–477.
11. Quillardet, P. and Hofnung, M. (1988) Ethidium bromide and safety. *Trends Genet.* **4**, 89.
12. Bensaude, O. (1988) Ethidium bromide and safety. *Trends Genet.* **4**, 89–90.
13. Anonymous. (No date) *Hazard Data Sheets.* BDH, Poole, UK.

CHAPTER 10

Analysis of Chromosomes with Restriction Endonucleases and DNase Hypersensitivity

*Joaquina de la Torre
and Adrian T. Sumner*

1. Introduction

The introduction of chromosome banding techniques about 20 years ago has not only provided a very powerful tool for chromosome identification, but has also highlighted structural and functional differences between different chromosomal segments *(1)*. Restriction endonucleases (RE) have been widely used to study some aspects of chromosome organization *(2–4)*. The original methods, involving digestion followed by Giemsa or ethidium bromide (EB) staining, lack both specificity and sensitivity. It is now clear that the Giemsa/EB staining does not necessarily represent the distribution of restriction sites along the chromosomes; other factors, such as the accessibility of the REs to the targets or the extractability of the DNA fragments produced, need to be considered.

More recently, another method with increased sensitivity and specificity has become available. In this method, sites of restriction endonuclease attack on chromosomes are identified by nick translation (RE/NT). The studies developed on this field have followed two different pathways: (a) the structural aspect; however, some of the problems observed with the RE/Giemsa technique still remain when using RE/NT (we shall come back to the point below) and (b) the functional aspect; these studies refer to the distinction between active and inactive regions on the basis of their differential sensitivity to DNaseI.

From: *Methods in Molecular Biology, Vol. 29: Chromosome Analysis Protocols*
Edited by: J. R. Gosden Copyright ©1994 Humana Press Inc., Totowa, NJ

1.1. Restriction Endonuclease/Giemsa
or Ethidium Bromide Staining

From a theoretical point of view, heavily stained regions after RE digestion and Giemsa or Ethidium staining would correspond to those regions that remain unattacked because they lack recognition sites for the enzymes. On the contrary, reduced staining of a particular region after digestion with certain enzymes could be correlated with the high degree of cutting by those enzymes and the subsequent DNA extraction from this region. However, this is certainly an oversimplification.

Restriction endonuclease banding has been applied to various organisms, from mammals to insects, including lower vertebrates and one species of plant. Essentially, three types of banding are obtained in mammals, although REs have been reported that give no banding at all. Those enzymes giving a C-positive or C-negative banding in humans do not necessarily produce a homogeneous differentiation of all the heterochromatic blocks (Fig. 1a and b). On the contrary, the RE banding permits the distinction of different types of heterochromatin, even within a particular heterochromatic block *(4–6)*.

There is another set of REs that produces G-banding on mammalian chromosomes (Fig. 1c). Some REs produce C- and/or G-like bands with both Giemsa and dyes that bind stoichiometrically to the DNA (e.g., *Alu*I, *Rsa*I, *Mbo*I, *Hae*III, *Eco*RII; *see* refs. *2–5,7*), whereas other REs induce G-like bands only with Giemsa *(3,8)*. It is noteworthy that no enzyme is reported in the literature to induce R-banding with Giemsa/or EB staining in spite of the wide variety of REs used. These points leave unanswered questions on the mechanism of action of the REs on fixed chromosomes.

In those organisms where no G-bands have been reported, such as insects, lower vertebrates, or plants, the REs only demonstrate heterochromatic bands. Most of the REs used produced a C-band-like pattern, whereas only a few of them failed to induce any banding at all *(9–14)*.

REs were also used to digest polytene chromosomes in *Drosophila melanogaster* and *D. virilis*. The authors found that specific bands were positively stained after digestion with *Alu*I and *Hae*III *(15,16)*.

Bianchi et al. *(17)* carried out experiments on Dipteran and human cells to analyze patterns of methylation on the basis of DNA extraction induced by REs that are inhibited or not by methylation of cytosine

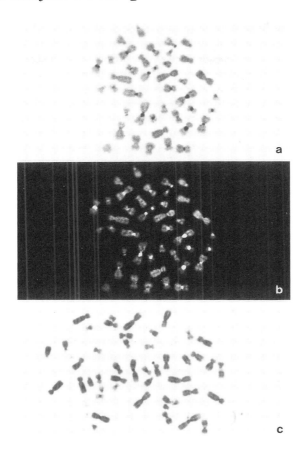

Fig. 1. Restriction endonuclease/Giemsa or ethidium bromide staining. C/G-like banding pattern induced by *Alu*I digestion of human chromosomes after Giemsa. (**a**) or ethidium bromide staining (**b**) G-banding pattern induced by *Msp*I digestion of human chromosomes and Giemsa staining (**c**) Figs. (a) and (b) were kindly provided by J. Gosálvez.

(*Hpa*II/*Msp*I). Although mosquito chromosomes were essentially unmethylated, a considerable proportion of methylated cytosine was found in human chromosomes.

REs also found their application in electron microscopy analysis. These studies permit us to go deeper into the mechanism of action of REs *(18,19)*. REs giving a similar pattern in the light microscope gave different results when used under the electron microscope, suggesting differences in chromatin conformation.

1.2. Restriction Endonuclease/ Nick Translation

Another method to detect the sites of RE attack on fixed chromosomes is the restriction endonuclease/nick translation technique (RE/NT). This procedure includes three different steps in the detection of specific nucleotide sequences on the chromosomes. First, chromosome preparations are digested *in situ* by using REs that recognize specific targets on the DNA. Second, the cuts generated by the REs are used as starting points for polymerization in the presence of biotinylated nucleotides. Third, the incorporated biotinylated nucleotides are detected by using different immunocytochemical methods.

It might be expected that results of nick translation would be the opposite of those obtained with Giemsa. However, this is not necessarily so.

The RE/NT technique has been applied to human and mouse chromosomes *(20–23)*. Recently, we have applied this technique on newt chromosome preparations obtained from the intestine and testes according to Herrero et al. *(24)*. This technique has also proven useful in grasshopper chromosomes *(25)*. The first work in this field was reported by Bullerdiek et al. *(26,27)* on human and Chinese hamster chromosomes, giving no conclusion about the patterns obtained. Adolph *(28)* applied the RE/Giemsa and RE/NT procedures to mouse chromosomes using the restriction enzymes *Ava*II and *Eco*RI. Both enzymes gave complementary results with nick translation and Giemsa staining as might have been expected. However, in an extensive study carried out in human chromosomes, Sumner et al. *(23)* found that the patterns obtained after RE/NT were not necessarily the reverse of those seen after RE/Giemsa staining. The authors concluded that the patterns obtained after RE digestion and Giemsa staining or nick translation depend not only on the distribution of the enzyme recognition sites on the chromosomes, but also on the accessibility of the REs and extraction of the chromosomal DNA. Similar conclusions were obtained by de la Torre et al. *(20)* on mouse chromosomes. The RE/NT technique was therefore proven to be a very powerful method for investigating the mechanisms of the RE-induced banding of chromosomes.

The RE/NT procedure was also applied for studying DNA methylation *in situ*. Much of the work has concerned differences between the X chromosomes in female mammals, but results have been inconsistent. Both the unmethylated and methylated status of the inactive X chromosome have been reported *(21)*, whereas other laboratories, as well as ourselves, have failed to find any differentiation of the inactive X *(22,29)*.

1.3. DNaseI Hypersensitivity

Since the work of Weintraub and Groudine *(30),* who first reported a differential sensitivity of active regions to DNaseI, and that of Gazit et al. *(31),* indicating that this property is maintained even in mitotic chromosomes, DNaseI has been used to map active genes on fixed chromosomes. Hypersensitive regions are preferentially nicked by DNaseI, thus becoming preferentially labeled after nick translation with labeled nucleotides, and can be visualized by using an appropriate detection method. Localization of DNaseI hypersensitive sites in mammals by *in situ* nick translation has indicated that they are distributed in a pattern that shows some resemblance to R-bands *(27,29,32–34).* Kerem et al. *(32)* used the term D-bands for the patterns of DNaseI hypersensitivity on chromosomes. There is also evidence of a differential labeling of the inactive X-chromosome *(35),* although Murer-Orlando and Peterson *(34)* found, as we did, no difference in the labeling of the inactive X compared with the rest of the chromosomes.

As we mentioned above, the DNaseI-induced patterns have been only analyzed in mammals. However, it would be interesting to extend the application of this technique to other species where no G/R-bands have been described.

2. Materials
2.1. Restriction Endonuclease/Giemsa or Ethidium Staining

1. RE solutions and buffers as supplied by the manufacturer.
2. Two percent Giemsa (Gurr R66, BDH) in phosphate buffer, pH 6.8, made from "Gurr" buffer tablets (BDH).
3. 0.04% Ethidium bromide in phosphate-buffered saline (PBS, made from Oxoid tablets).
4. 1% Sodium dithionite in PBS.

2.2. Restriction Endonuclease/Nick Translation

1. Nick translation buffer: 50 mM Tris-HCl, pH 7.8, 5 mM MgCl$_2$, 10 mM β-mercaptoethanol.
2. 5% Trichloracetic acid.
3. 10X Buffer 1: 121.0 g Tris base, 58.4 g NaCl, and 4.07 g MgCl$_2$ · 6H$_2$O made up to 900 mL with distilled water and 65 mL concentrated HCl added to bring the pH to 7.5. After autoclaving, 5 mL Triton X-100 are added when cool.
4. Buffer 2: 2% w/v bovine serum albumin (BSA), in buffer 1.
5. Streptavidin-horseradish peroxidase (SA-HRP) 1:250 in buffer 2 and H$_2$O: 4 μL SA-HRP stock solution (Vector Labs, Burlingame, CA), 96 μL buffer 2, 900 μL distilled water.
6. Phosphate-buffered saline (PBS) (made from Oxoid tablets, "Dulbecco A").
7. 0.5 mg/mL diameno-benzidine (DAB) (Sigma, St. Louis, MO) in PBS.
8. 1 vol Hydrogen peroxide.
9. 2.5 mM NaAuCl$_4$, pH 2.3.
10. 0.1M Sodium sulfide, pH 7.5.
11. Silver reagent: To 1 mL distilled water, add in order, with vortexing, 1 mL 0.013M ammonium nitrate, 1 mL 6 mM silver nitrate, 1.5 mM dodeca-tungstosilicic acid, 5 μL formaldehyde (0.6 μL/mL of 40% v/v), and 5 mL 0.24M sodium carbonate. Use as soon as the solution has become clear.
12. 1:50 Streptavidin-FITC (SA-FITC) in PBS (Vector Labs).
13. Citifluor (PBS/Glycerol solution).
14. Mouse antibiotin IgG (Dakopatts) in 0.05M Tris-HCl (1:50 v/v), pH 7.2.
15. 0.05M Tris-HCl, pH 7.2.
16. 1:50 v/v Peroxidase-labeled antimouse IgG (Sigma) in PBS.
17. 1:50 v/v Rabbit antimouse IgG fluorescein conjugate (Serotec, Oxford, UK) in PBS.
18. 2X SSC.
19. 4X SSC/TX: 0.05% Triton X-100 in 4X SSC.
20. 2 mg/mL Avidin-FITC (AV-FITC) (Vector Laboratories) stock solution.
21. 1:500 AV-FITC in 3% BSA/4X SSC.
22. 0.5 mg/mL Biotinylated goat antiavidin (BAA, Vector Laboratories) stock solution.
23. 1:100 BAA in 3% BSA/4X SSC.

2.3. DNase Hypersensitivity

1. Nick translation buffer (*see* Section 2.2.)
2. Deoxyribonuclease I, 0.2–200 ng/mL in the nick translation buffer, plus DNA polymerase I and nucleotides, as for restriction endonuclease/nick translation (*see* Section 3.2.1.).

3. Methods

3.1. Restriction Endonuclease/Giemsa or Ethidium Staining

Fixed chromosomes obtained from different sources (insects, fishes, amphibia, anura, birds, mammals, and plants) have been used by different authors and provide excellent results (references in *1* and *36*). This technique has been currently used for light microscopy. Preparations for chromosome analysis are obtained following standard procedures of fixation, and current techniques of spreading and squashing *(37)* (Chapter 1).

Digestion of fixed chromosomes with restriction endonucleases is always performed on fresh-dried preparations (no more than 12 h after having been prepared). The standard procedure was described by Mezzanotte et al. *(2,3);* however, slight deviations from this method, where different concentrations or digestion lengths are used, have also been tested. Digestion times and concentrations to be used are closely related with the amount of DNA extraction to be expected for a particular enzyme. On the other hand, we have to reach an equilibrium where chromosome morphology is still preserved.

1. One to 50 U of the RE diluted to 20–50 µL in the buffer recommended by the supplier are usually used per slide. The enzyme solution is placed on the slide and covered with a coverslip to spread the enzyme evenly.
2. Incubation is carried out in a humid box for the selected time and at the temperature specified by the manufacturer. For long incubations, the coverslip is sealed with rubber solution to prevent evaporation.
3. Control experiments are performed under identical conditions by treating cytological preparations with the incubation buffer without enzyme.
4. The reaction is stopped by washing the slides in running water.
5. Giemsa staining: Slides are stained for 30 min with Giemsa. After rinsing with distilled water, the stained slides are air-dried and mounted in DPX (Fig. 1a and c).
6. Ethidium bromide staining: Slides are stained for 1 h with ethidium bromide (BDH). After rinsing thoroughly in distilled water, the stained slides are dried, mounted in 1% sodium dithionite—PBS, and sealed with rubber solution (Fig. 1b).

3.2. Restriction Enzyme/Nick Translation

Chromosome preparations are obtained from cell cultures using standard procedures for fixation and spreading (*see* Chapter 1). As we mentioned above, the RE/NT technique includes three successive steps.

3.2.1. RE-Induced Nicking
and Synthesis of Labeled DNA

The digestion, as described above, must be long enough to induce specific cuts, but short enough to minimize DNA loss. Accordingly, short digestion lengths are commonly used (0–1 h); however, longer incubations have also been tested (including overnight digestion).

Full details of the *in situ* nick translation procedure were given by Sumner et al. *(23)* and de la Torre et al. *(20)*. Both radioactive and nonradioactive methods have been described; we shall concentrate here on various experimental conditions employing biotinylated-dUTP (bio-dUTP) as the incorporated signal.

1. After RE digestion (*see* Section 3.1.), the coverslip is removed and the slides washed in distilled water before proceeding to the subsequent nick translation procedure.
2. Five units of the DNA polymerase I (endonuclease-free) dissolved in 50 µL of the nick translation buffer complemented with 10 µ*M* each of dATP, dCTP, dGTP, and biotin-16-dUTP are added to each slide. All biochemicals are purchased from Boehringer (Mannheim, Germany). The slides are then covered by a 22 × 40 mm coverslip, and incubation at room temperature is resumed for 30–45 min.
3. The slides are washed for 5 min in 5% trichloracetic acid at 4°C to remove all unincorporated nucleotide triphosphates, followed by a rinse in buffer 1.
4. The chromosome preparations are blocked by incubation for 20 min at 42°C in buffer 2, followed by 10 min at room temperature in buffer 1.

3.2.2. Immunocytochemical Detection of Bio-dUTP

The incorporated biotinylated nucleotides are visualized by employing different detection methods as described below (Fig. 2).

3.2.2.1. STREPTAVIDIN-HORSERADISH PEROXIDASE
(SA-HRP) CONJUGATE

The biotinylated nucleotides are detected after binding of the streptavidin-horseradish peroxidase conjugate (SA-HRP, Bethesda Research Laboratories, Gaithersburg, MD), and the peroxidase substrate 3-3'-diaminobenzidine (DAB, Sigma tablets) is used to reveal the formed complexes (Fig. 2a).

1. A 1:250 solution of SA-HRP is used. One hundred microliters of the diluted solution are added per slide and covered with a 22 × 40 mm coverslip. The incubation at 37°C is resumed for 30 min in a humid box (paper towel soaked with PBS).

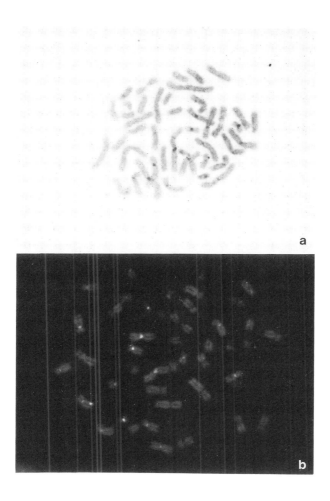

Fig. 2. Restriction endonuclease/nick translation. *Eco*RI digested human chromosomes after nick translation as visualized by the SA-HRP (**a**) and the SA-FITC (**b**) detection methods.

2. Slides are then developed by using 5 mL of DAB (Sigma) solution (0.5 mg/mL) in PBS to which 50 μL of 1 vol hydrogen peroxide are added immediately before use. Four hundred microliters of this solution are used per slide, and the slides incubated in the dark at room temperature for 45–60 min.
3. Slides are then washed thoroughly in distilled water, and rinsed twice in PBS and finally in distilled water.
4. The slides are then allowed to dry and mounted in DPX.

Before mounting, the DAB reaction can be intensified following the procedure of Gallyas et al. *(38)* as modified by Burns et al. *(39)*. The slides are sequentially incubated and washed at room temperature in the following solutions.

1. 2.5 mM NaAuCl$_4$, pH 2.3 for 5 min.
2. Distilled water for 5 min.
3. 0.1M Sodium sulfide (adjusted to pH 7.5 with 1M HCl) for 5 min.
4. Wash in distilled water for 5 min.
5. Incubate the slides at room temperature for 2–6 min in silver reagent.

3.2.2.2. STREPTAVIDIN-FLUORESCEIN ISOTHIOCYANATE CONJUGATE

The biotinylated nucleotides are detected after binding of the streptavidin-fluorescein conjugate (SA FITC; Amersham, Bucks, UK) (Fig. 2b). A 1:50 solution of SA-FITC in PBS is used.

1. One hundred microliters of the diluted solution are added per slide, and the slide covered with a 22 × 40 mm coverslip. The incubation is carried out at room temperature for 30 min.
2. After incubation, the coverslips are removed and the slides washed thoroughly in PBS.
3. After drying, the slides are mounted in Citifluor (PBS/glycerol solution) and sealed with rubber solution.

3.2.2.3. MONOCLONAL MOUSE ANTIBIOTIN/ANTIMOUSE HRP
OR MONOCLONAL MOUSE ANTIBIOTIN/ANTIMOUSE FITC

A two-step method is used for the detection of the biotinylated nucleotides.

1. One hundred microliters of a mouse antibiotin IgG (Dako Ltd., High Wycombe, UK) diluted 1:20 in 0.05M Tris-HCl, pH 7.2, are added and the slides are incubated at room temperature for 30 min.
2. The slides are washed once in 0.05M Tris-HCl, pH 7.2, and twice in PBS for 10 min each.
3. One hundred microliters of the second antibody, a peroxidase-labeled antimouse IgG (Sigma)—or a rabbit antimouse IgG fluorescein conjugate (Serotec)—diluted 1:50 in PBS, are added, and incubation is resumed for 30 min at room temperature.
4. Slides are washed twice in PBS, 10 min each.
5. Peroxidase-treated slides are then developed by using DAB as described before and finally mounted in DPX.
6. After drying, fluorescein-treated slides are mounted in Citifluor (PBS/glycerol solution) and sealed with rubber solution.

3.2.2.4. AVIDIN-FITC/BIOTINYLATED GOAT ANTIAVIDIN/AVIDIN-FITC

1. Prior to immunostaining, slides are washed twice for 5 min each in 2X SSC at room temperature, and once for 2 min in 4X SSC/TX (0.05% Triton X-100 in 4X SSC).
2. A 2 mg/mL stock solution of the first antibody, an avidin-fluorescein conjugate (AV-FITC, Vector Laboratories), is diluted 1:500 in 4X SSC containing 3% BSA (Sigma). Forty microliters of the diluted solution are added per slide, and the slides incubated at 37°C for 30 min.
3. The slides are washed three times, 2 min each, in 4X SSC/TX at room temperature.
4. A 0.5 mg/mL stock solution of the second antibody, a biotinylated goat antiavidin (BAA, Vector Laboratories), is diluted 100X in 3% BSA in 4X SSC. Forty microliters of the diluted solution are used per slide, and incubation at 37°C is carried out for 30 min, followed by three washes, 2 min each, in 4X SSC/TX at room temperature.
5. This process is repeated once more for the primary antibody followed by three further washes in 4X SSC/TX.
6. After drying, the slides are mounted in Citifluor and sealed with rubber solution.

3.3. DNase Hypersensitivity

Chromosome preparations are obtained from cell cultures fixed and spread according to standard procedures (Chapter 1). DNaseI/NT is performed on freshly spread preparations (no more than 12 h after preparation). The concentration of DNaseI used for detecting the hypersensitive sites is a very variable factor. Different authors have used different concentrations, varying from 0.2 ng/mL to 200 ng/mL. Different patterns are obtained with different amounts of enzyme (Fig. 3); moreover, chromosomes from different species require different concentrations of DNaseI to obtain optimal results *(33)*.

1. Pancreatic DNaseI (Sigma) is added to the nick translation mixture described above (Section 2.3.) to the required concentration. The reaction is carried out at room temperature for 5 min.
2. Further steps and washes are identical to those described in the *in situ* nick translation protocol (Section 3.2.).
3. Biotin incorporation is usually visualized after binding of the streptavidin-horseradish peroxidase complex by H_2O_2-mediated 3-3'-diaminobenzidine precipitation (*see* Section 3.2.).

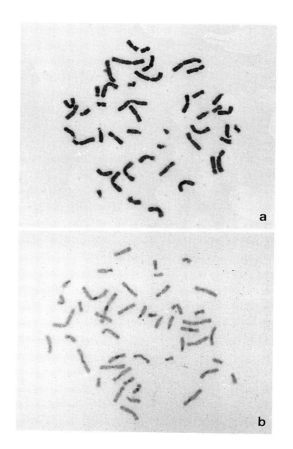

Fig. 3. Human metaphase plates obtained by *in situ* nick translation with DNaseI. Note the different reactions induced depending on the DNaseI concentration used: **a.** low concentration—0.125 ng/mL, **b.** high concentration—1 ng/mL.

4. Notes

1. The RE/Giemsa (EB) technique was based on the principle that any observed pattern would be the result of the distribution of the RE targets throughout the chromosome. As years go by, there is increasing information on the patterns obtained using these techniques in several species *(2–5,7,9–11,15,40,41)*, but the evidence indicates that this early hypothesis is not fully true; we still need to investigate the molecular mechanisms accounting for RE-induced banding.

   In order to understand the complexity underlying those mechanisms, we must consider the complicated structure of the eukaryotic chromosome. The highly condensed metaphase chromosome results from many different orders of packing, which would prevent by themselves RE access to the DNA targets. It is known that *Bst*NI cuts the mouse major satellite DNA into fragments of 234 bp *(42)*. However, when used on fixed chromosomes, *Bst*NI was not able to digest mouse centromeric heterochromatin regularly, unless the heterochromatin was decondensed as a result of culture in the presence of 5-azacytidine. Chromatin conformation was therefore proven to be an important factor in determining RE-induced banding patterns *(20)*.

On the other hand, even if RE attack actually occurs, there is still the possibility that the fragmented DNA cannot diffuse out of the compact chromosome. Miller et al. *(4)* estimated that DNA fragments larger than 1000 bp would be retained on fixed chromosomes, whereas Burkholder *(41)* showed that fragments up to 4000 bp could be lost from unfixed chromosomes after RE digestion. In any case, the RE/Giemsa (EB) method and, in general, any method based on DNA extraction appear to be rather inefficient for detecting sites of RE attack on chromosomes.

2. In theory, any pattern observed when using the RE/NT technique should reflect the distribution of the enzyme recognition sites along the chromosomes. In spite of the limitations referred to below and the greater complexity of the method, there is no doubt that the RE/NT is a much more reliable method than the RE/Giemsa staining for indicating the distribution on chromosomes of the recognition sites for REs. One of the most difficult problems to solve is that related to the accessibility of the REs to the DNA targets. Only by disturbing the complex chromosome structure with drugs, such as 5-azacytidine, is it possible for certain REs to gain access to their targets *(17,20)*.

Another important point to bear in mind is that spontaneous nicking and/or DNA loss is particularly undesirable in these experiments; thus, any method that helps to stabilize chromosome structure would be welcome. We have tested both formaldehyde and glutaraldehyde to reduce DNA loss, but these methods produced a reduction in sensitivity of the nick translation reaction.

In our hands, DNA polymerase I proved to be the most suitable enzyme for nick translation of RE-digested chromosomes. Nevertheless, Viegas-Péquignot et al. *(21)* obtained good results by using terminal transferase, an enzyme that might be expected to give a better signal, but was unsuccessful in our hands.

We have described above the different methods employed for the detection of the incorporated biodUTP. A summary of the advantages

Table 1
Comparison of the Different Detection Methods Employed
in the RE/NT Procedure

Detection Method	Signal/ Background	Reliability	Chromosome Morphology	Ease Speed
SA-HRP	Moderate (++)	Moderate (++)	Good (+++)	Reasonable (++)
SA-FITC	Good (+++)	Good (+++)	Good (+++)	Fast (+++)
Antibiotin Antimouse-HRP	Moderate (++)	Moderate (++)	Acceptable (++)	Reasonable (++)
Antibiotin/ Antimouse-FITC	Acceptable, but more background than with SA-FITC (++−)	Moderate— good (++−)	Acceptable (++)	Reasonable (++)
AV-FITC/BAA/ AV-FITC	Acceptable, but more background than with SA-FITC (++−)	Moderate— good (++−)	Acceptable (++)	Slow (+)

and disadvantages with respect to the signal/background ratio, the chromosome morphology, and the ease and reliability of each method is given in Table 1. In general, those methods including different steps in the detection of the bio-dUTP (i.e., the employment of primary/secondary antibodies and so on) lead to a reduction (although acceptable) in the preservation of the chromosome morphology, probably because of the incorporation of very many washes in between. On the other hand, these methods usually lead to an increase in the general staining of the chromosomes commonly appearing outlined with darker/brighter rings. This unspecific reaction was never observed after streptavidin-FITC (Fig. 2b) and only occasionally with the streptavidin-HRP detection method (Fig. 2a). With respect to the reliability of the detection methods employed, those employing a fluorescein-ligated conjugate have been proven more reliable than those using a peroxidase-ligated conjugate.

3. Some of the problems observed when using DNaseI/NT have been described in the previous section, and are related to the spontaneous nicking and/or DNA loss as well as the method for detecting the incor-

porated labeled nucleotides. Other problems arise from the particular action of the DNaseI compared to the REs. Although REs induce base-pair specific cuts for subsequent nick translation, the DNaseI/NT method does not depend on any base-pair specificity, but on the accessibility of the DNA to the DNaseI. In this sense, DNaseI follows a dynamic process, starting at those hypersensitive sites before digesting the active chromatin and finally the rest of the chromatin. We have mentioned already that the observed patterns are highly dependent on the concentration of DNaseI, the length of digestion, or the species being analyzed. Commonly, we observe changes in the DNaseI/NT pattern when changing any of these conditions (Fig. 3a and b). Thus, the optimal conditions for each experiment have to be achieved by trial and error.

References

1. Sumner, A. T. (1990) *Chromosome Banding.* Unwin Hyman Ltd., London, UK.
2. Mezzanotte, R., Ferrucci, L., Vanni, R., and Bianchi, U. (1983) Selective digestion of human metaphase chromosomes by AluI restriction endonuclease. *J. Histochem. Cytochem.* **31,** 553–556.
3. Mezzanotte, R., Bianchi, U., Vanni, R., and Ferrucci, L. (1983) Chromatin organisation and restriction endonuclease activity on human metaphase chromosomes. *Cytogenet. Cell Genet.* **36,** 562–566.
4. Miller, D. A., Choi, Y. C., and Miller, O. J. (1983) Chromosome localisation of highly repetitive human DNA's and amplified ribosomal DNA with restriction enzymes. *Science* **219,** 395–397.
5. Bianchi, M. S., Bianchi, N. O., Pantelias, G. E., and Wolf, S. (1985) The mechanism and pattern of banding induced by restriction endonucleases in human chromosomes. *Chromosoma* **91,** 131–136.
6. Babu, A., Agrawal, A. K., and Verma, R. S. (1988) A new approach in recognition of heterochromatic regions of human chromosomes by means of restriction endonucleases. *Am. J. Hum. Genet.* **42,** 60–65.
7. Kaelbling, M., Miller, D. A., and Miller, O. J. (1984) Restriction enzyme banding of mouse metaphase chromosomes. *Chromosoma* **90,** 128–132.
8. Mezzanotte, R., Manconi, P. E., Rozzo, C., Ennas, M. G., and Ferrucci, L. (1985) The banding pattern produced by restriction endonucleases in mouse chromosomes. *Basic Appl. Histochem.* **29,** 115–120.
9. Frediani, M., Mezzanotte, R., Vanni, R., Pignone, D., and Cremonini, R. (1987) The biochemical and cytological characterization of *Vicia faba* DNA by means of MboI, AluI and BamHI restriction endonucleases. *Theor. Appl. Genet.* **75,** 46–50.
10. Gosálvez, J., Bella, J. L., López-Fernández, C., and Mezzanotte, R. (1987) Correlation between constitutive heterochromatin and restriction enzyme resistant chromatin in *Arcyptera tornosi* (Orthoptera). *Heredity* **59,** 173–180.
11. Schmid, M. and Almeida, C. G. (1988) Chromosome banding in Amphibia. XII. Restriction endonuclease banding. *Chromosoma* **96,** 283–290.

12. Cau, A, Salvadori, S., Deiana, A. M., Bella, J. L., and Mezzanotte, R. (1988) The characterization of *Muraena helena* L. mitotic chromosomes karyotype, C-banding, nucleolar organizer regions, and *in situ* digestion with restriction endonucleases. *Cytogenet. Cell Genet.* **47,** 223–226.
13. López-Fernández, C., Gosálvez, J., Suja, J. A., and Mezzanotte, R. (1988) Restriction endonuclease digestion of meiotic and mitotic chromosomes in *Pyrgomorpha conica* (Orthoptera: Pyrgomorphidae). *Genome* **30,** 621–626.
14. López-Fernández, C., Gosalvez, J., and Mezzanotte, R. (1989) Heterochromatin heterogeneity in *Oedipoda germanica* (Orthoptera) detected by *in situ* digestion with restriction endonucleases. *Heredity* **62,** 269–277.
15. Mezzanotte, R. (1986) The selective digestion of polytene and mitotic chromosomes of *Drosophila melanogaster* by the AluI and HaeIII restriction endonucleases. *Chromosoma* **93,** 249–255.
16. Mezzanotte, R., Bianchi, U., and Marchi, A. (1987) In situ digestion of *Drosophila virilis* polytene chromosomes by AluI and HaeIII restriction endonucleases, *Genome* **29,** 630–634.
17. Bianchi, N. O., Vidal-Rioja, L., and Cleaver, J. E. (1986) Direct visualization of the sites of DNA methylation in human and mosquito chromosomes. *Chromsoma* **94,** 362–366.
18. Gosálvez, J. and Goyanes, V. (1988) Selective digestion of mouse chromosomes with restriction endonucleases. I. Scaffold-like structures and bands by electron microscopy. *Cytogenet. Cell Genet.* **48,** 198–200.
19. Gosálvez, J., Sumner, A. T., López-Fernández, C., Rossino, R., Goyanes, V., and Mezzanotte, R. (1990) Electron microscopy and biochemical analysis of mouse metaphase chromosomes after digestion with restriction endonucleases. *Chromosoma* **99,** 36–43.
20. de la Torre, J., Mitchell, A. R., and Sumner, A. T. (1991) Restriction endonuclease/ nick translation of fixed mouse chromosomes: a study of factors affecting digestion of chromosomal DNA *in situ*. *Chromosoma* **100,** 203–211.
21. Viegas-Péquignot, E., Dutrillaux, B., and Thomas, G. (1988) Inactive X chromosome has the highest concentration of unmethylated HhaI sites. *Proc. Nat. Acad. Sci.* **85,** 7657–7660.
22. Adolph, S. and Hameister, H. (1990) *In situ* nick translation of human metaphase chromosomes with the restriction enzymes MspI and HpaII reveals an R-band pattern. *Cytogenet. Cell Genet.* **54,** 132–136.
23. Sumner, A. T., Taggart, M., Mezzanotte, R., and Ferrucci, L. (1990) Patterns of digestion on human chromosomes by restriction endonucleases demonstrated by *in situ* nick translation. *Histochem. J.* **22,** 639–652.
24. Herrero, P., Bella, J. L., and Arano, B. (1989) Characterization of heterochromatic regions in two *Triturus alpestris* subspecies (Urodela:Salamandridae). *Heredity* **63,** 119–123.
25. de la Torre, J., López-Fernández, C., Herrero, P., and Gosálves, J. (1993) *In situ* nick translation of meiotic chromosomes to demonstrate homologous heterochromatin heterogeneity. *Genome* **36,** in press.

26. Bullerdiek, J., Dittmer, J., Faehre, A., Bartnitzke, S., Kasche, V., and Schloot, W. (1985) A new banding pattern of human chromosomes by *in situ* nick translation using EcoRI and biotin-dUTP. *Clin. Genet.* **28,** 173–176.

27. Bullerdiek, J., Dittmer, J., Faehre, A., and Bartnitzke, S. (1986) Mechanism of *in situ* nick translation of chromosomes using restriction endonucleases. *Cytobios* **47,** 33–44.

28. Adolph, S. (1988) *In situ* nick translation distinguishes between C-band positive regions on mouse chromosomes. *Chromosoma* **96,** 102–106.

29. de la Torre, J., Sumner, A. T., Gosálves, J., and Stuppia, L. (1992) The distribution of genes on human chromosomes as studied by *in situ* nick translation. *Genome* **35,** 890–894.

30. Weintraub, H. and Groudine, M. (1976). Chromosomal subunits in active genes have an altered conformation. *Science* **93,** 848–856.

31. Gazit, B., Cedar, H., Lerer, I., and Voss, R. (1982) Active genes are sensitive to deoxyribonuclease I during metaphase. *Science* **217,** 648–650.

32. Kerem, B. S., Goitein, R., Diamond, G., Cedar, H., and Marcus, M. (1984) Mapping of DNAseI sensitive regions on mitotic chromosomes. *Cell* **38,** 493–499.

33. Adolph, S. and Hameister, H. (1985) *In situ* nick translation of metaphase chromosomes with biotinlabelled d-UTP. *Hum. Genet.* **69,** 117–121.

34. Murer-Orlando, M. L. and Peterson, A. C. (1985) *In situ* nick translation of human and mouse chromosomes detected with a biotinylated nucleotide. *Exp. Cell Res.* **157,** 322–334.

35. Kerem, B. S., Goitein, R., Richler, C., Marcus, M., and Cedar, H. (1983) *In situ* nick translation distinguishes between active and inactive X chromosomes. *Nature* **304,** 88–90.

36. López-Fernández, C., Gosálvez, J., Ferrucci, L., and Mezzanotte, R. (1991) Restriction endonucleases in the study of eukaryotic chromosomes. *Genetica* **83,** 257–274.

37. Macgregor, H. and Varley, J. (1988) *Working with Animal Chromosomes,* 2nd. ed., Wiley, New York.

38. Gallyas, F., Gorcs, T., and Merchenthaler, I. (1982) High-grade intensification of the end-product of the diaminobenzidine reaction for peroxidase histochemistry. *J. Histochem. Cytochem.* **30,** 183–184.

39. Burns, J., Chan, V. T. W., Jonasson, J. A., Fleming, K. A., Taylor, S., and McGee, J. O. D. (1985) Sensitive system for visualising biotinylated DNA probes hybridised *in situ:* a rapid sex determination of intact cells. *J. Clin. Pathol.* **38,** 1085–1092.

40. Ferrucci, L., Romano, E., and De Stefano, G. F. (1987) The Alu-induced bands in great apes and man: implications for heterochromatin characterization and satellite DNA distribution. *Cytogenet. Cell Genet.* **44,** 53–57.

41. Burkholder, G. (1989) Morphological and biochemical effects of endonucleases on isolated mammalian chromosomes "in vitro." *Chromosoma* **97,** 347–355.

42. Southern, E. M. (1975) Long range periodicities in mouse satellite. *J. Mol. Biol.* **94,** 51–69.

CHAPTER 11

Automatic Karyotype Analysis

Jim Graham and Jim Piper

1. Introduction

1.1. A Warning to the Reader

This chapter differs from the majority in this book in that its subject matter is the application of computer image interpretation techniques to the analysis of metaphase chromosome spreads. Were we to follow the prescription of the remainder of the book, we might simply publish the code of a computer program together with a list of suitable equipment. This is not, however, a realistic option. The computer programs in current commercial systems for automated cytogenetics typically consist of approximately 100,000 lines of source code; in the case of automatic metaphase finders, the equipment may include proprietary mechanical or electronic components. Also, the rate of change in the performance and cost of cameras, displays, and computers are such that any list of equipment that is appropriate as we write in mid-1991 would most likely be nearing obsolescence by the time the book is published.

We have therefore decided to describe, in some detail, the main procedures that have to be implemented in software, and the minimum performance that would be required from commercially available computer and imaging hardware in order to run the software successfully. Both should be specified in sufficient detail that a working system could be built by an experienced computer programmer.

We will model our exposition on the best currently available technology. Commercially, we believe that this is represented by the Magiscan

From: *Methods in Molecular Biology, Vol. 29: Chromosome Analysis Protocols*
Edited by: J. R. Gosden Copyright ©1994 Humana Press Inc., Totowa, NJ

(Joyce Loebl, Gateshead, UK), Cytoscan (Image Recognition Systems, Warrington, UK) (both of these companies are now part of Applied Imaging International, Inc., Sunderland, UK) (the authors were, respectively, involved in the development of these two systems), AKS-2 (Amoco Technology Inc., Naperville, IL), Genetiscan (Perceptive Scientific Instruments Inc., League City, TX), and similar machines, together with recent developments that may well appear in commercial products in the near future.

However, we think it essential to warn readers contemplating making their own system that this is a big undertaking. The time and effort required depend, of course, on the skills and equipment available, but we cannot imagine that a simple but usable interactive karyotyping system (without automatic classification) could be programmed with less than six months of effort from an experienced programmer; an automatic karyotyper would require at least a year, as would an automatic metaphase finder. Polished, reliable, and ergonomic versions might increase these times by a factor of between two and ten! Those who think that these estimates are excessive should bear in mind the widely held belief that a competent computer programmer can, on average, produce just ten lines of correct, bug-free, and documented program code per working day. We believe that with modern operating systems and software tools, this figure is an underestimate; however, even a simple "no-frills" automatic karyotyping system would most likely require several tens of thousands of lines of code.

1.2. A Brief Introduction to Image Analysis

Automatic karyotyping involves the analysis by computer of two-dimensional light microscope images. In outline, such analysis involves the following stages.

1.2.1. Image Capture

Light transmitted through the microscope slide is focused onto the target of an electronic camera and sampled on a regular two-dimensional grid. The resulting brightness values or "pixels" are stored as numbers in computer memory (Fig. 1). The pixel values and their geometric positions are the basic data for all subsequent analysis. The natural unit of measurement in image analysis is the spacing between pixels in the image (the sampling interval), and unless stated other-

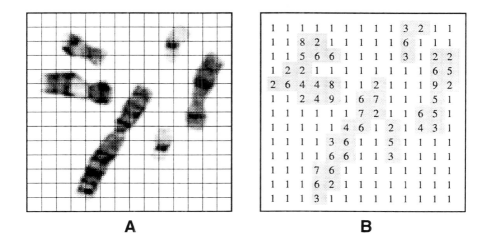

A   **B**

Fig. 1. **A.** A simulated image with sampling grid superimposed. **B.** The measured pixel values. The darker pixels (shaded) comprise several distinct connected components.

wise, measurements and geometrical constructions will be assumed to be based on this pixel spacing unit.

1.2.2. Segmentation

The set of pixels corresponding to a single chromosome must be determined so that they may be processed together in order to make measurements about the chromosome separately from the other objects in the field. This can be achieved, for example, by choosing a "darkness threshold" that is a little darker than the mean pixel value of the clear field between the chromosomes. Then pixels that are darker than the threshold "belong" to chromosomes, and individual chromosomes can be separated by finding connected subsets of the darker pixels (Fig. 1). Of course, this procedure is applicable to images other than metaphase cells, and sometimes other dark objects will occur even in metaphase fields, for example, interphase nuclei, so we will refer in general to such segmented sets of pixels as "image regions."

1.2.3. Feature Measurement

Feature measurements on each image region are made by applying mathematical formulae to the set of pixels; in many cases (e.g., for shape moments), the positional coordinates of pixels are also required. For example, the area of a chromosome may be estimated simply by counting the number of pixels. In practice, things are usually a little more complicated. In particular, in the case of chromosomes, most of the useful measurements depend on the position of the pixels relative not to the original Cartesian coordinate system of the pixel digitization grid, but to the chromosome's medial or symmetry axis, which may be imagined running between the chromatids, and so finding this axis is a necessary precursor to making such measurements, of which two obvious examples are the chromosome's length and centromeric index.

In order to make such feature measurements efficiently, each segmented image region or chromosome should be represented in an appropriate data structure. As will become clear in Section 3., the data structure must be capable of representing the arbitrary shapes, sizes, and orientations of chromosomes, and allow access to the pixel values so that computations may be made concerning the banding pattern. To describe such structures in detail is beyond the scope of this chapter, but examples may be found in refs. *1* and *2*.

1.2.4. Classification

Classification of image regions is typically made by applying statistical rules to a set of feature measurements. The rules are initially obtained either by introspection by the system designer, or more usually from a "training" or "design" set of image regions of predetermined class. Alternative classification schema, known variously as "syntactic" or "structural," are based on recognizing the "grammatical" arrangement of substructures of the image. More complicated systems based on artificial intelligence principles are the subject of current research.

1.2.5. Model

Crucially, a model or set of general principles that predict how a given biological entity, such as a metaphase chromosome, will be represented in digitized pixel values is essential to guide the search for meaning in the digitized image. The model has to accommodate both biological variability (for example, how to deal with touching chromosomes, bent chromosomes, the random position of chromosomes within the metaphase, or different metaphase contraction states), and image degradation on account perhaps of noise from the camera or a less than optimally set up microscope. Typically in chromosome analysis, the models are implicit rather than explicitly stated and are simplistic in the extreme, partly accounting for the widespread reliance on operator interaction for many of the nontrivial decisions.

1.3. Metaphase Finding

An essential component in any investigation involving chromosome analysis is the location of dividing cells of sufficient visual quality to permit the assessment of the chromosomes. The required cells may be at metaphase, prometaphase, or prophase, but the visual task does not vary greatly, and we will speak generically of "metaphase finding."

Unautomated metaphase finding involves visually scanning the microscope slide fairly rapidly at low magnification. When a metaphase is seen, it is examined carefully to assess its suitability for detailed analysis. If it appears suitably compact, well stained, and well spread, it may then be reexamined (either visually or automatically) at high magnification, when its quality can be completely determined and analysis performed as appropriate.

The proportion of the total analysis time and effort devoted to metaphase finding depends on the goals of the chromosome analysis and the material used. In "classical" (randomly induced) aberration scoring, for example, where the material is normally peripheral blood and the mitotic index is high, good-quality metaphases are easily found. The subsequent examination of individual cells, however, is very rapid, since dicentrics, acentric fragments, ring chromosomes, and so forth, are easily identified visually. The time spent locating new cells can therefore contribute significantly to the total analysis time. Karyotyping of bone marrow cells for leukemia diagnosis or treatment monitoring provides an example of a different type of task. The analysis of individual cells is a difficult, time-consuming exercise, but the visual quality of the metaphase cells may be so poor and the mitotic index so low that it may be necessary to locate all the dividing cells in a sample, involving a thorough search of the entire slide. In this case also, finding the metaphases is a significant proportion of the total task.

In clinical karyotyping using amniotic fluid or peripheral blood, metaphase finding contributes less significantly. Mitotic indices are high, and good-quality metaphases are fairly easily found in most routine material, although this is less true if direct chorionic villus samples are used. There are tasks of clinical interest, however, in which the metaphase finding component can be significant. Detection of fragile sites requires the examination of the order of 100 cells to be sure of correct diagnosis. The inspection of each cell can be fairly rapid, since the identification of the fragile site is often straightforward and the role of metaphase finding is similar to that in classical aberration scoring. Prophase analysis has similarities with cancer cytogenetics in the respect that a very thorough search might be necessary to locate a small number of cells in which the required bands can be identified on both homologous chromosomes.

1.3.1. Automatic Metaphase Finding

The central role of metaphase finding in all aspects of chromosome analysis and the fact that in some investigations it is a significant task in itself have led to the development of a number of automatic metaphase finders, some of which are associated with automated karyotyping systems. Finding metaphases automatically is a fairly typical image analysis task. However, the quantity of data is enormous. With the usual pixel size of about 1 μm^2, a coverslip area comprises about 10^9 pixels. Metaphase finders therefore aim to use simple, but fast, analysis methods.

It can be argued that metaphase finders have been more successful technically than karyotyping systems. Other than initial definition of the area of slide to be searched, they require no operator interaction and have been demonstrated to be highly efficient at identifying dividing cells *(3)*. Most metaphase finders also include a measure of metaphase quality that can be calculated when the cell is found, allowing the cells to be presented for analysis in ranked order. This is a useful feature in clinical karyotyping where only a small number of cells is required, but it is important that they should be of good visual quality. In particular, in prophase analysis, selection of cells in which the number of overlapping chromosomes is small may make a highly significant contribution to the efficiency of the overall process.

In the following paragraphs, we briefly discuss some of the features or properties of existing metaphase finders as they will be perceived by the user. In Section 3.1., we discuss some of the technical aspects of metaphase finding that influence these features. Detailed assessment of some of these features for metaphase finders in use in Europe has recently been made by Korthof and Carothers *(3)*.

1.3.2. Speed

At first sight, it appears that a high scanning speed is an essential feature of a metaphase finder. It is certainly the case that running the metaphase finder should not result in a significant time overhead for the busy cytogenetic laboratory. High scanning speeds can be achieved by applying highly optimized image acquisition methods (as used by Cytoscan, for example, *see* Section 3.1.1.). Machines based on less application-targeted hardware, which acquire their images using a television (TV) camera, scan more slowly. In the Korthof and Carothers survey, Cytoscan achieved scanning speeds of 88 s/cm^2 of slide on average over a range of material, whereas Magiscan took 596 s/cm^2 and other TV-based systems (no longer available commercially) took over 1000 s/cm^2. Also using line scanning, the recently developed Geneti-Scanner from Perceptive Scientific Instruments is reported to achieve scanning speeds of about 66 s/cm^2 *(4)*.

Speed is clearly important. All other things being equal, it is better to find metaphases quickly rather than slowly. However, TV-based systems may compensate for their lower scanning speeds by running metaphase finding overnight on a number of slides, which may be as beneficial, or more so, to clinical laboratory throughput as a scan of a few minutes on each slide as required. Performance comes at a cost, and the impact of fast scanning speed on the entire automated analysis package must be considered in assessing the benefit obtained.

1.3.3. Accuracy

We can consider accuracy in terms of false-negative rates (undetected metaphases), false-positive rates (nonmetaphases classed as metaphases), and ranking ability (the number of good-quality metaphases placed early in the analysis queue). For many clinical applications, the latter may be the only measure of interest to the user. If material with a low mitotic index is being analyzed, as in cancer cytogenetics, false-negative rates do become important. Fairly high false-positive rates may be tolerated, provided ranking is sufficiently good that nonmetaphases are only rarely presented to the user.

1.3.4. Adaptability

Slide preparation for karyotyping varies widely from laboratory to laboratory, and of course among different types of specimen. The parameters used by a metaphase finder should therefore be adjusted to provide optimal performance for each type of material for each laboratory. If these parameters are adjustable by the user, changes in laboratory practice, such as improvements in preparation techniques or introduction of new types of investigation, can be accommodated conveniently. The most suitable method of adjustment by the user is through system training, in which the metaphase finder is used on the new material and the trained operator labels each of the objects found according to its quality. The system then uses these quality scores to match the measured parameters to the desired properties.

1.3.5. System Considerations

Metaphase finding is never an end in itself. Automatic metaphase finding is always a component in some overall analysis task, and the features of a metaphase finder must be considered as part of the overall system. A slow metaphase finder as part of a stand-alone karyotyping system may enhance the overall system efficiency at fairly little additional cost. A laboratory with a large throughput may find a fast metaphase finder to be a useful central resource servicing a number of independent karyotyping stations. The Geneti-Scanner is clearly intended to be used in this way, since it can be loaded with up to 60 slides. After a setup period of about 30 min, these can be scanned unsupervised *(4)*.

The usefulness of a metaphase finder in any karyotyping environment depends not only on its basic performance characteristics, but also on its user interface. It is important not only that every cell presented to the operator for analysis is analyzable, but also that the operator interaction in loading the slides and specifying the scan parameters should be minimal and straightforward.

1.4. Automatic Karyotyping

Automatic karyotyping aims at describing the chromosome complement or karyotype of a metaphase cell and producing an annotated karyogram (an arrangement of images of the chromosomes in a prescribed pattern). In the early days of research in automated cytogenetics, the goal was to produce a completely automatic system.

However, the end product of the process of karyotyping is a statement about the genetic constitution of an individual from the point of view of his or her health. The consequences of that decision are of great importance to the individual. The decision is influenced by a number of factors, some of which involve detection of subtle signs in the image and some of which involve information not present in the image at all. For these reasons, it is clear that, for the foreseeable future, the assessment of the data leading to that clinical decision will be made by highly trained human beings and not by computer systems. Whatever level of computer assistance is provided, it will be in the form of an aid to human decision making. That is to say the system will be interactive.

A karyotyping system will be involved in either counting, or counting and fully analyzing, the chromosomes in a metaphase. However, the initial image obtained from the camera, and thresholded and segmented as described in Section 1.2., usually contains objects other than isolated chromosomes, notably chromosome clusters (both of touching and overlapping chromosomes), interphase nuclei, and noise of one sort or another (for example, stained cytoplasm, stain particles, or other dirt). In order to complete the classification and produce a karyogram, or even simply to perform a count, the objects that represent nonchromosomal material must be rejected, and the clusters resolved as far as possible into individual chromosomes. For karyotyping, the isolated chromosomes must be measured and classified. Methods for carrying out these procedures automatically are described in Sections 3.4.–3.6.

The current generation of image analyzers fall well short of performing these tasks with 100% reliability, either because the necessary algorithms cannot be run quickly enough on currently available computers, or because sufficiently sophisticated algorithms have not been developed. The result of this is that intervention by the operator is needed to resolve difficulties in the detailed analysis. From the point of view of the system developer, this is embarrassing, but because of the fact that karyotyping is inherently interactive, useful systems can be provided, albeit requiring rather more input from the user than is ideally desirable. The important features from the point of view of system usefulness are the number of interactions, the ease of interaction, and whether the interactions intrude on the user's interpretation of the image of the chromosomes.

1.5. Human–Machine Interaction

1.5.1. Interface Design

The process of interaction involves communication of knowledge between the user and the machine. For this communication to take place, it is necessary to have a physical medium on which messages are passed and an agreed vocabulary.

1.5.1.1. THE PHYSICAL INTERFACE

The physical components of the interface are displays, keyboards, and pointing devices, such as lightpens, mice, graphics tablets, or trackerballs. There has been some experimentation in karyotyping systems with voice input, but this technology is insufficiently advanced at this time to provide appropriate interaction.

The most important item to be displayed is the metaphase image, although other items, such as menus and textual information, need to be displayed also. The image display needs to be of high quality, since the final decision is often based on fairly subtle image features. The minimum specification acceptable for image display is 512×512 pixels of 64 gray levels. With earlier systems, the visual quality of such an image was generally believed to be poor compared to that obtained directly from the microscope or on a photograph, but probably sufficient for diagnostic purposes *(5–6)*. Nowadays, cameras and display monitors are available that are capable of considerably higher spatial and gray level resolution.

The display of nonimage information, such as menus or text, may be considered intrusive if it occupies the same area as the image. One answer to this is to use a separate display for this information. Alternatively, if high-resolution displays are used, a section of the display may be devoted to textual information without intrusion on the image. Many computer systems provide display management software using "windows," which allows information from several sources to be displayed and manipulated independently on the same screen. Thus, the areas of the screen to be used for different purposes may be altered interactively. Areas may be used temporarily for special purposes, such as magnification of selected regions of the image without altering the underlying display. The AKS-2 system, which is based on a MacIntosh computer, uses the high-resolution display and windows environment very effectively in this way.

Pointing devices are needed, since interaction usually involves specifying particular objects or parts of objects in the image, or selecting menu options. A mouse is preferred for this purpose, being inexpensive, robust, and easy to use. There is an advantage in using a lightpen for some types of interaction, particularly if careful drawing is required, but in general, lightpens are less satisfactory than mice. For karyotyping, trackerballs and graphics tablets appear to offer no particular advantage.

It is inevitable that some textual input will be required, such as sample identifiers or comments on a karyotype, and for this purpose, the keyboard is indispensable. However, it need have no other role in interaction, and its use should be kept to a minimum.

1.5.1.2. USER MODEL

By "user model" we mean the user's understanding of the objects displayed in the human–machine interface and his/her expectation of the system's behavior on interaction. A widely known example of a user model is that generated using the "desktop metaphor" employed by a number of office systems, where the user interacts with the system using concepts familiar from the everyday world, such as filing cabinets and wastepaper baskets. This model is successful, because it allows the user to express his/her requirements in terms of objects and activities that characterize the task, rather than the machine's implementation. In karyotyping, similarly, an appropriate interface should require the user to specify his/her requirements in terms of such objects as metaphases, chromosomes, centromeres, chromatids, or karyograms. It should not be necessary to require the user to think in terms of thresholds or pixels; these concepts are not difficult to cope with, but they introduce an element of opacity into a system that should be made as transparent as possible.

1.5.2. The Interaction Process

Here we outline some of the types of interaction that may be expected in automatic karyotyping systems.

1.5.2.1. SEGMENTATION

Inadequacies in segmentation algorithms generally show up as the inability to separate touching or overlapping chromosomes. In the case of touching chromosomes, it is easy for an operator to indicate with the pointing device the place where the composite object should be cut, either by drawing a separation line or indicating a few points around the cut location. Overlapping chromosomes call for more complex interaction, since the extent of each chromosome in the composite must be separately indicated. Cytoscan has a convenient method for achieving this by drawing a rough axis for each chromosome.

1.5.2.2. Axes and Centromere Positions

Defining a chromosome axis or centerline is a common step in extracting a number of important chromosome measurements (*see* Section 3.4.). For badly bent chromosomes, this may not be easy to define automatically. Centromere positions can also be difficult to measure, particularly in the case of highly elongated chromosomes. Since classification performance will be affected by errors in axis and centromere positions, correction of automatically generated positions may be required. This usually involves drawing a correct axis with the pointing device or indicating a correct centromere. However, it is often easier to accept errors of this type and correct the resulting classification errors at a later stage, and there is some evidence that this results in fewer interactions overall *(7)*.

1.5.2.3. Classification (Karyogram)

Classification errors occur whether or not all stages in the analysis of the image have proceeded correctly. All of these errors show up as misplaced chromosomes on the initially presented karyograms. Chromosomes may either be in the wrong locations on the display or allocated to a "reject" class. Since the chromosomes must be examined carefully at this stage, e.g., for small structural abnormality, interaction to correct these errors is not a serious overhead, provided that there are only a few corrections to be made. Such corrections are generally made by pointing to a chromosome on the display and indicating its correct position on the karyogram. Options will also be available for inverting a chromosome that has been presented the wrong way up or shifting chromosomes so that they are correctly aligned, in addition to other possible presentation facilities, such as rotation, chromosome straightening, or banding pattern enhancement *(8)*.

1.5.2.4. Counting

Counting chromosomes is the most easily described task in karyotype analysis, but it is one that is most difficult to automate. This is because the whole procedure must be carried out quickly (as quickly as the chromosomes can be counted by eye in the microscope). Using the types of computers appropriate for karyotyping systems, this precludes the use of highly sophisticated segmentation algorithms. Automated karyotyping systems approach this problem in various ways. In the Magiscan system, each image is digitized before any analysis takes place, and the user interacts with the image at all times via the screen. The Magiscan system provides semiautomated counting, in which an approximate count is presented to the operator, with all chromosomes marked, for correction by pointing at false chromosomes or missed chromosomes with the lightpen *(9)*. Since the user may wish to examine every chromosome at this stage in any case, it is frequently found more convenient to disable the automated counting phase and to have the operator simply mark each chromosome in turn. In this way, the operator is guaranteed to look at each chromosome in the image, and the count is generated as a byproduct. The Cytoscan system also provides interactive, screen-based counting. Again, however, except in particular cases (e.g., when counting hybrid cells with very many chromosomes), in typical use, counting is done entirely by "eyeball" analysis, in this case, of the metaphase directly in the microscope, because it is faster and easier for the operator, and not all counted cells need be analyzed further.

Having a mark reliably placed on the interior of each chromosome at the counting phase provides information that can be used to cut down the number of segmentation interactions required *(10)*. This indicates that the provision of interaction in karyotyping systems is a matter that should be considered at the system level and not merely as a local "fix" to a processing problem. The need for a large number of interactions does not necessarily signify an inefficient combination of operator and machine. Interactions that advance the operator's understanding of the image do no harm and could even be beneficial to the overall process. What should be kept to a minimum is interactions in which the user is performing low-level tasks because of the machine's lack of competence.

1.5.2.5. WHOLLY INTERACTIVE SYSTEMS

The Magiscan, Cytoscan, and AKS-2 systems are intended to be fully automatic systems, requiring interaction only to assist the automatic process. Other systems take a different approach. Genetiscan, for example, provides a completely interactive environment in which the operator indicates each chromosome with a pointing device and specifies its group, whereupon it is transferred to a karyogram. In systems of this kind, the method of isolating each chromosome varies, but may involve indicating several points to specify the axis of the chromosome. This style of interaction ensures that the operator examines the structure of the chromosomes. It may, however, require consideration of factors not normally of great interest to the operator, such as exactly where a chromosome bends, and can involve a large number of interactions for each image.

1.5.3. General Interaction Features

Whatever physical device is used to create the interface, and whatever the details of the user model, certain interaction features are essential to maintaining a "user-friendly" interface.

1.5.3.1. INSTANTANEOUS RESPONSE

Interaction frequently involves some new processing of the image or part of it following a user request. This processing should not be apparent to the user, who is interested only in the result. Being forced to wait for the response to a command can intrude on the course of an interaction, and it is important that responses should appear to be instantaneous. Thus, good user interaction can demand the use of a powerful computer.

1.5.3.2. VISUAL FEEDBACK

Many interactions involve indicating significant image regions by pointing or drawing. It is important that the user is kept aware of the machine's interpretation of interactive requests by suitably highlighting regions or lines, and indicating the type of interaction being undertaken. In the case of Cytoscan, as the pointer is moved around the screen by the mouse, the nearest chromosome (or other object) is highlighted by a box surrounding it, and it is this chromosome that is selected for any subsequent command. This method has the added advantage of immediately confirming whether a chromosome is separated or is part of a cluster. Visual feedback should take account of the context of the interaction, for example, by warning of illegal or ambiguous user requests. The need for instantaneous response is particularly important here.

1.5.3.3. UNDOING INTERACTIONS

A feature so useful as to be indispensable is the ability to undo the results of an interaction by returning to a previous state by at least one, but preferably several, steps. This is needed not only because interaction errors occur and need to be corrected, but also because it is sometimes unclear exactly what the outcome of an interaction should be. For example, it may be difficult to decide on the correct way to divide up a collection of overlapping chromosomes, and several trials may be needed.

1.5.3.4. CONSISTENT INTERFACE

It is much easier to interact efficiently if the style of interaction is kept as consistent as possible across different types of interaction. For example, all interactions might begin by selecting an object from the image. Many interactions involve drawing lines for different purposes. Line drawing should always be invoked and executed in the same way. If a mouse is used, the functions of the mouse buttons should be consistent. Interactions that are similar to each other should involve the user in similar actions.

1.5.3.5. USER ASSISTANCE

It should be possible to obtain on-line descriptions of the available options by the provision of a "help" facility at each interaction stage.

2. Materials

2.1. Equipment Required for Karyotype Analysis

The minimum equipment required by those intending to build their own karyotyping system comprises a microscope, a computer, a camera to acquire the images, and some means of display. The computer requires reasonable power and a good program development environment, ideally a scientific workstation running UNIX or a top-end PC. In either case, if the computer has a high-resolution monitor, then the display of images (digitized metaphase, karyogram) may be adequate without further equipment. The display should have at least 800×600 pixels and at least 6-bit (64 level) gray-scale resolution. Color is not particularly important, but some means for displaying graphical overlays is desirable. Some means of interactive control apart from the keyboard is needed; the ubiquitous mouse is ideal. Windows software is highly desirable, but not essential. You will need adequate disk space (at least 50 Mbyte) and some means of backing up images and software (e.g., magnetic tape or optical disk).

In order to digitize the image from the camera, a frame grabber will be required. In the past, these have had a display capability that required a separate monitor (in which case the requirements of the computer itself are obviously less in this respect than those specified above); nowadays, however, it is possible to display the digitized image directly in a window on the work station and possibly also the live image prior to digitization. The frame grabber will acquire a rectangular array of pixels by digitizing the camera signal; this frame should be at least 512×512 pixels, with 6-bit gray-scale resolution. It is desirable that the pixel spacing be the same in each direction (square or 1:1 aspect ratio).

The camera should be a high-quality monochrome camera, either vacuum tube (Chalnicon or Newvicon tubes are best) or a CCD with resolution (number of pixels) similar to the frame grabber. There are several important aspects to bear in mind. First, CCD cameras are usually most sensitive in the near infrared part of the spectrum, and an infrared filter either within the camera or on the microscope will be essential for good image contrast. Second, an electrical low-pass or antialias filter with a cutoff frequency of about 6 MHz should be included between the camera and frame grabber (unless either already incorporates one), in order to reduce high-frequency white noise, and the "aliasing" effects that can arise between a CCD camera and a frame store unless their pixel clocks are synchronized (which is usually not possible). Third, the sensitive area of most CCD cameras is smaller than that of "1-in." vacuum tube cameras, resulting in an apparently larger magnification of the digitized image and correspondly smaller field of view. If you intend to use a "$^2/_3$-in." tube or CCD camera, you should consider acquiring a 63× objective instead of (or in addition to) the 100×, which is more suitable for use with a 1-in. camera. An alternative is to use a zoom attachment, available for most good microscopes. The camera can be attached to a standard microscope by using a C-mount adaptor in the photography port. Fourth, you will need to experiment with microscope color filters in order to obtain the best contrast (e.g., of G-bands) with the chosen camera. It is worth bearing in mind that the camera will most likely be placed at the primary focus of the objective, where, depending on the microscope, the image may not be fully color-corrected, in which case a fairly narrow bandwidth filter may well improve the image sharpness.

A hard-copy device is essential for printing karyograms. There are two main types. Video printers attach directly to the composite video signal fed to a monitor; digital printers are capable of better resolution, but require a digital interface and will generally be slower in use. Relatively cheap video printers give reasonable results, with perhaps 64 levels of gray on thermal paper. Digital thermal printers are a little more expensive, whereas photographic laser printers (not to be confused with the widely used xerographic laser printers, which are unsuitable) are capable of superb reproduction quality, but are expensive to buy and to run.

2.2. Additional Hardware Requirements for Metaphase Finding

To search for metaphases autonomously, the metaphase finding computer must be in control of the microscope. That is, it must be able to move the microscope stage along its x and y axes with adequate speed and accuracy; it must maintain focus during its search and so must be able to move the stage along its z axis. This is usually achieved by using a microscope stage fitted with stepper motors that are driven from the computer. The step size of these motors should be no greater than about 5 μm. A stepper motor can be attached to the focus control and should be geared to produce movements of the stage in the z direction in steps of about 0.1 μm. It is also useful to have computer control of the microscope lamp to maintain a suitable constant illumination level during the search.

3. Methods
3.1. Metaphase Finding

In this section, we consider some of the technical issues that must be addressed in constructing a metaphase finder and that determine the system's performance characteristics.

3.1.1. Image Capture

As outlined in Section 2.1., image capture for karyotype analysis is generally done using a television camera, and this is also true of most metaphase finders. Scanning for metaphases involves moving the microscope stage in fixed size steps and allowing it to stabilize between image captures. An alternative approach has been adopted by Shippey et al. *(11)*, who exploited the fact that scanning is inherent to metaphase finding. The Fast Interval Processor, later to be made commercially available as the Cytoscan metaphase finder, uses a single-line CCD detector rather than the two-dimensional array of a television camera. The second image dimension is obtained from the continuous motion of the stage underneath the detector. A fast hardware preprocessor analyzes the input line by line and generates descriptions of the imaged objects that are passed on to a computer for analysis. Although inherently less flexible than systems using TV cameras, this strategy provides very high speeds of data capture and processing in scanning tasks. Line scanning is also used in the Geneti-Scanner *(4)*.

3.1.2. Features Used for Metaphase Recognition

Each image that is captured as the stage is moved must be analyzed to detect potential metaphases. A metaphase can be recognized as a region of rather granular image texture of a certain expected size. These regions may be automatically identified in various ways, and since each field needs to be analyzed rather quickly, the method used in any machine tends to exploit the strengths of that machine's particular hardware. However, the image properties that are measured are essentially the same from one system to another. A number of separate objects must be found within a predictable size range and with some optimum separation.

The image analysis problem is to estimate the properties of object number, size, and separation given that individual chromosomes are not well resolved by the approx $1\text{-}\mu m^2$ sized pixels typically used for metaphase finding. The method adopted by Graham and Pycock *(12)* and implemented in the Magiscan system was to threshold a suspected metaphase region using a locally determined threshold and to use methods from the field of Mathematical Morphology *(13)*, involving erosion and dilation of the binary image, to estimate the sizes and separations of individual touching objects (Fig. 2). Regions are selected for this analysis according to the output of a rapid local texture measurement applied over the entire image and tuned to the variation in brightness expected within the region of a metaphase.

Automatic Karyotype Analysis 159

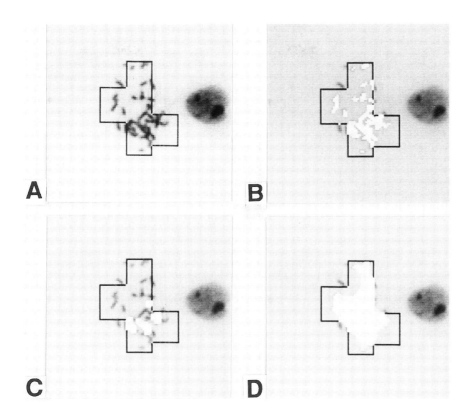

Fig. 2. Analysis of a suspected metaphase using morphological sizing *(12)*. **A.** Extent of an irregular area with image texture appropriate for a metaphase. **B.** Result of applying a locally determined threshold within the area to detect the chromosomes. **C.** The detected regions have been subjected to an opening (erosion + dilation) operation. Most isolated objects have been removed, but clumpy areas remain. Application of this operation with differently sized erosion/dilation structuring elements allows a size distribution of possibly touching objects to be determined. **D.** The detected regions from (B) have been subjected to a closing (dilation + erosion) operation. The areas between the detected regions have been filled in, allowing object separation and overall object size to be measured. (Reproduced by permission of Science Printers and Publishers Inc., St. Louis, MO.)

A method of achieving essentially the same measures appropriate for linear scanning is described by Shippey et al. *(11)*. The clustering in this case uses measured distance between detected "limbs" (simply connected above threshold regions that may touch each other).

Both of these systems assign a quality index to the detected metaphase. Graham and Pycock *(12)* assign a figure of merit consisting of a weighted sum of measured parameters, such as number of objects, image brightness, and object separation, the weights being determined by training on samples of the material to be used. Shippey et al. *(11)* use a similar measure, applying a box classifier *(see* Section 3.6.1.) to eliminate at an early stage objects that are highly unlikely to be useful metaphases.

3.1.3. Autofocus

Reliable metaphase detection is dependent on the ability of the system to keep the microscope slide in good focus. Regular measurements must be made from which the focus can be determined and adjusted if necessary. A number of image properties may be measured for this purpose, such as average image density or gradient. The effectiveness of several different focus functions has been assessed by Groen et al. *(14)* and by Firestone et al. *(15)*.

In the continuous scanning system of Shippey et al. *(11)* the focus can be continuously monitored by using two additional linear detectors set slightly out of focus in either direction with respect to the principal linear detector array. The average image intensity from each of these three detectors can be used to determine the stage position for optimal focus. Usually in TV-based systems, focus is maintained by driving the stage through the focus position at regular intervals in the scan area to find the best value of the focus measure. Graham and Pycock *(12)* use a method of determining a sparse grid of correct focus positions before scanning for metaphases and interpolating between neighboring grid points as the scan proceeds.

3.1.4. Building Your Own

Commercially available metaphase finders are generally based on fairly specialized computers. These may have been designed specifically to optimize scanning processes, such as Cytoscan, or may be machines intended to address a wider range of image processing tasks. In either case, the machines are architecturally rather specialized and therefore expensive.

Up to about the time of writing this chapter, this use of specialized processors was necessary to allow the application of sufficient computing power to achieve realistic scanning speeds. This situation has changed recently by the introduction of very powerful, inexpensive personal computers and scientific work stations. These machines deliver sufficient performance for image processing, while retaining a general-purpose architecture. This chapter is intended in part to act as a guide to those who wish to build their own systems, and these developments open up the possibility of a do-it-yourself metaphase finder built of commercially available components.

The performance that might be expected from such a system can be judged by the recent implementation of a metaphase finder on a MacIntosh IIfx computer by Vrolijk and his colleagues at the University of Leiden *(16)*. They have used commercially available hardware for image acquisition and microscope control, and achieved scanning speeds of about 360 s/cm². The method of detection and assessment of metaphases used by these workers is similar to that described in *(12);* regions detected by a specially designed texture filter are measured and ranked using a combination of mathematical morphology operators. The caveat of our introduction should, however, be particularly emphasized here. To achieve the scanning speeds they report, these workers have used their long experience in this field to develop methods that are not only highly specific to the images, but also highly optimized for the particular computer architecture they chose. Any laboratory considering an *ab initio* implementation of a metaphase finder should bear in mind the investment in time and expertise necessary to build a working system with reasonable performance.

3.2. High-Resolution Image Capture

For karyotype analysis, it is particularly important that the quality of the image captured by the camera is as high as possible. To this end, care should be taken with the optical setup of the microscope lamp and condensor, cleanliness of the lenses, the level of illumination, the filter color (both of the latter may need to be different for the camera than for the human eye), and the overall magnification, taking the camera pixel size into account. As mentioned above, an infrared filter is essential for a CCD camera, and an electrical antialias filter is recommended. Image degradation can be caused by incorrect electrical termination of video signals and also by electrical noise pickup. To reduce radio-frequency noise, it is wise to link all metal components, *including the microscope frame,* to a common earthing point.

A number of factors can be optimized by appropriate image analysis programs. Light level can be measured by identifying the background peak in a histogram of digitized pixel gray values; the lamp should be adjusted so that this peak lies near the "white" end of the frame grabber's range of pixel gray values. Focus is best adjusted by looking at the live image as seen by the frame grabber (since the camera and eyepieces may not be parfocal). Most microscopes show nonuniform illumination, in that they are typically less bright toward the edge of the field; this can be compensated for by taking a "shading map" of a clear field and using it for shading correction, and also to compensate for any camera nonuniformity.

Captured images will comprise a large amount of data, typically between 250 and 500 kbyte. Storing such images will soon fill up whatever disk storage is available. Since most of the image is "background" (clear field), removing background (segmentation; *see* Section 3.) before storing to disk may reduce file sizes by about 90%. Your operating system may provide a file compression program; this can typically reduce the size of the thresholded images by a further 30%.

There will always be some exceptionally well-spread metaphases that do not fit within the camera frame. The solution is to fuse parts of multiple digitized fields under software control; here again, it is sensible to use segmented images as the basis of the operation.

3.3. Metaphase Image Segmentation

3.3.1. Initial Image Segmentation

This is invariably done by thresholding; a darkness value is chosen, and "background" pixels lighter than this threshold value are discarded. Finding the connected sets of darker pixels results in an initial division into image regions that may represent individual chromosomes, chromosome clusters, or unwanted objects, such as stain particles and interphase nuclei.

The threshold may be chosen automatically, by analysis of the histogram of density values (Fig. 3). Such a histogram has a pronounced "background" peak, and the threshold must be chosen at a value a little above the upper end of the background region.

Some authors *(9)* have described methods of local thresholding to take account of a nonuniform background, caused, for example, by slight cytoplasm staining. However, the most usual cause of nonuniform back-

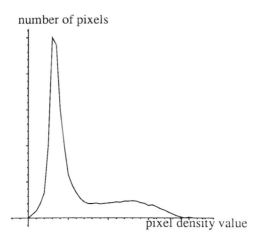

number of pixels

pixel density value

Fig. 3. Histogram of pixel densities from a digitized metaphase image. The pronounced peak comes from the large area of clear background, whereas the chromosomes give rise to the relatively small number of darker pixels.

ground is uneven microscope illumination; this and any camera non-uniformity is best compensated for by preliminary shading correction *(8,17)* (Section 3.2.). In an unpublished experiment, one of us (J. P.) found that local thresholding led to significant deterioration of the per-class coefficients of variation of relative chromosome size compared with simple global thresholding.

In an interactive system, the operator should have control over the final detection level, whether obtained from global or local analysis. As noted in Section 1.5., it is inappropriate for the operator to be asked to specify a threshold numerically. A rapid visual method can easily be provided if the display facilities include a look-up table (LUT). The effect of any particular threshold choice (specified, say, by pointing at a "slider bar") may be simulated by setting LUT values below the proposed threshold to some uniform, non-natural color such as mid-gray or pale blue. The visual effect on the metaphase image is as if the operator had a bird's eye view of the tide rising or falling around a number of islands. If the automatic threshold selection has been done properly, then interactive adjustment should in any case be required only rarely. After setting the threshold, the values of the remaining pixels may be "stretched" to make use of the full dynamic range of the display, resulting in a useful increase in image contrast.

3.3.2. Interactive Segmentation

The user interface has been described above (Section 1.5.2.). From the programming point of view, the requirement is then quite straight-forward, namely, to take an image region and some graphical object generated by the interaction system (such as a polygon along the desired split path), and return the image regions of the segmented chromosomes. Further discussion on semiautomatic segmentation can be found in Note 1.

3.4. Feature Measurement

The purpose of feature measurement is to obtain information in numerical form that is useful for classification of a chromosome into its correct class, or to decide that it is abnormal in some way. The features commonly used include relative size, centromeric index, and some numerical description of the banding pattern.

3.4.1. Chromosome Size

To a cytogeneticist, size usually means the length of a chromosome, and the relative length is, of course, an important discriminator of chromosome class. However, it has been found that chromosome area is an equally reliable size measure, which has the advantage of being easy to compute, simply by counting the number of pixels, and in particular, does not depend on correctly locating the chromosome's axis.

3.4.2. Relative Density

Some chromosomes are, overall, paler than others, and the relative density of a chromosome may be obtained simply by adding its pixel values and dividing by the area.

3.4.3. Medial Axis, Orientation, and Polarity

For all the other measurements that we wish to make, whether the chromosome is bent or straight, or whatever its orientation in the metaphase plate is irrelevant, and such geometric variation is compensated for by making all measurements in a non-Euclidean coordinate frame determined by the chromosome's axis of symmetry or centerline. Since one aim of a karyotyping system is to produce a karyogram presentation of the metaphase, the orientation must also be found explicitly, so that the chromosome can be displayed vertically in the karyogram. Finally, it is conventional to display the short arm uppermost, and so the chromosome polarity (which arm is the short arm) must also be determined.

Although in principle the chromosome orientation could be defined as the average direction of the medial axis, it turns out that finding the orientation is rather more reliable than finding the axis, and indeed, most axis-finding methods rely on an initial estimate of orientation. Possible methods include taking second-order moments of gray values *(18)*, finding the least-squares straight line fit to boundary coordinates *(9)*, or finding the minimum width enclosing rectangle (MWR) *(7)*. The MWR method makes use of the fact that the MWR is parallel to one chord of the convex hull or minimum enclosing convex polygon. Assuming an appropriate data structure for the chromosome image, the convex hull can be found extremely rapidly *(19)*, and finding the MWR is then straightforward and rapid.

Axis finding is still an unsolved problem; looked at another way, existing methods are prone to error in a significant number of cases. The consequence of finding a curve that is not in fact the chromosome's symmetry axis is that subsequent measurement of length, centromere position, and banding features may well be erroneous. Since the system under discussion is intended to be automatic, such errors will not be apparent until the chromosome is misclassified and presented in the wrong location in the karyogram. Axis errors are an important cause of classification errors, and as was mentioned in Section 1.5.2., in some systems, the operator is given the opportunity to correct the axis interactively.

Given the orientation, the axis can be found initially as a straight line *(9,18)*. Of course, very few chromosomes are truly straight, and a curved axis is usually required. For relatively straight, well-formed chromosomes, the set of midpoints of chords perpendicular to the major orientation direction (Fig. 4) suffices *(7)*. In the case of more seriously bent chromosomes, various methods have been proposed: fitting a cubic to the chord midpoints *(9)*, a piece-wise linear fit *(18)*, or use of the "skeleton" of the chromosome image region *(7)*.

As yet, no known method copes well with metaphase chromosomes that have an acute bend at the centromere (or elsewhere), since the true centerline of the chromosome no longer corresponds to the midline of the segmented "shape" of the object. The problem could be solved if it were known *a priori* that the object was an acutely bent chromo-

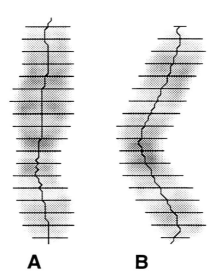

A   **B**

Fig. 4. The axis derived from the midpoints of chords perpendicular to the major orientation of a chromosome is usually satisfactory in the case of relatively straight chromosomes **A,** but can be significantly in error at (particularly) the ends of bent chromosomes **B.** For clarity, only every fourth chord has been shown.

some. However, even visually, such an object can often only be recognized as a single chromosome, because, in effect, its two arms are recognized independently as belonging to the same chromosome class. In an automatic system, recognition follows segmentation and axis finding, and such circular reasoning has not yet been proven possible *(20)*. Similarly, chromosomes whose chromatids are not parallel will typically confuse an axis algorithm. These are illustrations of a general principle that an automated system for biomedical image analysis will only work satisfactorily if care is taken to ensure that the biological preparation is of the highest possible quality and conforms to the system's implicit model of such material.

3.4.4. Profiles

Having obtained the chromosome's symmetry axis, the first stage in obtaining the remaining features is to reduce the two-dimensional chromosome image to a one-dimensional form known as a profile. A profile represents the distribution of some property of the chromo-

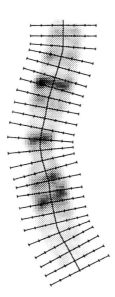

Fig. 5. Non-Euclidean coordinate system for computing profiles, based on lines perpendicular to the chromosome axis. For clarity, the scale used has been reduced by 4×.

some, for example, its width or the intensity of staining, as it varies along the chromosome in a direction determined by the medial axis. More precisely, we define a non-Euclidean coordinate space (Fig. 5) and make measurements at points in this space. The points of interest are obtained in the following way.

First, points are found on the medial axis that are unit distance (one pixel spacing) apart. Note that such points themselves do not usually have integer coordinates. Next, at each such point, a line is constructed perpendicular to the axis, and points are found on each such line at unit distance spacing (Fig. 5). Again, these points do not have integer coordinates, nor are they usually at unit distance from all of their neighbors. At each such point, an appropriate pixel intensity value is computed from the values of the neighboring original pixels. This can be done most simply by finding the nearest original pixel and choosing its value (nearest-neighbor method, Fig. 5), but it has been shown that values obtained by bilinear interpolation among the four surrounding original pixels (Fig. 5) lead to more accurate measurement *(21)*, and this is now the commonly used technique.

Profiles are used both to represent the banding pattern and also to reduce the chromosome's shape to a one-dimensional representation, in order to find the centromere. For band pattern representation, the "integrated density" profile is computed by taking the sum of all pixel values inside the chromosome boundary on each of the transverse lines across the chromosome (Fig. 6). Shape may be represented by the "width" profile (Fig. 6), computed by finding the number of connected pixels with above-threshold values in each transverse slice *(9)*. The width may well either be noisy on account of closely adjacent chromosomes or stained cytoplasm, or the width at the centromere may not be significantly less than elsewhere. An alternative profile that partly overcomes these problems by integrating information across the chromatid structure is the moment or "shape" profile *(7,22)*, computed as shown in Fig. 7. Shape profiles are compared with width profiles in Fig. 8.

3.4.5. Centromere

Usually, a metacentric chromosome's centromere appears as a pronounced minimum in either the width or shape profile, whereas that of an acrocentric is represented only by a smaller than usual gradient at one end of the profile (Figs. 6 and 8). Since it is not known *a priori* whether a particular chromosome is in fact metacentric or acrocentric, the essential problem to be solved is how to compare the properties of the gradient at an end of the profile with properties of a profile minimum. Various solutions have been proposed, none of which is entirely satisfactory:

1. Groen et al. *(18)* used the width profile, truncated at either end, and chose the overall minimum width. The assumption is that this will be at the correct end in the case of an acrocentric.
2. Graham *(9)* found the end with lower gradient if there was no profile minimum in the central 60% of the width profile.
3. Piper *(22)* took the convex envelope of the profile and found the most "significant" chord. The centromere was then assumed to be at the point furthest beneath this chord.
4. Piper and Granum *(7)* deliberately constructed minima at either end of the profile and then chose the "best" minimum, which in the case of metacentric chromosomes was expected not to be one of those at the end.

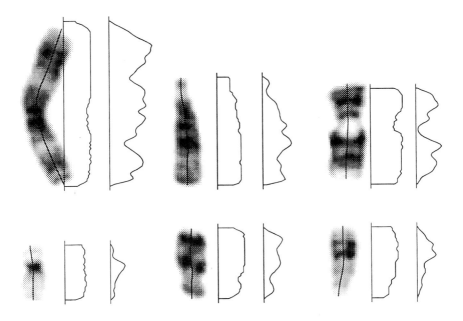

Fig. 6. Chromosome width (left) and density profiles, determined from the central axes shown.

3.4.6. Shape Features

Centromeric index is the most useful shape measure yet discovered. It may be computed on the basis of length, area, or total pixel intensity. Although the former two are highly correlated, the last introduces some additional information about the chromosome. In order to compute the centromeric indices by area and total pixel intensity, the chromosome image must be divided by a line perpendicular to the medial axis that passes through the centromere, and pixels on either side of this line must be determined.

In ref. 7, some other shape features were proposed, computed by applying Granum's weighted density distribution (WDD) functions (23) to the shape profile. However, these tend either to be quite highly correlated with centromeric index or to have rather little class discrimination ability. The centromere position is the best-known automatic determinant of chromosome polarity (which end is the short arm),

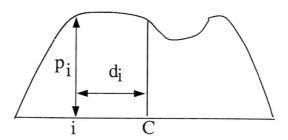

Fig. 7. Computation of single point of "shape" profile. The profile shown is of the distribution of pixel values of a single "slice" across the chromosome (Fig. 5), perpendicular to the axis. If C is the centroid of the slice, and point i at distance d_i from C has pixel density p_i, then the profile value for this slice is $\Sigma p_i |d_i| \Sigma p_i$.

which in turn is required for the computation of some of the following band pattern features.

3.4.7. Band Pattern Features from Density Profile

Band pattern features divide into two overall classes, "global" and "local." A global feature is a single number computed from the entirety of the density profile by a uniform arithmetical procedure. On the other hand, a local feature describes some particular structure in the density profile, for example, the location of the most intense band. For comparison, the area of a chromosome is also a global feature, whereas the centromeric index is a local feature, determined by the centromere position.

The view has long been held that local band pattern features will be required in order to detect and describe abnormality in banding patterns, and attempts at local band pattern descriptions have been made for more than two decades. However, from the point of view of classification of normal chromosomes into the normal classes, it has been found that the global features are superior. Active research continues in a number of laboratories into local description methods.

3.4.7.1. Global Band Pattern Features

Two approaches are used to obtain single numbers that represent some aspect of an entire density profile. First, the profile values may be treated as samples from a distribution, and parameters of the distri-

Fig. 8. Width (left) and "shape" profiles of metacentric and acrocentric chromosomes.

bution estimated *(7)*. A variation is that the density differences between adjacent profile points are taken as the sample *(23)*.

    The second main method is to multiply the profile by each of a set of basis functions, resulting in a corresponding set of feature values. If appropriate sinusoidal basis functions are used, then the resulting set comprises the Fourier transform of the profile *(24)*. However, the lack until recently of affordable floating point hardware has led to widespread adoption of Granum's WDD basis functions, which are triangular rather than sinusoidal *(23)*. Typically, the first four functions are used. Granum *(23)* recommends the use of these functions both on the entire profile, and also on the p and q portions separately in order to obtain further features. The usefulness of the latter may, however, not be great in a system in which the machine-found centromere is left uncorrected. Piper and Granum *(7)* showed that two additional WDD functions (Fig. 9) were also valuable. They also showed that if the WDD basis functions were applied either to the

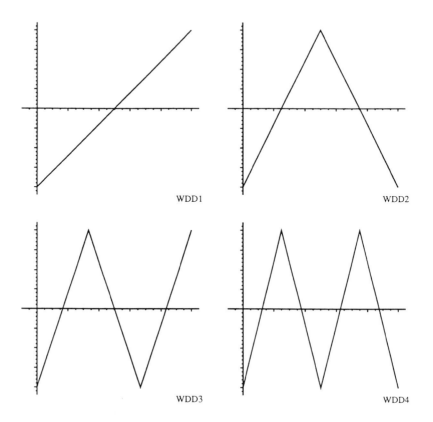

Fig. 9. The first four weighted density distribution functions *(23)*.

"shape" profile or to the profile of differences between adjacent points of the density profile, then further valuable features resulted.

3.4.7.2. LOCAL BAND PATTERN DESCRIPTION

By analogy with the centromere, it is possible to use the location of certain landmark bands as classification features. Thus, the locations of the darkest band in either arm, and of the dark bands nearest to the centromere and to the telomeres provide usable features *(17,18)*. Thus far, such features have been used with a conventional statistical classifier, but together with a structural/syntactic classifier, they could well provide the means of detecting some band pattern abnormalities. A more rigorous approach to addressing that problem is provided by the work of Granum and his associates *(25)* in the use of hidden Markov models for chromosome band patterns; so far, however, they have only presented data from normal material.

3.5. Feature Normalization

In a prometaphase cell, a number 1 chromosome may be two or three times longer than a number 1 in a midmetaphase. Indeed, the midmetaphase number 1 may be shorter than, say, a chromosome 10 in the prometaphase cell. Thus, "raw" size is not a very helpful measure. What remains true is that in either cell the length of a number 1 comprises about 8% of the length of a haploid set.

The transformation to relative size by, perhaps, division by the sum of the sizes of all chromosomes in a cell is an example of a process known as normalization *(7,9,18,23)*. Unfortunately, for the majority of features except size, there is no clear theoretical reason to justify normalization or to guide how to perform it. Centromere index varies only slightly with cell contraction and is usually left unnormalized. Other features may be normalized by standardizing the distribution within a cell (i.e., obtaining zero mean and unity standard deviation) *(7)*, and in many cases, this appears to improve their discrimination capability, but the reason for this improvement is not well understood in most cases.

3.6. Classification

In Sections 3.4. and 3.5., we described ways in which attributes of chromosomes may be measured and represented numerically by an automated karyotyping system. Here we describe how these measurements can be used to produce an automatic classification. This subject is often referred to as Pattern Recognition. We will begin with a brief introduction to Pattern Recognition methods and then consider how these are applied to chromosome classification.

3.6.1. Pattern Recognition

This is a necessarily brief introduction to a highly developed subject, and the reader is referred to one of a number of excellent texts for a full account (e.g., *26,27*). In any classification or pattern recognition task, objects are to be assigned to classes on the basis of a set of measured attributes, or features, such as those described in Section 3.4. Features should be numeric (i.e., they must be measurements), they should have some discriminating power (i.e., the features measured from objects in different classes should be different), and they should ideally be independent (i.e., they should represent truly different properties of the classes).

Consider a case where we measure two features x and y (say chromosome length and centromeric index, as used for the classification of unbanded chromosomes), and we wish to distinguish three classes. There are a number of methods that may be applied to discriminate the classes on the basis of these features. To determine which method to choose and the appropriate parameters, features must be collected from a representative set of objects, and these objects assigned to their classes by an expert in the appropriate domain (a cytogeneticist in our case), in a process known as "classifier training." We can plot the feature values on a space whose axes correspond to the features (Fig. 10). This space is known as a *feature space*. The feature values (x,y) for a particular object constitute its *feature vector.* The task of the classifier is to partition the feature space, so that when the feature vector for a new (unknown) object is plotted, it can be assigned to one of the classes. Figure 10 shows some common methods of partitioning the space.

Fig. 10. *(opposite page)* Scattergrams representing the two-dimensional feature vectors for a number of training examples of three classes. Depending on the distribution of these vectors in feature space, different strategies may be applied for allocating an unknown object with feature vector (x',y') to a class. **A.** Box classifier: The classes can be distinguished by thresholds on each of the feature axes. The thresholds may define upper and lower bounds for class membership. In the example shown, a single threshold on each of the axes is sufficient to partition the feature space. **B.** Linear discriminant: In this case, the classes would be poorly discriminated by thresholds, but can be easily separated by straight lines in feature space. An unknown vector is assigned to one of the classes according to its position with respect to these lines, i.e., according to the value of $A_1x' + B_1y' + C_1$ and $A_2x' + B_2y' + C_2$. **C.** Parametric classifier: The feature vectors of the training set form recognizable clusters that may overlap and so cannot be separated by a decision line. The clusters may be modelled by a bivariate (in general, multivariate) normal distribution. The ellipses represent the area contained within one standard deviation of the mean values of these distributions. An unknown feature vector is assigned to the class according to its distance from each of the class means, the distance being weighted by the covariance of the appropriate class. **D.** Nearest neighbor classifier: If the feature vectors in the training data are few in number, or not well clustered, a new vector may be assigned to the class of the nearest vector in the training data.

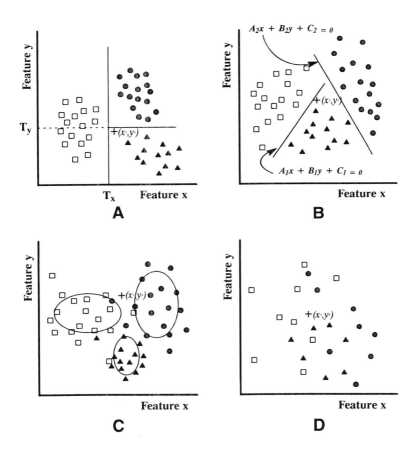

3.6.1.1. BOX CLASSIFIER

This is the simplest form of partition. "Boxes" are defined around each cluster by setting thresholds on the feature values. A new object will be classified according to which "box" its feature vector falls into. The advantages of a box classifier are its simplicity and ease of computation. Its principal disadvantage is that it requires the clusters to be well separated along at least one of the dimensions of feature space. This is rarely the case.

3.6.1.2. LINEAR DISCRIMINANT

If classes cannot be separated by thresholds on the features, they may be separated by a straight line in feature space. If the line $Ax + By + C = 0$ separates the classes, then a measure of $Ax_1 + By_1 + C$ for some new object with feature vector (x_1,y_1) will be greater than zero for (x_1,y_1) on one side of the line and less than zero on the other. If more than two classes are present, several lines can be used.

3.6.1.3. PARAMETRIC CLASSIFIER

In this case, the clusters arising from the classes are represented in some parametric form. Commonly, the clusters are modeled by multivariate normal distributions (bivariate in the two-dimensional case considered here). The classes are parameterized by the mean and variance of the corresponding clusters along each of the dimensions. A new object may be assigned to one of the classes by measuring its distance from the mean vector of each class, weighted by the variance of that class. In general, this measure can be used to assign a likelihood of a new object belonging to each of the classes. The likelihood that an object with feature vector (x,y) belongs to class i is given by:

$$[1/2\pi(\sigma_{xi}^2 + \sigma_{yi}^2)^{1/2} \exp -^1/_2] \{[(x - \mu_{xi})^2/\sigma_{xi}^2] + [(y - \mu_{yi})^2/\sigma_{yi}^2]\} \quad (1)$$

Since, in general, the object will be assigned to the class with highest likelihood, this method is often referred to as a maximum likelihood classifier.

As described above and in Fig. 10, the features are assumed to be independent. This assumption is usually unrealistic and can be dispensed with by including the covariances in the calculation of distances. This, however, adds greatly to the computational cost, but has been shown to add little to the overall classification accuracy, at least for classification of chromosomes *(28,29)*.

3.6.1.4. NEAREST NEIGHBOR CLASSIFIER

If the feature vectors do not fall into compact clusters or the training set is very small, none of the above methods may be suitable. In this case, an unknown feature vector may be assigned to the class of the nearest object in the training set or, more robustly, to the class to which the majority of the k nearest objects belong (a k-NN classifier). The k-NN classifier can be highly effective, its principal disadvantage being that the entire set of training data must be available and searched for each classification.

3.6.2. Classifying Chromosomes

3.6.2.1. CLASSIFIER CAPABILITY

Karyotyping is a rather challenging classification problem. There are few other applications in which it is necessary to assign objects to as many as 24 classes. In current implementations, the assignment may be based on anything from five to 16 features *(7,9,18);* that is to say that the two-dimensional feature spaces shown in Fig. 10 should be visualized in up to 16 dimensions. The topic of automatic selection of suitable features is considered in Note 2. To our knowledge, all currently available karyotyping systems use maximum likelihood classification. In the case of the Magiscan and Cytoscan, the likelihood estimates are based on a parameterization of the observed distribution of the training set as in Fig. 10 C. In the AKS-2 system, the probability density functions are estimated directly from the training set, rather than being expressed as a small number of parameters *(18)*.

Because of a number of factors, perfect chromosome classification is never achieved in practice. Errors in feature measurement, inadequacies in the feature sets used, and imperfect separation of the classes in feature space result in misclassification rates on the order of 5–20% for routine quality preparations of material used for clinical karyotyping *(7,30,31)*. We should be a little careful about what we mean by classification error rates. The percentage misclassifications just quoted give us a measure, over several different studies, of the total number of chromosomes not assigned to their correct classes by an automatic classifier. However, if we examine classifier performance from a system point of view, this is not necessarily the most meaningful number we could derive. In a working karyotyping system, a classification error will be corrected interactively by the operator. This is much more easily done if the misclassified chromosomes can be identified and placed together in a special group, rather than being assigned to the wrong groups and scattered all over the karyogram. This can be achieved to some extent by the inclusion of a "reject class" to which chromosomes are assigned if their likelihood of belonging to any real group is below some threshold. There will, of course, remain a number of chromosomes that are wrongly classified with high likelihood, and these are the most serious classification errors from a system standpoint. Lundsteen et al. *(30)* find that their residual misclassification rate is reduced from 9.0 to 5.5% by the inclusion of a reject class. We should, of course, be somewhat circumspect about this. We could easily achieve near-zero error rates by setting the likelihood threshold high enough at the expense of rejecting most of the chromosomes.

3.6.2.2. CONSTRAINTS ON CHROMOSOME CLASSIFICATION

The classification rates reported above refer to context-free classification; that is to say, the class to which a chromosome is assigned depends entirely on the features measured for that chromosome, with no account being taken of the features or classification likelihoods of other chromosomes in the cell (other than by normalization; Section 3.5.). The fact that almost all chromosomes in a cell will be paired as homologs of very similar appearance provides constraints on classification that can be exploited to improve the overall classification performance. (This is of use in most cases, although when karyotyping cells from bone marrow or solid tumors it is often the case that not all chromosomes in a cell are visible or the cell is in any case highly aneuploid, and this type of constraint is of limited use.)

The most useful constraint arising from this source is the knowledge that no class should contain more than two chromosomes (except in the rare, but important case of numerical abnormality). Context-free classification may well assign more than two chromosomes to the same class on the basis of their maximum likelihoods. The classification must therefore be "rearranged" by assigning some chromosomes to "second choice" classes, possibly displacing other chromosomes from these classes, and so on. Piper *(32)* tested a number of algorithms for achieving such a rearrangement and showed that the overall classification rate can indeed be improved in this way. All of the methods improve classification, but none guarantee an optimal rearrangement in the sense that the maximum overall likelihood is obtained subject to the constraint. Tso and Graham *(33)* showed that an optimal assignment of chromosomes to classes can be achieved using a method derived from Operations Research. An efficient algorithm for performing this assignment has recently been described and tested *(34)*. Application of this technique results in a further small improvement in assignment over the suboptimal methods in ref. *32*. It should be noted, however, that the overall performance improvement obtained by the use of such rearrangement algorithms is small, of the order of 2–3% in a misclassification rate of 5–20% *(32,34)*. This change alone would almost certainly pass unnoticed by the user of a karyotyping system. The methods do, however, result in an increase in the number of cells in which no misclassifications occur or in which there is only one misclassification. These cells will be exactly those of high visual quality, which should be specifically selected by a competent metaphase finder. Thus, the effects on the efficiency of the system will be greater than might be expected from consideration of misclassification rates alone.

Some consideration has also been given to the fact that two homologous chromosomes assigned to the same class should look similar. Zimmerman et al. *(35)* showed that chromosomes could be matched to their homologs with high accuracy. Recently, this constraint has been incorporated into a classifier with promising results, but the high computational cost makes it unsuitable at present for inclusion in a practical automated karyotyping system *(36)*.

Karyotyping, as we have said, is a difficult classification task, and looked at in isolation, existing chromosome classifiers do not do particularly well by pattern recognition standards, but in combination with other system components, they can contribute to useful semiautomatic cytogenetic analysis systems. Some further aspects of karyotyping classification are considered in Notes 3 and 4.

4. Notes

1. Semiautomatic segmentation: Although the purely interactive segmentation methods described in Sections 1.5.2. and 3.3.2. are adequate, at least some automation is highly desirable, particularly when analyzing difficult material, such as bone marrow preparations. Fully automatic segmentation is still an area of active research, and existing techniques are both not particularly accurate and extremely complex, so that only the barest outline will be given here, since a detailed review would comprise a long chapter all by itself. However, even rather straightforward automatic strategies can assist considerably, and a few of these will be mentioned here. The problem may be regarded as consisting of two stages, (a) recognition of objects, i.e., individual chromosomes, clusters, nuclei, or other nonchromosome material, and (b) resolution of clusters. Since nonchromosomal material may be involved in clus-

ters, the two stages may iterate. The operator must still be allowed to review and change a machine decision, or initiate an action that the machine has not suggested.

In some material, there is a large amount of particulate debris that appears in the image as many small spots. These may be highlighted in some way and classified as noise, unless the operator cancels the highlighting. The operator's involvement remains essential, since frequently the satellites of a D-group chromosome will have been separated by the initial segmentation by thresholding. Similarly, large objects cannot possibly be isolated chromosomes. If these are also highlighted and the operator prompted that something must be done about them, then the scope for missing some necessary decisions is reduced.

There are two different possible approaches to the resolution of clusters. Either the cluster detection and segmentation can both be automatic, with operator review of the final result *(10,37,38)*, or the operator can be relied on to point at an object, which is then resolved automatically *(39,40)*. In either case, the system will make errors in a substantial proportion of cases (usually fewer in "better" material), so some means of highlighting machine actions is important so that the operator can review and correct the decisions.

Automatic cluster recognition and decomposition can be based on one of two techniques. Graham thresholded the image at two levels, and found an optimal grouping of the higher-threshold particles by a region-based split and merge technique that is guided by the expected position of chromosomes obtained by a previous count-by-pointing phase *(10)*.

The other approach to cluster recognition and segmentation is largely based on an analysis of the shape of the boundary compared with the expected shape of a single chromosome. Those boundaries with complex curvature are most likely to belong to clusters, and concavities on the boundary are likely end points for a path that separates the cluster. Such an analysis may be used both for cluster recognition *(37,38,41)* and for splitting *(39,40)*. The more successful systems construct splitting paths by "valley following" (regarding pixel value as topographical height) and compare several potential splitting paths, choosing the most probable on the basis of a set of measured features *(39,41)*.

2. Feature selection for classification: Not all features have the same discriminating power, and in some circumstances, a feature may contribute little or nothing. Consider, for example, the case of the band-pattern features if classifying homogeneously stained chromosomes. In such cases, inclusion of a feature may make the classification error rate higher,

whereas omitting it will also reduce the computational cost. Thus, it makes sense to evaluate the discriminating power that each feature contributes, in order to select a useful subset.

Methods for automatic feature selection for chromosome classification are discussed and illustrated in refs. *7,23,* and *28.* Essentially, these depend on both the discrimination capability of the feature taken alone, which may be estimated from the classifier training data by a simple formula, and on the correlation between a particular feature and others already selected as "useful," since the inclusion of an additional feature that is highly correlated with one already selected will most likely contribute little.

Alternatively, one can run full classification experiments with the training data (split into separate "training" and "test" sets *[7]*), using a variety of different, but plausible sets of features, and choose the best on the basis of minimum error rate. However, to do this thoroughly is extremely (computer) time-consuming, since the number of possible feature sets explodes combinatorially as the number of features increases.

3. Future classifier developments:

Classifier design: Classifiers and their associated feature sets in current systems were designed for use with fairly contracted metaphase chromosomes. The tendency in cytogenetics laboratories to analyze cells with longer chromosomes, showing more bands, may result in decreasing performance of these classifiers. Two areas of development in classifier design address this problem. Granum and his coworkers *(25)* have developed an approach to chromosome classification based on syntactic analysis, that is a structural description of the banding pattern, which is in principle extendible to high resolution banding. The application of an artificial neural network to chromosome classification has been described by Errington and Graham *(42).* Classification performance is similar to that which can be obtained using statistical classifiers, and the flexibility inherent in neural networks should make them easily adaptable to changes in the appearance of cells being analyzed.

Automatic detection of abnormalities: Another notable feature of the current generation of classifiers is that they are designed only to classify normal cells. In the main, they have no inherent definition of any specific abnormality. At first sight, this appears curious, since the object of karyotyping is to identify specific abnormalities. It can be understood by noting that a cytogeneticist spends most of his/her time examining normal cells. Since karyotyping systems are intended to be used interactively, a normal cell classifier is a useful system component.

This is not to say that a classifier capable of recognizing abnormalities is undesirable, but only that its design would be more difficult and that little work has been done in this area. Lundsteen et al. *(43)* discuss some possible ways of approaching this and include a description of a small pilot study suggesting that analysis of the feature values for banded chromosomes in a corrected karyotype could provide an indication of the existence of abnormalities that are difficult to perceive by eye. Carothers et al. *(44)* showed that it is theoretically possible in a multiple-cell karyotyping system *(see* Note 4 *below)* to detect numerical abnormalities completely automatically by processing 16–32 cells from a particular specimen, assuming the use of a classifier whose performance is not very different from those in current systems. If enough cells are analyzed, an aneuploidy should be detectable above the noise of the system error rate. The use of such a system would require a regime in which tests for aneuploidies would be carried out separately from analysis for structural abnormalities. This would involve a radical change in the normal practice of most cytogenetic laboratories.

4. Multiple cell karyotyping: It has been suggested several times during the development of automated cytogenetics systems that multiple-cell karyotyping would be a highly useful application of computer technology. The original idea, in the era when chromosome analysis research aimed at complete automation, was that the final karyotype (description of the chromosome complement) would be produced in a statistical fashion from several cells *(45,46)*. Alternatively, it has been proposed that the chromosomes in each group from all cells be displayed together *(47)*. In either case, the aim is not only to provide a useful means of presenting the information from several cells, but also to reduce the need for operator interaction. Those analysis errors resulting in incorrect segmentations or wrongly positioned axes or centromeres would simply be ignored, and result in objects that would be either wrongly classified or impossible to classify. Provided the number of these errors is fairly small, there should be enough examples of correctly identified chromosomes in each class to generate a karyotype.

Carothers et al. *(44)* have specified the conditions under which a fully automatic system could be successful. Lundsteen et al. *(43)* have shown that a multiple-cell karyotyping display system can be made to work, in which the only interactions required are the initial interactive count for each cell and an inspection of the final composite karyogram. The interesting point here is that all the interactions involve the operator understanding the chromosomes. This kind of interactive facility is not yet offered by any of the suppliers of karyotyping systems, but is well within the capability of current technology. Its introduction would require a change in the working practice of cytogenetics laboratories, which may not be possible until there is a wider acceptance of machine-assisted karyotyping.

References

1. Piper J. and Rutovitz D. (1985) Data structures for image processing in a C language and Unix environment. *Patt. Recog. Letts.* **3,** 119–129.
2. Graham J., Taylor, C. J., Cooper, D. H., and Dixon, R. N. (1986) A compact set of image processing primitives and their role in a successful application program. *Patt. Recog. Letts.* **4,** 325–333.
3. Korthof, G. and Carothers, A. D. (1991) Tests of performance of four automatic metaphase finding and karyotyping systems. *Clin. Genet.* **40,** 441–451.
4. Castleman, K. R. (1992) The PSI automatic metaphase finder. *J. Radiation Research,* **33 (suppl.),** 124–128.
5. Martin, A. O. (1985) My life with two automated systems. Automated Chromosome Analysis Workshop, Leiden.
6. Daker, M. (1985) The detection of chromosome abnormalities using Magiscan 2. Automated Chromosome Analysis Workshop, Leiden.
7. Piper, J. and Granum, E. (1989) On fully automatic feature measurement for banded chromosome classification. *Cytometry* **10,** 242–255.
8. Lloyd, D., Piper, J., Rutovitz, D., and Shippey, G. (1987) Multiprocessing interval processor for automated cytogenetics. *Appl. Optics* **26,** 3356–3366.
9. Graham, J. (1987) Automation of routine clinical chromosome analysis. I. Karyotyping by machine. *Anal. Quant. Cytol. Histol.* **9,** 383–390.
10. Graham, J. (1989) Resolution of composites in interactive karyotyping, in (Lundsteen, C. and Piper, J., eds.) *Automation of Cytogenetics* Springer-Verlag, Berlin, pp. 191–203.
11. Shippey, G., Carothers, A. D., and Gordon, J. (1986) Operation and performance of an automatic metaphase finder based on the MRC fast interval processor. *J. Histochem. Cytochem.* **34,** 1245–1252.
12. Graham, J. and Pycock, D. (1987) Automation of routine clinical chromosome analysis. II. Metaphase finding. *Anal. Quant. Cytol. Histol.* **9,** 391–397.
13. Serra, J. (1982) *Image Analysis and Mathematical Morphology.* Academic, London, UK.
14. Groen, F. C. A., Young, I. T., and Ligthart, G. (1985) A comparison of different focus functions for use in autofocus algorithms. *Cytometry* **6,** 81–91.
15. Firestone, L., Cook, K., Culp, K., Talsania, N., and Preston, K. (1991) Comparison of autofocus methods for automated microscopy. *Cytometry* **12,** 195–206.
16. Vrolijk, J., Sloos, W. C. R., Verwoerd, N. P., and Tanke, H. J. (1991) A MacIntosh based system for metaphase finding. Poster contribution to EC Concerted Action on Automated Cytogenetics Workshop, Leiden, September 2–3.
17. van Vliet, L. J., Young, I. T., and Mayall, B. H. (1990) The Athena semi-automated karyotyping system. *Cytometry* **1,** 51–58.

18. Groen, F. C. A., ten Kate, T. K., Smeulders, A. W. M., and Young, I. T. (1989) Human chromosome classification based on local band descriptors. *Patt. Recog. Letts.* **9,** 211–222.
19. Rutovitz, D. (1975) An algorithm for in-line generation of a convex cover. *Computer Graphics Image Processing* **4,** 74–78.
20. Piper, J. and Lundsteen, C. (1987) Human chromosome analysis by machine. *Trends in Genet.* **3,** 309–313.
21. Groen, F. C., Verbeek, P. W., Zee, G. A., and Oosterlinck, A. (1976) Some aspects concerning computation of chromosome banding profiles, in *Proceedings of the 3rd International Joint Conference on Pattern Recognition,* Coronado, CA, pp. 547–550.
22. Piper, J. (1981) Finding chromosome centromeres using boundary and density information, in *Digital Image Processing.* (Simon, J.-C. and Haralick, R. M., eds.) D. Reidel, Dordrecht, Netherlands, pp. 511–518.
23. Granum, E. (1982) Application of statistical and syntactical methods of analysis and classification to chromosome data, in *Pattern Recognition Theory and Applications.* (Kittler, J., Fu, K. S., and Pau, L. F. eds.) NATO ASI (Oxford 1981), Reidel, Dordrecht, pp. 373–398.
24. Caspersson, T., Lomakka, G., and Moler, A. (1971) Computerised chromosome identification by aid of the quinacrine mustard fluorescence technique. *Hereditas* **67,** 103–109.
25. Thomason, M. G. and Granum, E. (1986) Dynamic programming inference of markov networks from finite sets of sample strings. *IEEE-Transactions on Pattern Analysis and Machine Intelligence (PAMI)* **8,** 491–501.
26. Devijver, P. A. and Kittler, J. (1982) *Pattern Recognition, A Statistical Approach.* Prentice-Hall International, London, UK.
27. Duda, R. O. and Hart, P. E. (1973) *Pattern Recognition and Scene Analysis.* Wiley, New York.
28. Piper, J. (1987) The effect of zero feature correlation assumption on maximum likelihood based classification of chromosomes. *Sign Proces.* **12,** 49–57.
29. Kirby, S. P. J., Theobald, C. M., Piper, J, and Carothers, A. (1991) Some methods of combining class information in multivariate normal discrimination for the classification of human chromosomes. *Statistics in Medicine* **10,** 141–149.
30. Lundsteen, C., Gerdes, T., and Maahr, J. (1986) Automatic classification of chromosomes as part of a routine system for clinical analysis. *Cytometry* **7,** 1–7.
31. Piper, J. (1992) Variability and bias in experimentally measured classifier error rates. *Patt. Recog. Letts.* **13,** 685–692.
32. Piper, J. (1986) Classification of chromosomes constrained by expected class size. *Patt. Recog. Letts.* **4,** 391–395.
33. Tso, M. K. S. and Graham, J. (1983) The transportation algorithm as an aid to chromosome classification. *Patt. Recog. Letts.* **1,** 489–496.
34. Tso, M., Kleinschmidt, P., Mittereiter, I., and Graham, J. (1991) An efficient transportation algorithm for automatic chromosome karyotyping. *Patt. Recog. Letts.* **12,** 117–126.

35. Zimmerman, S. O., Johnston, D. A., Arrighi, F. E., and Rupp, M. E. (1986) Automated homologue matching of human G-banded chromosomes. *Comput. Biol. Med.* **16,** 223–233.

36. Piper, J., Carothers, A., and Guest, E. (1991) Chromosome classification incorporating similarity constraints. *Digest of the World Congress on Medical Physics and Biomedical Engineering, Kyoto, Japan, 1991, Medical and Biological Engineering and Computing* **29 (suppl),** 221.

37. Wu, Q., Snellings, J., Amory, L., Suetens, P., and Oosterlinck, A. (1989) Model-based contour analysis in a chromosome segmentation system, in *Automation of Cytogenetics,* (Lundsteen, C. and Piper, J., eds.,) Springer-Verlag, Berlin, pp. 217–229.

38. Vossepoel, A. M. (1989) Separation of touching chromosomes in *Automation of Cytogenetics,* (Lundsteen, C. and Piper, J., eds.) Springer-Verlag, Berlin, pp. 205–216.

39. Ji, L. (1989) Intelligent splitting in the chromosome domain. *Patt. Recog.* **22,** 519–532.

40. Ji, L. (1989) Decomposition of overlapping chromosomes, in *Automation of Cytogenetics,* (Lundsteen, C. and Piper, J., eds.) Springer-Verlag, Berlin, pp. 177–190.

41. Ji, L. (1991) Fully automatic chromosome segmentation. *Cytometry,* in press.

42. Errington, P. A. and Graham, J. (1993) Application of artificial neural networks to chromosome classification. *Cytometry,* in press.

43. Lundsteen, C., Gerdes, T., and Maahr, J. (1989) Cytogenetic analysis by automatic multiple cell karyotyping, in *Automation of Cytogenetics* (Lundsteen, C. and Piper, J., eds.) Springer-Verlag, Berlin, pp. 263–274.

44. Carothers, A. D., Rutovitz, D. and Granum, E. (1983) An efficient multiple-cell approach to automatic aneuploidy screening. *Anal. Quant. Cytol.* **5,** 194–200.

45. Granlund, G. H., Zack, G. W., Young, I. T., and Eden, M. (1976) A technique for multiple-cell chromosome karyotyping. *J. Histochem. Cytochem.* **24,** 160–167.

46. Hilditch, C. J. (1969) The principles of a software system for karyotype analysis, in *Human Population Cytogenetics* (Jacobs, P. A., Price, W. H., and Law, P., eds.) Edinburgh University Press, Edinburgh, Scotland, pp. 297–325.

47. Lundsteen, C. (1978) A proposed format for system output: the combined karyotype. *Proceedings of the 1978 European Workshop on Automated Human Cytogenetics.* Electronics Laboratory, Technical University of Denmark, Lyngby, pp. s3.3,s3.4.

CHAPTER 12

Bivariate Chromosome Analysis Using a Commercial Flow Cytometer

Nigel P. Carter

1. Introduction
1.1. Flow Cytometer Requirements and Operation

The bivariate analysis of human chromosomes in flow using the fluorochromes Hoechst 33258 (with specificity for AT-rich DNA) and Chromomycin A3 (with specificity for GC-rich DNA) was first described by Gray et al. in 1979 *(1)*. Chromosomes stained with these two dyes can be resolved on the flow cytometer not only by their DNA content, but also by base pair ratio (*see* Fig. 1). Although other dye combinations have been used (e.g., refs. *2–4*), Hoechst and Chromomycin are the most widely used DNA fluorochrome pair for the bivariate analysis of human chromosomes.

Hoechst and Chromomycin have excitation maxima (365 and 425 nm, respectively) that are well separated and can be excited efficiently by the UV and 457.9-nm lines of the Argon Ion laser. However, the emission spectra of the two dyes have a considerable degree of overlap, so that it is necessary to use two laser beams spatially separated within the flow chamber or stream in order to obtain independent measurements of Hoechst and Chromomycin fluorescence (*see also* Note 1). The separation of the excitation beams translates to a spatial separation of the fluorescence emissions within the detection light path. This enables a half mirror to be used to direct the Hoechst and

From: *Methods in Molecular Biology, Vol. 29: Chromosome Analysis Protocols*
Edited by: J. R. Gosden Copyright ©1994 Humana Press Inc., Totowa, NJ

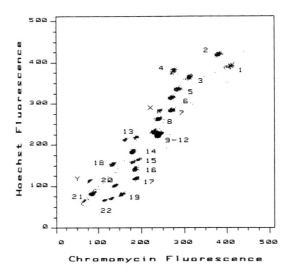

Fig. 1. A bivariate flow karyotype of human chromosomes stained with Hoechst 33258 and Chromomycin A3. The chromosome numbers (types) corresponding to the clusters of events on the karyotype are indicated.

Chromomycin fluorescence to separate detectors. However, the consequence of this optical arrangement is that as a chromosome passes through the flow system, a time delay is generated between the signal pulses produced at the two detectors. Delay compensation electronics are therefore necessary to allow correct correlation of measurements.

Most high-resolution bivariate flow karyotypes have been produced on flow cytometers specifically designed and built for chromosome analysis (e.g., refs. *5,6*). Typically such instruments feature high-power lasers capable of producing over 1 W of UV wavelengths, elliptical laser beam shaping optics, a quartz flow chamber, and advanced signal processing and digital electronics. Such systems have been utilized by groups at the Lawrence Livermore National Laboratory (Livermore, CA), Los Alamos Flow Cytometry Resource (Los Alamos, NM), and the University of California.

Until recently, bivariate karyotypes produced on commercial flow cytometers have seldom displayed the resolution of those from custom-designed instrumentation. However, advances in laser technology, in signal processing, and in chromosome preparation and staining techniques *(7)* have enabled high-resolution flow karyotypes to be produced routinely on unmodified commercial flow cytometers *(8)*.

In this chapter, I will describe the important features and requirements for bivariate flow karyotype analysis on an unmodified commercial flow cytometer. Although this will be based on experience with FACStar Plus instruments (Becton Dickinson, Rutherford, NJ), the information presented should be of relevance to instruments from other manufacturers.

1.2. Chromosome Preparation and Staining

The basic features of the preparation of a suspension of chromosomes for flow cytometric analysis involve the use of inhibitors of mitotic spindle formation to accumulate cells in metaphase, swelling of the cells in a hypotonic solution to aid the separation of individual chromosomes, and the use of detergents to release the chromosomes into a buffer designed to stabilize the structure of the chromosomes. The buffers most commonly used for bivariate chromosome analysis use either polyamines or magnesium ions for the final stabilization of the chromosomes. I have found that modifications of the polyamine buffer procedure of Sillar and Young *(9)* and the HEPES/magnesium sulfate buffer of van den Engh et al. *(10)* have proven very reliable for the preparation of chromosome preparations from many cell types while retaining good bivariate resolution. Examples of bivariate karyotypes of the same lymphoblastoid cell line prepared using these two isolation buffers are shown in Fig. 2.

2. Materials
2.1. Flow Cytometer Requirements and Operation
2.1.1. Minimum Cytometer Requirements—A Check List

1. Dual laser optical bench with necessary prism/mirror adjustments for laser beam spatial separation at the detection point (*see* Note 2).
2. Two 5-W or greater argon ion lasers with power output feedback control, one laser with UV mirrors and high-field magnet capable of maintaining a minimum of 250 mW UV multiline, and one laser tuned to the 457.9-nm line maintaining a minimum of 250 mW output (*see* Note 3).
3. Dual beam delay signal compensation electronics.
4. A minimum of 10-bit analog-to-digital converters (1024-channel resolution).
5. Two photomultiplier tubes for fluorescence detection.
6. Point-focused collection optics with half-mirror steering assembly.

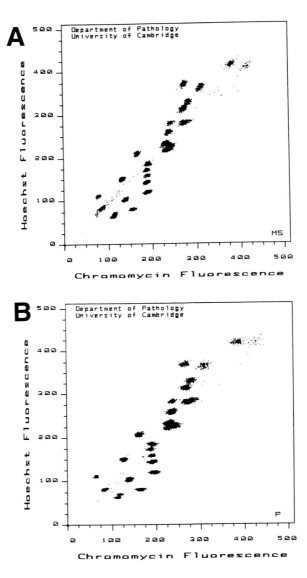

Fig. 2. **A.** Flow karyotype of chromosomes prepared using the magnesium sulfate/HEPES buffer. **B.** Flow karyotype of chromosomes from the same cell line prepared using the polyamine buffer.

2.1.2. Reagents

Sheath buffer: 100 m*M* sodium chloride, 10 m*M* Tris (hydroxy-methyl) methylamine, 1 m*M* EDTA—adjust pH to 7.2 with HCl, autoclave, and store at room temperature (stable for at least 1 mo).

2.2. Chromosome Preparation and Staining

2.2.1. Tissue Culture Reagents

1. RPMI 1640 medium supplemented with 16.6% fetal bovine serum, 2 mM L-glutamine, and penicillin-streptomycin (100 U/mL and 100 mg/ mL, respectively).
2. HAMS F10 medium supplemented with 10% fetal bovine serum, 2 mM L-glutamine, and penicillin-streptomycin (100 U/mL and 100 mg/mL, respectively).
3. Colcemid solution 10 µg/mL (Gibco BRL, Gaithersburg, MD).
4. Histopaque 1119 (Sigma, St. Louis, MO).
5. Versine.
6. Trypsin/EDTA.
7. Phytohemagglutinin (HA17, Wellcome Diagnostics, Dartford, UK).

2.2.2. Chromosome Isolation Buffers

1. HEPES/magnesium sulfate buffer: 45 mM potassium chloride, 5 mM HEPES, 10 mM magnesium sulfate, 3 mM dithiothreitol, pH 8.0. Prepare on the day of chromosome isolation as detailed in Section 3. Do not store.
2. Polyamine buffer (10X stocks):
   a. 75 mM Tris(hydroxymethyl)methylamine, 20 mM EDTA, pH 8.0.
   b. 75 mM Tris(hydroxymethyl)methylamine, 5 mM EGTA, pH 8.0.
   c. 800 mM Potassium chloride.
   d. 200 mM Sodium chloride.
      Make solutions a–d using sterile distilled water, and filter through a sterile 0.22-µm filter before storage at 4°C. Stable for 1 mo.
   e. 0.4M Spermine.
   f. 1.0M Spermidine.
      Store in 100-µL aliquots at –20°C. Stable but do not refreeze.
3. 100 mM Magnesium sulfate: 7H$_2$O (sterile filter and store at 4°C). Stable for 1 mo.
4. 100 mM Tri-sodium citrate (make on the day of running sample).
5. 250 mM Sodium sulfite (make on the day of running sample).
6. Hoechst 33258: 1 mg/mL in sterile distilled water (sterile filter and store in the dark at 4°C). Stable.
7. Chromomycin A3: 2 mg/mL dissolved in absolute ethanol (store at –20°C in small aliquots). Stable.
8. Turck's stain: 0.01% gentian violet in 1% glacial acetic acid.

3. Methods

3.1. Flow Cytometer Operation

3.1.1. Cytometer Configuration

1. The lasers should be arranged such that the chromosomes pass first through the UV beam and then through the 457.9-nm beam (*see* Note 1). The spatial separation between the two beams should be set according to the manufacturer's recommended procedure.
2. Hoechst fluorescence excited by the UV beam is collected by the first detector through a UV blocking filter (400-nm long pass) combined with a 480-nm short pass filter. Chromomycin fluorescence is reflected by a half mirror to the second detector and collected through a 490-nm long pass filter. Signals from the first detector are passed through dual beam delay compensation circuitry.
3. If available, the laser beam focusing lens is selected to maximize the light intensity experienced by the chromosomes (*see* Note 3). On the FACStar Plus, the 2-in. focal length lens is selected without the lateral beam expander.

3.1.2. Cytometer Operation

1. Slowly bring the lasers up to operational power (e.g., 300 mW UV, 300 mW 457.9 nm) selecting power (light output) feedback control. Allow lasers to run for 2 h or until stable. Adjust for minimum plasma tube current.
2. Replace sterile sheath buffer and sheath-line 0.2-μm filter before each run. Allow sheath to stabilize.
3. For cytometers using "stream in air" analysis, ensure that the jet is orthogonal to the laser beam and detection optic light paths.
4. Run fluorescence microspheres (e.g., Fluoresbrite #18338, Polysciences) and tune cytometer for minimum peak coefficient of variance for the Hoechst fluorescence channel. Adjust the alignment of the second laser beam to achieve minimum peak coefficient of variance for the Chromomycin fluorescence channel.

3.2. Cell Culture and Procedures Prior to Chromosome Isolation

3.2.1. Epstein-Barr Virus Transformed Lymphoblastoid Human Cell Lines (Suspension Culture, See Figs. 1 and 2)

1. Grow the cell line just to confluency in 20 mL of supplemented RPMI medium at 37°C in a gassed incubator (4–5% CO_2). Gently shake flask,

and allow cell clumps to settle. Add 30 mL of fresh medium, gently break up clumps, and culture for 24 h.

2. Add 0.5 mL of colcemid (10 µg/mL), resuspend the cells gently breaking up clumps, and culture for 5–6 h.

3. Remove cells and medium into a 50-mL tube, and estimate the cell concentration using a hemocytometer. Each culture should yield approx 2×10^7 cells with a mitotic index better than 50%.

3.2.2. Human Fibroblast Cell Lines
(Monolayer Culture, see Fig. 3)

1. Grow cells to near confluency in 50 mL of supplemented HAMS F10 medium in a 175 cm^2 flask at 37°C in a gassed incubator (4–5% CO_2). Subculture by versine wash and trypsinization into five T150 flasks to give a cell density of approx 15–20% of confluency, and incubate for 48 h. At this time the cells should have reached approx 60–75% of confluency.

2. Remove medium, and replace with 50 mL of fresh medium to which is added 0.5 mL of colcemid solution. Incubate for 12–16 h (overnight).

3. Gently shake the flasks, and remove the medium into a 50-mL tube. Each flask should yield approx 5×10^5 cells with a mitotic index better than 80%. Centrifuge at 200g for 10 min. Discard supernatant, and pool cell pellets in 20 mL of supplemented HAMS F10 medium. Calculate cell concentration using a hemocytometer.

3.2.3. Human Peripheral Blood Cultures (See Fig. 4)

1. Add 0.5 mL of heparinized peripheral blood to a tube containing 10 mL of supplemented RPMI medium containing 10 U/mL of heparin and 15 µL/mL of phytohemagglutinin. Incubate in a gassed incubator at 37°C for 96 h. Invert the tube at least once during each 24-h period. If possible, set up a minimum of four tubes.

2. Add 0.1 mL of colcemid solution to each tube, mix gently, and incubate for 12–16 h (overnight).

3. Gently mix the tube with a Pasteur pipet and underlayer with 3 mL of Histopaque 1119. Centrifuge at 800g for 20 min.

4. Transfer the cell layer formed at interface into a fresh tube, and resuspend in 10 mL of supplemented RPMI medium containing 0.1 µg/mL of colcemid. Centrifuge at 400g for 5 min, discard supernatant, pool cell pellets, and resuspend in a further 10 mL of medium. Calculate cell concentration using a hemocytometer. Each tube should yield approx 5×10^5 cells with a mitotic index of approx 50%.

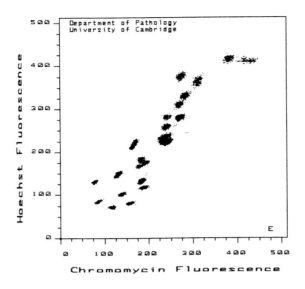

Fig. 3. Flow karyotype of chromosomes prepared from a human fibroblast cell line.

3.2.4. Chinese Hamster and Somatic Cell Hybrid Cell Lines

Adherent rodent cell lines are cultured as for human fibroblast lines, except that the fetal bovine serum in the supplemented HAMS F10 medium is reduced to 8.3%. Since the doubling time for these cell lines is on average between 12 and 15 h, confluent cultures are subcloned to a density of 25% confluency, incubated for 8–12 h, and 0.1 µg/mL of colcemid added for a further 4 h. The cells are then harvested using mitotic shakeoff as for human fibroblast cell lines.

3.3. Chromosome Isolation Procedures
3.3.1. Magnesium Sulfate / HEPES Buffer

1. Prepare the buffer on the day of chromosome isolation. For 100 mL of isolation buffer, dissolve 335 mg of potassium chloride and 119 mg of HEPES in 85 mL of sterile distilled water. Add 10 mL of 100 m*M* magnesium sulfate solution and pH to 8.0 using 0.1*M* potassium hydroxide. Add 46 mg of dithiothreitol, and adjust volume to 100 mL. Transfer 10 mL of the buffer to a universal tube, and add 250 µL of Triton X-100 using a positive displacement pipet. Dissolve the detergent by placing the universal tube on a rotating wheel for 15 min or until dissolved.

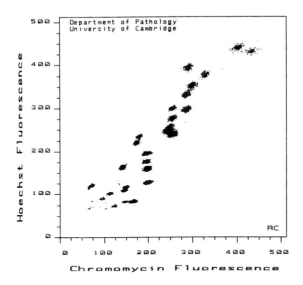

Fig. 4. Flow karyotype of chromosomes prepared from a human peripheral blood culture (routine blood culture prepared by the East Anglian Regional Genetics Service, Cambridge, UK).

2. Centrifuge the cell preparation for 5 min at 200g. Discard supernatant, and place tube inverted on an absorbent paper towel for a few seconds. Resuspend the cell pellet in isolation buffer to give a cell concentration of approx 4×10^6/mL. Incubate at room temperature for 10 min.
3. Swelling can be monitored by staining 10 μL of the cell suspension with an equal volume of Turck's stain and viewing in a hemocytometer by phase-contrast microscopy. The mitotic index of the sample can also be determined easily in this way.
4. Add a $^1/_{10}$ vol of 2.5% Triton X-100 in magnesium sulfate-HEPES, and incubate on ice for 10 min.
5. Vortex for 10 s at a speed that produces a swirling film of suspension on the tube wall.
6. Remove 10 μL of suspension onto a microscope slide, and add 1 μL of Hoechst stain. Check that most chromosomes are free in suspension and not clumped using the fluorescence microscope. Vortex for further intervals of 5 s until few clumps are apparent. Overvortexing will result in increased numbers of broken chromosomes.
7. Store chromosome suspension at 4°C until required.

3.3.2. Polyamine Buffer

1. Make hypotonic potassium chloride (75 mM) using sterile distilled water.
2. Make a 1X strength buffer from the four 10X stocks with sterile distilled water on the day of chromosome isolation. Add a $1/2000$ vol of spermidine stock solution, a $1/2000$ vol of spermine stock solution, and a $1/1000$ vol of β-mercaptoethanol. Adjust pH to 7.2 using 0.1M hydrochloric acid. Add Triton X-100 using a positive displacement pipet to give a final concentration of 0.25%.
3. Centrifuge the cell preparation for 5 min at 200g. Discard supernatant, and place tube inverted on an absorbent paper towel for a few seconds. Add 10 mL of hypotonic potassium chloride to the cell pellet, and resuspend gently using a Pasteur pipet. Incubate for 15 min at room temperature.
4. Swelling can be monitored by staining 10 µL of the cell suspension with an equal volume of Turck's stain and viewing in a hemocytometer by phase-contrast microscopy. The mitotic index of the sample can also be determined easily in this way.
5. Centrifuge at 400g for 5 min.
6. Discard the supernatant, and place tube inverted on an absorbent paper towel for a few seconds. Resuspend the cell pellet in polyamine/ Triton X-100 buffer at a cell concentration of 4×10^6/mL, and incubate on ice for 10 min.
7. Vortex for 10 s at a speed that produces a swirling film of suspension on the tube wall.
8. Remove 10 µL of suspension onto a microscope slide, and add 1 µL of Hoechst stain. Check that most chromosomes are free in suspension and not clumped using the fluorescence microscope. Vortex for further intervals of 5 s until few clumps are apparent. Overvortexing will result in increased numbers of broken chromosomes.
9. Store chromosome suspension at 4°C until required.

3.3.3. Chromosome Staining (See Note 4)

1. Centrifuge 850 µL of chromosome suspension at 100g for 1 min. Transfer 740 µL of the supernatant to a fresh tube. (This step is omitted if determination of chromosome numbers under each peak is required.)
2. Add 20 µL of stock Chromomycin A3 solution to 740 µL of chromosome suspension, and mix immediately.
3. Add 20 µL of 100 mM magnesium sulfate solution, and mix immediately.
4. Add 20 µL of a $1/10$ dilution of stock Hoechst 33258 solution, and mix immediately.
5. Incubate at 4°C for at least 2 h before analysis.

6. Add 100 µL of stock sodium citrate and 100 µL of stock sodium sulfite 15 min prior to analysis.

3.4. Chromosome Analysis and Display

The stained chromosome suspension is analyzed on the flow cytometer by acquiring a bivariate plot of Hoechst fluorescence (*y* axis) vs Chromomycin fluorescence (*x* axis). If possible, the sample should be maintained at 4°C. Best resolution for analysis is obtained by using slow sample flow rates (e.g., 300 chromosomes/s), but for many chromosomes, resolution is adequate to allow sorting at flow rates of up to 2000/s (*see* Notes 5 and 6). Fluorescence measurements will drift during the first few minutes of running a fresh sample. Best resolution is obtained by running the sample, and monitoring the mean fluorescence intensity of one of the Hoechst and one of the Chromomycin peaks until stable conditions are obtained (usually within 5–10 min).

The efficient analysis and display of bivariate flow karyotypes require specialist software as yet unavailable as standard with commercial flow cytometers. However, within the limitations of the standard software, karyotypes are best displayed as simple dot plots or as contour plots where the lowest contour can be set to exclude low-frequency events from debris, chromosome fragments, and clumps. A more detailed discussion of analysis and display options will be found in Note 7.

4. Notes

1. Although the fluorescence differences between Hoechst and Chromomycin are in most part determined by their AT and GC base pair specificities *(1,11,12)*, resonance energy transfer occurs between the two dyes when used in combination *(13,14)*. In consequence, the fluorescence measured after UV excitation is a composite of true Hoechst fluorescence with a small amount of Chromomycin fluorescence stimulated by energy transfer from the Hoechst fluorescence. Because of these spectral interactions, the order of excitation of the dyes has an effect on the separation of chromosomes in the bivariate plot. The best separation is achieved when the chromosomes pass through the UV beam first (G. J. van den Engh, personal communication).
2. Vibration of the optical bench can have a considerable detrimental affect on measurement resolution. The most likely source of vibration is the passage of water through the lasers. This can be reduced by operating

the lasers at the minimum water flow rate. Other sources of vibration, such as air compressors, vacuum pumps, and laser power supplies, should be located as far from the optical bench as possible. Improvements can also be obtained by isolating the optical bench from its support by standing it on antivibration feet (or on rubber bungs of appropriate size and compliance).

3. To achieve high-resolution flow karyotypes, it is essential that variations in illumination intensity contribute as little as possible to the measured fluorescence. Since the lasers generally display (in TEM 00) a Gaussian light intensity distribution across the beam, chromosomes taking different trajectories through the beam will be exposed to different intensities of excitation. One approach to minimize this effect is to expand the laser beam laterally so that the Gaussian distribution of the beam is flattened and chromosomes will be exposed to more even illumination. Alternatively, at laser excitation powers high enough to achieve sufficient dye saturation and/or photobleaching, fluorescence becomes increasingly independent of illumination intensity. This approach has proven to be most effective on the FACStar Plus, where this phenomenon becomes apparent for Hoechst fluorescence at laser powers >250 mW UV multiline using the standard 2-in. focusing lens. For each installation, calibration curves of relative fluorescence vs laser illumination power for chromosomes should indicate the minimum laser power necessary for high-resolution measurements. Similarly, dye concentration should be titrated to determine the saturation point.

4. The DNA fluorochromes rapidly saturate sample tubing as the chromosome preparation is analyzed. Simple washing of the tubing, even using bleach, will not remove all of this dye. Cells run in such tubing will slowly take up these dyes and become stained. I have found it necessary at least to replace all of the sample tubing before running cells stained by immunofluorescence. Ideally, a complete nozzle/sample tube assembly should be reserved exclusively for this purpose.

5. Very fine adjustments of the flow cell or jet position and of the second laser light path can be used to achieve the best resolution. However, care must be used, since it is easy to lose resolution completely, requiring rerunning of fluorescent microspheres to correct.

6. During long analysis or sorting periods, differential sedimentation of chromosomes will take place. Gentle agitation of the sample at regular intervals will avoid this problem.

7. The display of bivariate flow karyotypes using the analysis software available on commercial instruments generally produces disappointing results. One reason for this is that in order to distinguish chromosome

peaks clearly, it is usually necessary to remove the low-frequency events owing to debris and chromosome clumps from the display (Fig. 5A). A standard way of achieving this is to use contour plots of the data setting the lowest contour above the low-frequency noise level. Unfortunately, because of the limitations of computer displays and hardware currently supplied with flow cytometers, the data resolution is often reduced to 64×64 channels, even if the data have been collected with 1024 channel resolution (Fig. 5B). Some software programs, e.g., LYSIS 2 (Becton Dickinson) will allow areas of the contour plot to be viewed at a higher resolution (zoomed), and although this achieves good discrimination between peaks, the whole karyotype cannot be viewed (Fig. 5C). Simple dot plots of the data usually produce better resolution of peaks, although it is seldom possible to filter out the low-frequency events with such software, and again data reduction is often used to match screen pixel resolution (Fig. 5A). Again, viewing of a reduced area of the plot at greater resolution can aid in peak discrimination, but with the same criticisms as for zoomed contour plots (Fig. 5D). Some groups have overcome these limitations by writing their own software using higher resolution dot plots with background subtraction (Fig. 5E) or higher resolution contour plots (Fig. 5F). However, such software should still retain the ability to display low-frequency events if required, so that the quality of the chromosome preparation can be assessed.

Similarly, the analysis of bivariate flow karyotypes is difficult to perform using the software supplied with commercial instruments. The analyses normally required are (a) to estimate the number of events in each peak for chromosome aneuploidy determination and (b) to estimate the DNA content of aberrant chromosomes.

The number of events in a peak can usually only be determined in commercial software by drawing a window around the peak using a mouse or other pointer device. Although this procedure will supply frequency data, repeating this procedure for each peak (there are usually more than 20 peaks) in a karyotype is tedious and often limited by the number of windows available at one time.

Measurement of the DNA content of a chromosome from a bivariate plot is based on determining the Hoechst fluorescence and Chromomycin fluorescence coordinates for each peak. After adjusting for the relative contributions of each dye to the overall DNA measurement and relating the sum of all chromosomes to the known DNA content of the human genome, the relative DNA content of any one peak can then be estimated. Although mean peak fluorescence coordinates can be determined easily from the windows set for frequency analysis,

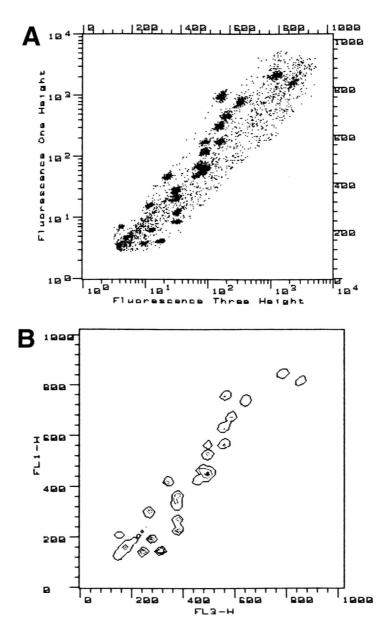

Fig. 5. Different displays of the same bivariate flow karyotype data. **A.** Dot plot display (FACStar Plus Research Software, Becton Dickinson). **B.** Contour plot (FACStar Plus Research Software, Becton Dickinson).

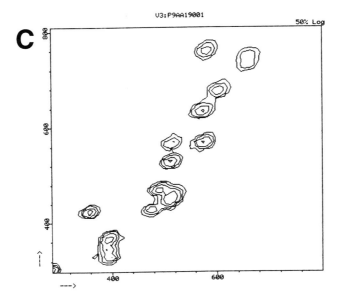

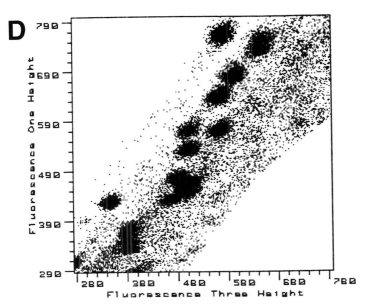

C. Zoomed contour plot (LYSIS II, Becton Dickinson). **D.** Zoomed dot plot (FACStar Plus Research Software, Becton Dickinson).

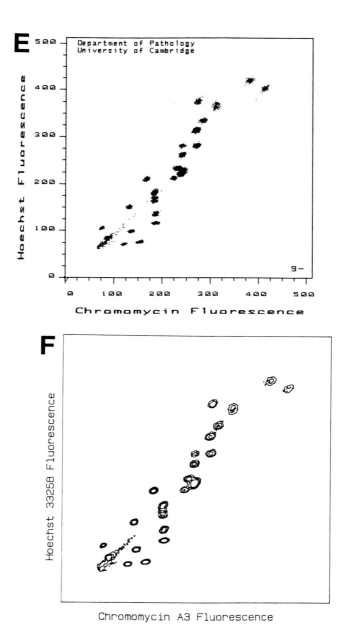

E. Higher resolution dot plot (CAP1, N. P. Carter, Cambridge University). **F.** Higher resolution contour plot (ANALIST, G. van den Engh, Lawrence Livermore National Laboratory).

again this procedure is time-consuming as are the subsequent calcula-tions. These limitations have led several groups to write their own analy-sis programs (e.g., ref. *8,15–17*).

I have found the techniques described in detail by van den Engh *(15)* and Trask et al. *(16)* to be very robust in the analysis of bivariate flow karyotypes. In brief, the basic features of the analysis require that the data first be normalized. This is achieved by determining the mean Hoechst fluorescence and Chromomycin fluorescence peak coordinates for each chromosome (directly by summation or by curve fitting), cal-culating mean fluorescence values for summed peaks, and scaling all data to arbitrary predefined and equal mean values. Data points are then projected onto a line passing through the origin and the peak of normal chromosome 4 (at an angle α of approx 50°), where the distance from the origin along this line is directly proportional to DNA content (the angle was determined by direct comparison of data projected onto the line and univariate karyotypes produced using staining with Propidium iodide). The distance from the origin to the point of projection along the line is calculated by:

$$d = CA \times \cos(\alpha) + HO \times \sin(\alpha) \qquad (1)$$

where d is the distance from the origin to the point of projection, CA is the Chromomycin mean peak fluorescence channel number, and HO is the Hoechst mean peak fluorescence channel number. The relative DNA content for all the peak means can be calculated in this way. The accu-racy of this approach has been independently demonstrated by differ-ent groups who showed a high degree of correlation between chromosomal DNA content measured from bivariate flow karyotypes and as determined by CYDAC absorption measurements *(8,16)*.

References

1. Gray, J. W., Langlois, R. G., Carrano, A. V., Burkhart-Schultz, K., and Van Dilla, M. A. (1979) High resolution chromosome analysis: one and two parameter flow cytometry. *Chromosoma* **73**, 9–27.
2. Lebo, R. V., Globus, M. S., and Cheung, M.-C. (1986) Detecting abnormal human chromosome constitutions by dual laser cytogenetics. *Am. J. Med. Genet.* **25**, 519–529.
3. Lebo, R. V., Gorin, F., Fletterick, R. F., Kao, F.-T., Cheung, M.-C., Bruce, B. D., and Kan, Y. W. (1984) High resolution chromosome sorting and DNA spot-blot analysis assign McArdle's syndrome to chromosome 11. *Science* **225**, 57–59.
4. Langlois R. D. (1989) DNA stains as cytochemical probes for chromosomes, in *Flow Cytogenetics* (Gray, J. W., ed.) Academic, London, UK, pp. 61–81.

5. Dean, P. and Pinkel, D. (1978) High resolution dual laser flow cytometry. *J. Histochem. Cytochem.* **26,** 622–627.
6. Lebo, R. V. and Bastain, A. (1982) Design and operation of a dual laser chromosome sorter. *Cytometry* **3,** 213–219.
7. van den Engh, G., Trask, B., Lansdorp, P., and Gray, J. (1988) Improved resolution of flow cytometric measurements of Hoechst and Chromomycin A3 stained human chromosomes after addition of citrate and sulfite. *Cytometry* **9,** 266–270.
8. Carter, N. P., Ferguson-Smith, M. E., Affara, N. A., Briggs, H., and Ferguson-Smith, M. A. (1990) Study of X chromosome abnormality in XX males using bivariate flow karyotype analysis and flow sorted dot blots. *Cytometry* **11,** 202–207.
9. Sillar, R. and Young, B. D. (1981) A new method for the preparation of metaphase chromosomes for flow analysis. *J. Histochem. Cytochem.* **29,** 74–78.
10. van den Engh, G. J., Trask, B. J., Gray, J. W., Langlois, R. G., and Yu, L.-C. (1985) Preparation and bivariate analysis of suspensions of human chromosomes. *Cytometry* **6,** 92–100.
11. Latt, S. and Wohlleb, J. (1975) Optical studies on the interaction of 33258 Hoechst with DNA, chromatin and metaphase chromosomes. *Chromosoma* **51,** 297–316.
12. Langlois, R. G., Carrano, J. W., Gray, J. W., and Van Dilla, M. (1980) Cytochemical studies of metaphase chromosomes by flow cytometry. *Chromosoma* **37,** 229–251.
13. Langlois, R. G. and Jensen, R. H. (1979) Interactions between pairs of DNA specific fluorescent stains bound to mammalian cells. *J. Histochem. Cytochem.* **27,** 72–79. Erratum p. 1559.
14. van den Engh, G. J., Trask, B. J., and Gray, J. W. (1986) The binding kinetics and interaction of DNA fluorochromes used in the analysis of nuclei and chromosomes by flow cytometry. *Histochemistry* **84,** 501–508.
15. van den Engh, G. J., Hanson, D., and Trask, B. (1990) A computer program for analyzing bivariate flow karyotypes. *Cytometry* **11,** 173–183.
16. Trask, B., van den Engh, G., Nussbaum, R., Schwartz, C., and Gray, J. (1990) Quantification of the DNA content of structurally abnormal X chromosomes and X chromosome aneuploidy using high resolution bivariate flow karyotyping. *Cytometry* **11,** 184–196.
17. Dean, P. N., Kolla, S., and Van Dilla, M. A. (1989) Analysis of bivariate flow karyotypes. *Cytometry* **10,** 109–123.

CHAPTER 13

Chromosome Sorting
by Flow Cytometry

Production of DNA Libraries and Gene Mapping

Judith A. Fantes, Daryll K. Green,
and Andrew Sharkey

1. Introduction

Bivariate flow cytometry is now able to resolve the majority of chromosomes of the human karyotype (*1,2* and Chapter 12). When this is coupled to a sorting facility, specific chromosomes can be separated and purified in small, but useful quantities. These chromosomes have been used for the production of chromosome-specific DNA libraries *(3);* each human chromosome, sorted from lymphoblastoid cell lines or somatic cell hybrids, has been cloned into λ or plasmid vectors, and these libraries are now available from the American Type Culture Collection *(4).* Chromosome abnormalities, such as balanced translocations, deletion, or marker chromosomes, can also be distinguished in a flow karyotype *(5,6),* and these have provided alternative starting material for more restricted DNA libraries *(7,8).*

In the past, such libraries have been a useful source of DNA sequences for the scientific community, but together with fluorescence *in situ* hybridization, they now have an additional role in delineating or painting individual chromosomes in metaphases or interphase nuclei *(9).* Chromosome painting is proving a useful tool for identifying complex translocations *(10)* and in radiation dosimetry *(11).*

From: *Methods in Molecular Biology, Vol. 29: Chromosome Analysis Protocols*
Edited by: J. R. Gosden Copyright ©1994 Humana Press Inc., Totowa, NJ

Another application for sorted chromosomes is gene mapping, where specific chromosome homologs are sorted onto nitrocellulose filter paper and hybridized with DNA probes of interest *(12)*. A positive signal from a particular chromosome maps the probe to that chromosome, and then translocation or deletion chromosomes (if detectable) can be used to refine the map position further *(13,14)*.

Useful though these techniques are, they require considerable expenditure of time to sort the purified material. For example, it can take 4 d to sort the 2×10^6 chromosomes required for a DNA library and 1–2 d to sort 30,000 chromosomes of each chromosome homolog for a gene-mapping experiment. It is often difficult to achieve the necessary optimal performance from the flow cytometer for such a long period of time. The recent introduction of the polymerase chain reaction for amplifying stretches of DNA directly *(15)* has made a considerable difference to many sorting projects. Far fewer chromosomes need to be sorted; 10,000 chromosomes are enough for a chromosome-specific DNA library *(16)*, 500 chromosomes are sufficient to prepare an *Alu* PCR painting library *(17)*, and a specific sequence can be detected with as few as ten chromosomes *(18)*. The balance in sorting can now be shifted from throughput and speed toward quality and purity of the sorted material. Such techniques can now be applied in situations where the production of large quantities of isolated chromosomes was almost impossible (tumor material; plants) or where sorting large quantities of a particular chromosome (one particular translocation chromosome) was very time-consuming.

Nevertheless, the success of a chromosome-sorting project still depends heavily on the quality of the isolated chromosome preparation. Techniques for preparing isolated chromosomes containing high-mol-wt DNA have been presented in vol. 5 of this series *(19)* and are further discussed in this volume. The careful adjustment of a clean flow cytometer to give maximum laser power, good chromosome resolution, and defined sorting windows is also vital, and methods of achieving this are described in this chapter.

We present here a protocol for extracting the DNA from sorted chromosomes to provide the starting material for cloning into plasmid, λ, or cosmid vectors or for a PCR-amplified library. Methods are described for gene mapping either by hybridization to sorted chromosomes on filters or using PCR amplification of specific sequences on sorted chromosomes.

2. Materials

1. RBS 25 detergent: 2% in filtered distilled water. Warm to 37°C before use.
2. Phosphate-buffered saline sheath fluid: Oxoid Dulbecco "A" tablets dissolved in distilled water per instructions. Filter through 0.2 μm filter before use. Store at 4°C, and use within 7 d.
3. Alternative sheath fluid for PCR: 10 mM Tris-HCl, 0.1M NaCl, 1 mM EDTA, pH 7.5. Filter and autoclave before use. Store at 4°C, and use within 7 d.
4. Chromosome dialysis buffer: 15 mM Tris-HCl, 2 mM EDTA, 0.5 mM EGTA, 80 mM KCl, 20 mM NaCl, pH 7.2. Store at 4°C, and use within 7 d.
5. DNA extraction buffer: 10X concentration is 1.5M NaCl, 100 mM EDTA, 100 mM Tris-HCl, pH 8.0. Autoclave and store at –20°C.
6. Rat tRNA: 10 mg/mL in sterile distilled water.
7. SDS: 20% in distilled water. Store at room temperature.
8. Proteinase K: Stock solution is 100 mg/mL in distilled water. Store at –20°C.
9. Phenol, phenol:chloroform 50:50 v/v, chloroform:isoamyl alcohol 50:50 v/v.
10. Microdialysis thimble filters from Schleicher and Schuell (Keene, NH).
11. Absolute alcohol.
12. TE: 10 mM Tris-HCl, pH 7.4, 1 mM EDTA, pH 8.0. Autoclave and store at 4°C.
13. 3M Sodium acetate.
14. Dextran mol wt >2 × 10^6: 100 μg/mL in distilled water. Store in aliquots at –20°C.
15. Nitrocellulose filters from Schleicher and Schuell.
16. 20X SSC: 3M NaCl, 0.3M tri-sodium citrate.
17. Swinnex filter holders from Millipore (Bedford, MA).
18. Denaturation fluid: 0.5M NaOH, 1.5M NaCl.
19. Neutralizing buffer: 0.5M Tris-HCl, 0.5M NaCl, pH 7.4.
20. *Taq* polymerase and 10X *Taq* buffer from Promega (Madison, WI). Store at –20°C.
21. Deoxyribonucleotides: 50X stock solution is 10 mM mixture. Store at –20°C.
22. Mineral oil from Sigma (St. Louis, MO).

3. Methods

3.1. Flow Cytometer

Chromosome sorting will for the most part be carried out with a commercial flow cytometer, which, depending on usage, will need varying amounts of attention before sorting begins. Routine use at least usually guarantees regular performance checks. Time spent on checking the cytometer adjustments and experimenting with the effect that each one has on the measurement CV (coefficient of variation) will give credence to the cytometer performance when disappointing results raise doubts about the overall performance of the sample/cytometer. Fluorescent beads tend to produce contamination of the sorted fractions, and hence, it is useful to use an actual sample of suspended chromosomes to adjust the cytometer. Use chromosomes harvested every 2 or 3 wk from a lymphoblastoid cell line as a "stock suspension" for cytometer adjustment. It will be assumed that the mechanics of setting sort windows over the display of accumulated data, and the adjustment of droplet cluster, phase, and delay are understood. An invaluable reference source regarding the technical and biological aspects of chromosome analysis and sorting by flow cytometry can be found in *Flow Cytogenetics (20)*. Figure 1 shows a schematic layout of the front end of an "in air" flow cytometer and may be a useful reference for the sections that follow. A checklist is also shown in Fig. 2, where the important factors in preparing a flow cytometer for chromosome analysis are highlighted.

3.1.1. Preparation of Flow Cytometer

Flow cytometers are unavoidably contaminated by the sample material of each experiment. It is therefore essential to flush out the flow cytometer, even following another chromosome-sorting session, with solutions that clean, but do not clog. Before introducing the first cleaning solution (warm detergent), check that the flow nozzle size is suitable for chromosomes, 70 μm or less for "in air" cytometers. This is less critical for enclosed flow chambers, where the measurement CV is unaffected by nozzle size. After 30 min of warm detergent flushing, continue with a further 30 min of distilled water flushing, and finally introduce the sheath fluid intended for chromosome sorting. Organic solvents should be avoided for flushing purposes, since although these will fix any contamination, they will also cause contamination to be fixed to the flow tubing, only to be dislodged later at the most crucial stage of chromosome sorting. During the flushing process, inspect the nozzle with the instrument viewing telescope for small obstructions. Large obstructions will cause obvious disruption of the flow stream; small ones will only become apparent when suspicious droplet formation and poor chromosome resolution are observed, and this could be well into the experiment.

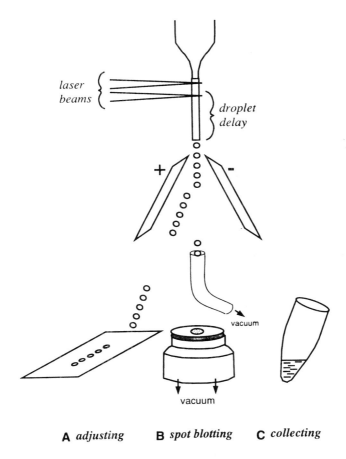

A *adjusting*   **B** *spot blotting*   **C** *collecting*

Fig. 1. Schematic layout of a "charged droplet deflection" sorting mechanism showing the deflection components and a variety of sorted object collection devices. Undeflected droplets are shown falling into a vacuum exhaust tube. A microscope slide is shown with a series of sorted deposits for calibration, a nitrocellulose filter paper is shown fixed, by vacuum, to a Swinnex filter base for spot blotting, and a centrifuge tube is shown containing a measured quantity of buffer for collecting a predetermined number of chromosomes.

3.1.2. Adjustment of Flow Cytometer

Dual-beam flow cytometry and the instrument alignment procedures that should be followed have been discussed in an earlier volume of this series *(19)*. The experimenter's aim should be to achieve two well-aligned laser beams, which give rise to two well-shaped

Cleaning	* Detergent - 1/2h * Distilled water - 1/2h * Buffer - 1/2h
Aligning	* Centre UV beam * Position 458nm beam * Position emission detectors * Re-adjust both laser beams
Delivering	* Use motor syringe if possible * Purge sample stream with buffer and fluorochromes for 10min. * Follow purge buffer imediately with stained chromosome suspension
Sorting	* Set aside a collection of 10,000 chromosomes into 0.25ml buffer for each sorting window for later identification of sorted product.

Fig. 2. List of important points to note when preparing and using a flow cytometer for chromosome sorting.

and intense fluorescence emission signals from the Hoechst 33258 and Chromomycin A3 dyes. Gating on forward and orthogonal light scatter signals does not enhance the resolution of fluorescence signals and should therefore be ignored. The master trigger for capturing the fluorescence intensities of each chromosome should be one of the fluorescence signals. Use a freshly prepared chromosome suspension as a sample for alignment, where the chromosomes were either harvested from a cell line maintained for this purpose or taken from the suspension about to be analyzed, the latter only if the user is fairly certain of the sample integrity from the mitotic index and microscopic examination of the chromosomes. Begin by centering and focusing the UV laser beam by minimizing the width and maximizing the intensity of the Hoechst fluorescence. Follow the same procedure for the 458-nm blue laser beam, taking care to adjust only those components that affect the alignment of the blue laser and the corresponding fluorescence emission. It is a good idea to practice the fine adjustments, which ideally are one for each laser beam, so that good resolution can be easily maintained throughout the experiment.

3.1.3. Sample Analysis

During the initial stages of an experiment, a period of equilibration between sample and sheath occurs, which causes fluctuations in fluorochrome intensities. Stabilization of these fluctuations occurs more rapidly if prior to introduction of the stained chromosome, suspension of a "dummy" sample containing everything but the chromosomes is passed through the sample stream for 10 min. Control of the flow rate, which is normally by adjustment of gas pressure, is much more manageable if a motorized syringe driver is installed. The benefits of a syringe driver are that:

1. The exact concentration of chromosomes in the suspension can be determined;
2. The flow rate can be quickly adjusted to suit the sorting requirements and determined requirements; and
3. The amount of time a sample will last is exactly predictable, assuming that all other factors remain stable.

3.1.4. Sorting Mechanics

The properties of the charged droplet deflection system should be calibrated before an experiment begins. The most sensitive of these parameters is the droplet delay, the time (measured in fractions of droplets) between signal detection and droplet charging. Optimizing this delay is best performed by sorting a few thousand fluorescent beads onto a microscope slide at a series of droplet delays around the estimated optimum followed by a quick search of the series of "puddles" under the fluorescence microscope for the one most dense in sorted beads. From the point of view of catching the sorted chromosomes and the health and safety of the experimenter, the undeflected stream is best drawn away by suction into a closed container. The same vacuum pump can be used to hold a filter paper in place and draw off any surplus liquid when sorting chromosomes for spot-blotting experiments. The base of a Swinnex filter can be utilized for supporting the filter paper in this situation. The condition for collecting chromosomes into a tube, in terms of which buffer and how much is placed in the tube before sorting, depends on the experiment. Sorting chromosomes for a polymerase chain reaction would, for example, require a quantity of PCR buffer to be placed in the tube. Here, the important factor is maintaining a low level of contamination of the PCR buffer with sheath liquid. In practice, contamination >1–2% of the total reaction volume causes problems with the amplification of DNA. It is only necessary to know the volume of sheath liquid produced by one sorted chromosome to calculate the upper limit of sorted chromosomes above which contamination exceeds 1–2%. In the section on PCR, it will be seen that, in our hands, sorting 500 chromosomes into 80 µL of PCR buffer followed by topping up with reaction ingredients to 100 µL gives rise to a successful amplification.

3.1.5. Sorting Windows

When specific chromosomes were sorted for DNA library construction, which usually implies at least 2 million sorted chromosomes, a generous electronic sorting window was set in order to keep the throughput of sorted chromosomes high. One of the disadvantages of this approach is that contamination from adjacent chromosomes will inevitably occur, and a quantity of background debris proportional to the sorting window size will also be present. Sorting chromosomes for amplification by PCR, where only a few hundred chromosomes are needed, requires only a few seconds of sorting instead of several days. Stretching the few seconds to a few minutes by virtue of setting a tight sorting window, covering only the center of a specific chromosome fluorescence distribution, is easily tolerated. The rewards in terms of increased sorted fraction purity more than justify the extra time.

3.2. DNA Preparation
from Sorted Chromosomes

This protocol describes the preparation of DNA from small quantities of sorted chromosomes for the production of DNA libraries. An initial dialysis step is required to remove bound DNA fluorochromes, Hoechst 33258, and particularly Chromomycin A3, which have been shown previously to interfere with subsequent steps. The protocol is based on a method described by Fuscoe et al. *(21)*. The main problem is the small amount of material since 2 million average-sized chromosomes only contain 500 ng of DNA; care is needed to avoid any loss, especially at such steps as ethanol precipitation. Volumes should be kept as small as possible. If any step is inefficient because of impurities (e.g., cutting DNA with restriction enzymes), the number of recombinant clones obtained will be drastically reduced. The DNA has to be especially pure, so two separate dialysis steps are included in the preparation procedure. Once clean restricted DNA is obtained, it can be ligated into any suitable vector.

1. Sort at least 5×10^5 chromosomes; if necessary, pool sorted chromosomes from 2 d sorting.
2. Dialyze against 1 l of dialysis buffer for at least 16 h. At least one change of buffer is necessary.
3. Carefully remove the chromosome suspension from the dialysis tubing. Wash tubing thoroughly with fresh dialysis buffer to minimize chromosome loss.
4. Take an aliquot of chromosomes to check on the purity. This can be a simple chromosome identification check after spinning the chromosomes down onto a slide either by banding analysis *(19)* or by *in situ* hybridization with chromosome-specific alphoid centromeric sequences (*see* Chapter 25).
5. Pellet the chromosomes by centrifugation at 2000*g* for 15 min at 4°C. Remove as much residual buffer as possible.
6. Store at –20°C.
7. Thaw the pellet, and thoroughly disperse the metaphase chromosomes. Add 10X extraction buffer to give 1X final concentration.
8. Add 2 µg of rat tRNA from stock. This acts as carrier for the DNA through later stages. It does not interfere with restriction enzyme cutting and is itself not clonable.
9. Make the suspension 0.5% in SDS. The vol should be <100 µL.
10. Add proteinase K to a final concentration of 1 mg/mL. Incubate for at least 5 h, or preferably overnight, at 37°C.
11. Extract the 100 µL with 100 µL of phenol. Extract the supernatant with phenol/chloroform and finally with chloroform/isoamyl alcohol. Each extraction should be back-extracted with 20–30 µL of TE.
12. Dialyze against 4 L of TE using a microdialysis filter for at least 5 h or preferably overnight. The dialysis filter should be preincubated with 1 mL of TE containing 5 µg tRNA, to block the membrane and prevent subsequent adsorption of the DNA sample.
13. Remove DNA from dialysis thimble, and cut for 4 h with an appropriate restriction enzyme and buffer.
14. Repeat the series of extractions as detailed in step 11. The volume at this stage should be 200–300 µL.

15. Repeat the dialysis step as in step 12.
16. Precipitate the DNA using 1/10 vol of 3*M* sodium acetate, 100 µg/mL Dextran, and 2 vol of absolute alcohol. Incubate at –20°C for 2 h.
17. Spin down at 30,000*g* for 1 h.
18. Wash the pellet in 70% alcohol, and spin again.
19. Dry the DNA pellet briefly; do not overdo this step.
20. Resuspend DNA in a small volume of TE or ligation buffer ready for ligation into chosen vector (*see* Notes 1–3).

3.3. Gene Mapping by Spot Blotting

Cloned genes or single-copy DNA sequences can be mapped to human chromosomes that have been sorted onto nitrocellulose filter paper. A panel of filters containing 30,000 chromosome of each type can then be hybridized to a radiolabeled DNA probe, and the probe assigned to a particular chromosome. Rearranged or deleted chromosomes that occupy a different position in the flow karyotype from the original chromosomes can then be used to sublocalize the probe to a particular region of the chromosome. Care must be taken to concentrate the chromosomes onto a tight spot or ellipse to give a large hybridization signal. An example of spot blotting is shown in Fig. 3.

1. Prewash nitrocellulose filters in 20X SSC, and air-dry before use to decrease the spreading of the sample on the filter.
2. Mark the filter so the correct orientation can be preserved; place the filter on the base of a Swinnex filter, and apply a gentle vacuum to concentrate the sorted chromosomes onto a small area.
3. Sort 30,000 chromosomes of each chromosome of interest on filters; two chromosomes that sort at a similar rate can be sorted on the same filter. Remember to sort 12,000 chromosomes for the 9, 10, 11, and 12 peak to ensure all chromosomes are represented to the same extent.
4. Denature the chromosome DNA by placing the filters, chromosome side up, on Whatman 3MM filter paper saturated with 0.5*M* NaOH and 1.5*M* NaCl for 5 min.
5. Neutralize by transferring the filters to paper saturated with 0.5*M* Tris-HCl, pH 7.4, 0.5*M* NaCl (two changes) and 2X SSC.
6. Bind the DNA to the nitrocellulose by baking at 80°C under vacuum for 2 h.
7. Store the filters in a sealed polythene bag at –20°C.
8. Hybridize to a radiolabeled probe under appropriate conditions (*see* vol. 2 of this series).

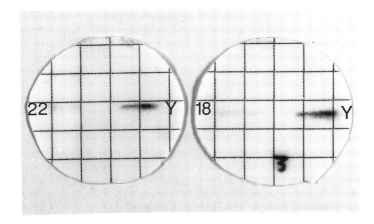

Fig. 3. Nonradioactive hybridization of a biotin-labeled probe for the hetero-chromatic region of the Y chromosome to sorted fractions (10,000 chromosomes) of Y, 18, and 22. The hybridization signals were detected by incubation with streptavidin alkaline phosphatase and a subsequent color reaction. Large hybrid-ization signals are seen on the sorted Y chromosomes; faint signals on the 18 and 22 result from nonspecific binding.

3.4. Gene Mapping Using
the Polymerase Chain Reaction

Reliable amplification of a specific sequence defined by oligo prim-ers from 500 or fewer chromosomes is possible when the chromo-somes are sorted directly into tubes containing *Taq* polymerase buffer, and the amplification reaction is performed in the same tubes *(22)*. A known volume of sheath fluid is sorted with a given number of chro-mosomes, and small amounts of some sheath fluids (polyamine buffer, for example) can inhibit the amplification reaction. We use a Tris/NaCl/EDTA sheath fluid (filtered and autoclaved before use) and calculate for our nozzle that 500 chromosomes are sorted in 1.2 μL of sheath liq-uid. We use 100 μL reaction vol, rather than the more commonly used 50 μL vol, for the amplification step to reduce further any inhibitory effect of the sheath fluid. Chromosomes prepared by the polyamine method usually amplify better than those stabilized by magnesium; this is either because of the decreased nicking of DNA in polyamine chromosomes or the adverse effect of a high-magnesium concentration on the amplification reaction. Amplification is also reduced by incubating the chromosomes overnight in fluorochrome dyes and by using stored chromosomes. Gloves should be worn at all times and precautions taken to reduce contamination; for example, cleaning the flow cytometer before each sorting run. An example of mapping using PCR and sorted chromosomes is shown in Fig. 4.

1. Prepare PCR tubes containing 10 μL of 10X *Taq* buffer and 70 μL of distilled water. We use Promega *Taq* polymerase enzyme and buffer.
2. Set the flow cytometer to sort 500 chromosomes, or calculate the time needed to sort this number.
3. Sort 500 chromosomes into each tube.
4. Close tube lid tightly, and vortex the contents to ensure all the chromosomes are collected from the side of the tube. Centrifuge briefly to collect.
5. Freeze the tubes for storage.
6. Bring the tubes to room temperature and add oligonucleotide primers to 1 μM and deoxyribonucleotide triphosphates to 0.2 mM. Make the vol up to 100 μL with distilled water; vortex and centrifuge briefly. Add 80 μL of mineral oil to prevent evaporation.
7. Prepare a positive control (total human DNA) and a negative control (no DNA).
8. Transfer the tubes to an automated thermal cycler. An initial denaturing step of 10 min at 94°C is necessary for chromosomes, and this is followed by the addition of 2.5 U of *Taq* polymerase. Times and temperatures for subsequent annealing and extension steps are dependent on the base composition of the primer and the length of the target DNA to be amplified. Refer to a standard PCR text for details of exact calculations *(23)*.
9. At the end of the amplification, take a 10-μL aliquot from each tube, add 1 μL of gel-loading buffer, and run on a 2% agarose gel.
10. If a sequence defined by the primers is present on a particular chromosome, then it will be amplified in the tubes containing that chromosome, and a band of the defined size will be seen on the gel. Tubes containing other chromosomes should give a blank lane on the gel.
11. Primers for *Alu* sequences will give a complex pattern of bands on the gel. This amplified DNA should be purified from contaminating nucleotides and proteins before using for labeling or cloning.

4. Notes

1. Most people clone into λ vectors, because they obtain more recombinants per microgram of input DNA. However, they can be more awkward to use later when screening the library and preparing inserts. The

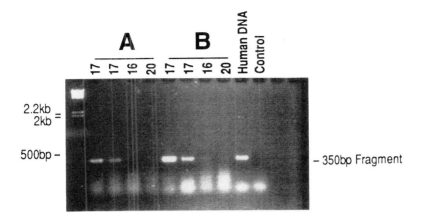

Fig. 4. Agarose gel electrophoresis of the products of PCR amplifications using a pair of primers that amplifies a 350-bp fragment of the p53 gene. Fractions of 500 chromosomes (17, 16, and 20) were sorted from chromosome suspensions stabilized either with magnesium (**A**) or polyamines (**B**). The amplified fragment is seen only in fractions containing chromosome 17 and a positive control, human DNA. Size markers are indicated at the left-hand side.

efficiency of cloning in plasmids has increased to the point where it is quite possible to clone small quantities of DNA from sorted chromosomes into plasmids, and these may be easier to work with.

2. Using *Alu* PCR on the sorted chromosomes (*see* Chapter 26), followed by cloning of the resulting material, can provide a way of producing a library of a particular chromosome in which the content of clones containing *Alu* repeats has been substantially reduced.

3. It is also possible to make cosmid libraries with a large insert size from sorted chromosomes *(24)*. Extra care must be taken to keep the DNA as large as possible by using freshly prepared chromosomes, adding extra EDTA, and transferring sorted chromosomes directly into agarose plugs or beads rather than freezing them.

References

1. Langlois, R. G., Yu, L.-C., Gray, J. W., and Carrano, A. V. (1982) Quantitative karyotyping of human chromosomes by dual beam flow cytometry. *Proc. Natl. Acad. Sci. USA* **79,** 7876–7880.
2. Boschman, G. A., Rens, W., Van Oven, C. H., Manders, M. M., and Aten, J. A. (1991) Bivariate flow karyotyping of human chromosomes: evaluation of variation in Hoechst 33258 fluorescence, Chromomycin A3 fluorescence and relative chromosomal DNA content. *Cytometry* **12,** 559–569.

3. Krumlauf, R., Jeanpierre, M., and Young, B. D. (1982) Construction and characterisation of genomic libraries of specific human chromosomes. *Proc. Natl. Acad. Sci. USA* **79**, 2971–2975.
4. Van Dilla, M. A. and Deaven, L. L. (1990) Construction of gene libraries for each human chromosome. *Cytometry* **11**, 208–218.
5. Lalande, M., Schreck, R., Hoffman, R., and Latt, S. A. (1985) Identification of inverted duplicated #15 chromosomes using bivariate flow karyotype analysis. *Cytometry* **6**, 1–6.
6. Lebo, R., Golbus, M., and Cheung, M.-C. (1986) Detecting abnormal chromosome aberrations by dual label flow cytogenetics. *Am. J. Med. Genet.* **25**, 519–529.
7. Lalande, M., Kunkel, L. M., Flint, A., and Latt, S. A. (1984) Development and use of metaphase chromosome flow-sorting methodology to obtain recombinant phage libraries enriched for parts of the human X chromosome. *Cytometry* **5**, 101–107.
8. Sharkey, A. M., McLaren, L., Carroll, M., Fantes, J., Green, D., Wilson, D., Scambler, P. J., and Evans, H. J. E. (1992) Isolation of anonymous DNA markers for human chromosome 22q11 from a flow sorted library, and mapping using hybrids from patients with DiGeorge syndrome. *Hum. Genet.* **89**, 73–78.
9. Lichter, P., Cremer, T., Borden, J., Manuelidis, L., and Ward, D. C. (1988) Delineation of individual human chromosomes in metaphase and interphase cells by in situ suppression hybridization using recombinant DNA libraries. *Hum. Genet.* **80**, 224–234.
10. Cremer, T., Lichter, P., Borden, J., Ward, D. C., and Manuelidis, L. (1988) Detection of chromosome aberrations in metaphase and interphase tumor cells by in situ hybridization using chromosome-specific library probes. *Hum. Genet.* **80**, 235–246.
11. Cremer, T., Popp, S., Emmerich, P., Lichter, P., and Cremer, C. (1990) Rapid metaphase and interphase detection of radiation-induced chromosome aberrations in human lymphocytes by chromosomal suppression in situ hybridisation. *Cytometry* **11**, 110–118.
12. Lebo, R. V., Gorin, F., Fletterick, R. J., Kao, F., Cheung, M., Bruce, B. D., and Kan, Y. (1984) High resolution chromosome sorting and DNA spot-blot analysis assign McArdle's syndrome to chromosome 11. *Science* **225**, 57–59.
13. Delattre, O., Grunwald, M., Bernard, A., Grunwald, D., Thomas, D., Frelat, F., and Aurias, A. (1988) Recurrent t(11;22) breakpoint mapping by chromosome flow sorting and spot-blot hybridisation. *Hum. Genet.* **78**, 140–143.
14. Carter, N. P., Fergusson-Smith, M. E., Affara, N. A., Briggs, H., and Fergusson-Smith, M. A. (1990) A study of X chromosome abnormality in XX males using bivariate flow karyotype analysis and flow sorted dot blots. *Cytometry* **11**, 202–207.
15. Saiki, R. K., Scharf, S., Faloona, F., Mullis, K. B., Horn, G. T., Erlich, H. A., and Arnheim, N. (1985) Enzymatic amplification of B-globin genomic sequences and restriction site analysis for diagnosis of sickle cell anemia. *Science* **230**, 1350–1354.

16. Vooijs, M., Yu, L.-C., Tkachuk, D., Pinkel, D., Johnson, D., and Gray, J. W. (1993) Libraries for each human chromosome constructed from sorter-enriched chromosomes by using linker-adaptor PCR. *Am. J. Hum. Genet.* **52,** 586–597.

17. Cotter, F. E., Das, S., Douek, E., Carter, N. P., and Young, B. D. (1991) The generation of DNA probes to chromosome 11q23 by *Alu* PCR on small numbers of flow-sorted 22q- derivative chromosomes. *Genomics* **9,** 473–480.

18. Fantes, J. A. (1991) Unpublished data.

19. Fantes, J. A. and Green, D. K. (1990) Human chromosome analyses and sorting, in *Methods in Molecular Biology,* vol. 5 (Pollard, J. W. and Walker, J. M., eds.) Humana, Clifton, NJ, pp. 529–542.

20. Gray, J. W. (ed.) (1989) *Flow Cytogenetics.* Academic, London.

21. Fuscoe, J., Clark, L. M., and Van Dilla, M. A. (1986) Construction of fifteen human chromosome specific DNA libraries from flow-purified chromosomes. *Cytogenet. Cell Genet.* **43,** 79–86.

22. Cotter, F., Nasipuri, S., Lam, G., and Young, B. D. (1989) Gene mapping by enzymatic amplification from flow-sorted chromosomes. *Genomics* **5,** 470–474.

23. Erlich, H. A. (ed.) (1989) *PCR Technology: Principles and Applications for DNA Amplification.* Stockton, New York.

24. Nizetic, D., Zehetner, G., Monaco, A. P., Gellen, L., Young, B. D., and Lehrach, H. (1991) Construction, arraying, and high density screening of large insert libraries of human chromosomes X and 21: their potential use as reference libraries. *Proc. Natl. Acad. Sci. USA* **88,** 3233–3237.

CHAPTER 14

Electrophoretic Karyotype Analysis

Pulsed Field Gel Electrophoresis

John Maule

1. Introduction

Electrophoretic karyotyping is a term first introduced by Carle and Olson in 1985 *(1)* to describe the use of the new technique of pulsed field gel electrophoresis (PFGE) to visualize whole chromosomes from unicellular organisms. Conventional agarose gel electrophoresis has a useful upper size limit of about 20 kilobases (kb). PFGE extends this limit to at least 5.7 megabases (Mb) *(2)* and may be up to 12 Mb *(3)*, encompassing the size range of chromosomes from many bacteria, fungi, and protozoa. Chromosomes from most of these organisms fail to condense sufficiently during mitosis to allow karotyping by light microscopy and, prior to the advent of PFGE, estimates of genome size and chromosome number were based on genetic linkage analysis, DNA reassociation kinetics, and in some cases, electron microscopy.

The first full electrophoretic karyotype to be published was performed on the common yeast *Saccharomyces cerevisiae* by Carle and Olson *(1)*, in which they described the existence of 16 chromosomes ranging in size from 200 kb to over 2 Mb. More recently, a complete physical map of this yeast has been published by Link and Olson *(4)*, in which they accurately sized each chromosome by summing the sizes of individual *Not*1 and *Sfi*1 fragments. Electrophoretic karyotypes are now available for many other yeasts *(5)*, including *Schizosaccharomyces pombe (2)* and *Candida albicans (6)* as well as

From: *Methods in Molecular Biology, Vol. 29: Chromosome Analysis Protocols*
Edited by: J. R. Gosden Copyright ©1994 Humana Press Inc., Totowa, NJ

fungi, such as *Neurospora crassa (3), Aspergillus nidulans (7),* and *Phytophthora megasperma (8).* The accurate sizing of chromosomes from *S. cerevisiae* and *S. pombe,* based on rare cutter restriction enzyme mapping, means that chromosomes from these two yeasts can be used as size markers on pulsed field agarose gels. Protocols for the preparation of chromosomes from these two organisms are described in Sections 3.1. and 3.2. Some of the most useful and versatile molecular-size standards used with conventional agarose gels are "ladders" consisting of multiple repeats of an accurately sized molecule. Concatemers based on bacteriophage λ provide such a broad, uniform distribution of band sizes for pulsed field gels and extend in multiples of 48.5 kb (for wild-type λ) up to about 1 Mb. A protocol for the formation of λ concatemers is described in Section 3.4.

Two associated techniques have contributed to the success of PFGE as a separation method for DNA macromolecules. The first is a method for embedding intact DNA in agarose plugs, which are then loaded directly onto a gel. The agarose serves to protect the DNA from shearing forces, which would normally break the molecules into fragments of ≤ 200 kb in size. The second consists of adapting existing protocols to permit the digestion of DNA, in agarose plugs, by restriction endonucleases. Both these techniques are presented in Sections 3.6. and 3.7.

Accurate sizing of very large chromosomes, especially those >1 Mb, is dependent on digestion by restriction enzymes to produce fragments that can be easily separated by PFGE. A whole new generation of rare cutter restriction enzymes has become available, which fulfills this criterion. This approach has been particularly successful in electrophoretically karyotyping bacteria and, to date, as many as 42 bacterial species have been analyzed in this way *(9).* Bacterial DNA, in agarose plugs, can be used as an important substrate for assaying rare cutter restriction enzymes. The frequency with which these enzymes cut bacterial DNA is influenced by the G + C content and the methylation status of the substrate, as well as the presence of certain groups of nucleotides, which occur rarely in bacteria, in the recognition sequence of the enzymes *(10).* The preparation of agarose plugs containing *Escherichia coli* DNA (G + C = 50%) is described in Section 3.3.

In addition to karyotyping microorganisms, PFGE has been used extensively as a technique in the construction of long-range restriction maps in eukaryotes *(11)*. Digestion of DNA with rare cutter restriction enzymes, in single and double digests, can be used to map mutations and chromosome rearrangements, such as insertions, deletions, translocations, and inversions. In some cases, distantly spaced markers can be linked on a single rare cutter restriction fragment. The success of these mapping approaches is very much dependent on the efficient transfer of restriction fragments from pulsed field gels onto nylon or nitrocellulose membranes and subsequent hybridization to radiolabeled probes. Hints on optimizing these techniques are provided in Sections 3.9. and 3.10.

The exact mechanism by which DNA is separated by PFGE is not completely understood. Basically, the technique differs from conventional agarose gel electrophoresis in that the direction (and sometimes the intensity) of the electric field periodically changes relative to the gel. Smaller DNA molecules respond quicker to this perturbation than larger ones and therefore migrate faster. Observations of individual DNA molecules undergoing electrophoresis have provided some important insights into this process *(12)*. Several types of equipment have been designed to provide the appropriate conditions for PFGE. Earlier equipment generated nonuniform electric fields, and suffered from the disadvantage that DNA migrated in different directions and speeds depending on its position in the gel *(13,14)*. Lane-to-lane comparisons were often difficult. More recent models produce uniform fields, in which tracks run straight and comparisons between lanes are easier *(15–22)*. One of the most successful instruments is the CHEF (Contour-clamped Homogeneous Electric Fields) *(15)*, in which the field switches in direction through 120°. The CHEF can provide a versatile, reliable, high-sample-capacity apparatus, ideal for both analytical and preparative gels. At least two CHEFs are available commercially, or enthusiasts can build their own machine *(23)*. Many interactive variables determine the operational characteristics of pulsed field machines, and in Section 3.8., some details of the successful operation of the CHEF are described.

2. Materials

The following materials are common to several of the methods described in Section 3.:

1. YPD medium: 20 g bactopeptone (Difco, Surrey, UK), 10 g yeast extract (Difco), 1 L distilled water. Autoclave, and then when cool, add 50 mL 40% sterile glucose. For YPD agar, add 1.5% agar to the above medium.

2. LB medium: 10 g bactotryptone (Difco), 5 g yeast extract (Difco), 5 g sodium chloride. Adjust pH to 7.2 (with 5M sodium hydroxide solution) and finally make up the vol to 1 L. Autoclave. For LB agar, add 1.5% to the above medium.
3. 1% NDS solution: 0.45M EDTA, 10 mM Tris-HCl pH 9, 1% sodium *N*-lauroyl sarcosine (Sigma, St. Louis, MO). Mix solid EDTA and Tris with 29 g sodium hydroxide pellets in 900 mL water. Adjust pH to 9 by adding 5M sodium hydroxide solution and finally make up to 1 L with distilled water. Autoclave. Add sodium *N*-lauroyl sarcosine to 1%.
4. Proteinase K (Boehringer, Mannheim, Germany): Make up at 20 mg/mL in 1% NDS solution. Store frozen at –20°C.
5. Low melting temperature agarose: Several different brands of agarose are suitable for plug formation, but make sure the sulfate content is < 0.15%. Gibco BRL (Gaithersburg, MD) ultrapure low melting temperature agarose has given consistently good results. FMC Incert (Rockland, ME) agarose is designed for plug formation, but is considerably more expensive than the BRL product.
6. Zymolyase: An enzyme used to digest yeast cell walls is available from ICN Biomedicals (High Wycombe, UK) in two strengths, 100T (100,000 U/g) and 20T (20,000 U/g). Other enzymes that are suitable are lyticase (Sigma L5263), lyticase (Boehringer), and yeast lytic enzyme (ICN Biomedicals). The unit definition differs among these various products.
7. Nunc (Roskilde, Denmark) 10-µL plastic disposable inoculating loops are ideal for maneuvering agarose plugs.
8. Fine-tip Pasteur pipets (Pastets) are available, in sterile packs, from several manufacturers specializing in disposable plastic laboratory ware. The tip orifice is comparable in diameter to a standard 10–200 µL Eppendorf plastic tip and is therefore ideal for aspirating liquid surrounding an agarose plug, and avoids the possibility of sucking the plug up into the pipet.
9. Hemocytometer—improved Neubauer design, counting cell depth: 0.1 mm.
10. TE: 10 mM Tris, 1 mM EDTA, pH 8. Make up as 10X stock and autoclave.

2.1. S. cerevisiae *Chromosome Preparation*

1. 0.125M EDTA, pH 7.5. Dilute 1/2.5 to give 50 mM solution.
2. Cell wall digestion solution: 2 mL SCE (1M sorbitol, 0.1M trisodium citrate, 60 mM EDTA pH 7—autoclave), 0.1 mL 2-mercaptoethanol, 2 mg zymolyase 100T (*see* Section 4.1., Note 5).
3. ETM: 0.45M EDTA, 10 mM Tris-HCl, pH 8, 7.5% 2-mercaptoethanol. (Autoclave and allow to cool before adding the last compound.)

2.2. S. pombe *Chromosome Preparation*

1. 0.125M EDTA, pH 7.5: Dilute to 50 mM for washing cell pellets.
2. CPES: 40 mM citric acid, 120 mM Na_2HPO_4, 20 mM EDTA, 1.2M sorbitol, 5 mM dithiothreitol, pH 6. Autoclave and add latter reagent just prior to use.
3. Novozym 234—Calbiochem (La Jolla, CA). This is a cell-wall digestion enzyme.
4. 0.1% Sodium dodecylsulfate (SDS).
5. 0.125M EDTA, 0.9M sorbitol, pH 7.5—autoclave.

2.3. E. coli *Chromosome Preparation*

1. Chloramphenicol: Make up at 30 mg/mL in ethanol and store at –20°C.
2. TN: 10 mM Tris-HCl, pH 7.5, 1M sodium chloride. Autoclave.
3. EC lysis solution: 6 mM Tris-HCl, 1M NaCl, 100 mM EDTA, pH 7.5. Autoclave. Then add 0.5% Brij 58 (polyoxyethylene 20 cetyl ether— Sigma), 0.2% sodium deoxycholate (Sigma), and 0.5% sodium N-lauroyl sarcosine. Prior to use, add 1 mg/mL lysozyme and 20 μg/mL RNase A. Make up RNase A in 10 mM Tris-HCl, pH 7.5, 15 mM NaCl at 10 mg/mL. Heat to 100°C for 15 min. Allow to cool to room temperature, and then freeze.

2.4. λ *Concatemers Preparation*

1. Lysogen N1323(λ) *(24)* carries a temperature-sensitive repressor (cIts), and so can be induced at the nonpermissive temperature of 43°C. The S gene product is required for cell lysis, and this strain carries an amber mutation in this gene, which is not suppressed. This results in the accumulation of several hundred phage per cell, following induction and subsequent incubation. The cells can then be concentrated by centrifugation prior to lysis with chloroform; *lop*8 is a ligase overproducing mutation *(25)* that may be beneficial in the repair of single-strand breaks following induction and prolonged incubation.
2. RNase A (*see* Section 2.3., step 3.).
3. DNase 1 (Sigma) made up at 20 mg/mL. Store at –20°C.
4. EDTA pH 8: Make up at 0.5M and autoclave. Dilute to 0.1M for Section 3.4., step 18.

2.5. *Mammalian Chromosome Preparation*

1. PBS: Dissolve 0.2 g KCl, 0.2 g KH_2PO_4, and 8 g NaCl in 800 mL water. Adjust pH to 7.2, and make up to 1 L with water.

2.6. Agarose Plug Preparation

1. A plug mold can be made from a rigid polystyrene flat-bottomed 96-well microtiter plate (ICN Flow catalog number 76-307-05) by milling off the base or drilling out the individual wells. A Titertek plate sealing strip (ICN Flow catalog number 77-400-05) is secured across the top, and the plate is inverted so that the base is now uppermost.
2. The mixture of cells and molten agarose is poured into a reagent trough (ICN Flow catalog number 77-824-01) prior to dispensing.

2.7. Digestion of Agarose-Embedded DNA

1. PMSF is a potent inhibitor of certain enzymes, including proteinase K. Great care must be taken in handling this substance. The solid becomes electrostatically charged, so use a wooden spatula while weighing out and wear gloves throughout. Add 1 mL of propan-2-ol to 20 mg of the solid, and dissolve by incubating at 50°C for 5 min. This solution is unstable, so prepare just prior to use, and deactivate any unused material by making alkaline and incubating at 50°C for a few hours, before pouring down the drain.
2. Triton X-100: Prepare as a 10% stock solution and autoclave.
3. BSA (bovine serum albumen): Boehringer, special molecular biology grade, supplied at 20 mg in 1 mL.
4. Stop buffer: 0.5X TAE, 10 mM EDTA, 2 mg/mL Orange G (Sigma); 0.5X TBE should be substituted for the TAE if the plugs are to be electrophoresed in this buffer.
5. Restriction enzyme buffers: Since considerable volumes are required for equilibrating plugs, it is wise to prepare 10X stock solutions and autoclave. Boehringer now supplies 5-mL quantities of its 10X restriction buffers.

2.8. Separating DNA Using the CHEF

1. TAE: Prepare as a 20X stock solution containing 800 mM Tris, 400 mM sodium acetate, and 20 mM EDTA. Adjust the pH to 8.2 with acetic acid.
2. TBE: Prepare as 5X TBE containing 450 mM Tris, 450 mM boric acid, and 10 mM EDTA.
3. Agarose: The standard medium EEO (electroendosmosis) agarose used for conventional gels can be used for PFGE. Special PFGE agaroses are available that exhibit high gel strength and low EEO and, therefore, can be used at low concentrations. Under these conditions, faster separation times are possible. The following PFGE agaroses are currently available: FMC Fastlane and Seakem Gold, Bio-Rad (Richmond, CA)

Chromosomal Grade, Boehringer Multipurpose agarose, Stratagene (La Jolla, CA) Pulsed field grade agarose, Clontech (Palo Alto, CA) Kilorose and Megarose agaroses, and Gibco BRL Rapid agarose. These products tend to be more expensive than standard-grade agaroses.

4. Ethidium bromide is a mutagen and should be handled with care. Always wear gloves. Bio-Rad sells ethidium bromide tablets (each tablet makes 11 mL of 1 mg/mL solution), which reduce the danger of spillage of the solid during preparation of the solution.

5. Commercially available CHEF apparatus is available from Bio-Rad (CHEF DR-II) and Pharmacia (Brussels, Belgium) (Pulsaphor system with hexagonal electrode kit).

6. Cooling systems: The Pulsaphor has the most straightforward arrangement for buffer cooling—chilled water from an accompanying cooling unit circulates through heat-exchanger tubes beneath the gel. The Bio-Rad apparatus, as well as homemade equipment, require an external heat exchanger system. The main requirement is that electrically live gel running buffer must not come in direct contact with the cooling water. This problem can be solved in two ways:

   a. The buffer can be circulated through polythene tubing that is coiled within a reservoir of cooled water.

   b. Buffer can be circulated through a glass cooling coil that is surrounded by a jacket containing circulating chilled water. A single coil condenser of the type used in water distillation equipment can be adapted for this purpose. Glass is a good conductor of heat, so this form of heat exchanger is very efficient. Consideration should be given to the consequences of condenser breakage, which might bring live buffer in contact with cooling water. The inclusion of a residual current circuit breaker (RCCB) in the electrical supply to this equipment is a prudent safety measure.

7. A safe and reliable buffer circulating pump, for use with a homemade CHEF, is available from Totton Pumps Ltd., Southampton Road, Cadnam, Southampton, Hampshire, SO4 2NF, UK. Specify model EMDP 35/3.

2.9. Southern Transfer

1. HCl: Make up as $5M$ (86 mL of concentrated HCl made to 200 mL with water) and dilute 1/20 prior to use.

2. Denaturant: $0.5M$ NaOH, $1.5M$ NaCl.

3. Neutralizer: $1M$ Tris, $2M$ NaCl. Adjust pH to 5.5 with HCl. (*see* Section 4.9., step 3).

4. SSC: 20X solution is $3M$ NaCl, $0.3M$ trisodium citrate, pH 7.4.

5. Stratalinker (Stratagene) is ideal for UV crosslinking membranes.

2.10. Hybridization and Autoradiography

1. FMC Seakem GTG agarose: specially pure agarose for preparative gels. Note: This is not low melting temperature.
2. Spin-X centrifuge filter units (Costar, Cambridge, MA): 0.22 μm, cellulose acetate.
3. 3*M* Sodium acetate, pH 5.5: Dissolve sodium acetate, and adjust to pH 5.5 with glacial acetic acid. Make up to the final volume and autoclave.
4. Random·primed DNA labeling kit—Boehringer.
5. Deoxycytidine 5'-[α-^{32}P] triphosphate (~3000) Ci/mmol—Amersham (Bucks, UK) PB 10205.
6. Whatman (Maidstone, UK) GF/B 2.4-cm filter circles.
7. Trichloroacetic acid (TCA): Make up as 50% stock solution, and dilute 1/10.
8. NICK columns (Pharmacia): prepacked with Sephadex G-50.
9. 10X TNE: 100 m*M* Tris-HCl, pH 8, 10 m*M* EDTA, 2*M* NaCl. Autoclave.
10. Sonicated salmon sperm DNA—Sigma (D 1626): Make up at 10 mg/mL in water by stirring overnight at 4°C. Sonicate sufficiently to achieve a size of 600 bp. Store at –20°C. This reagent is used as a blocking agent to reduce nonspecific hybridization. Yeast RNA (Boehringer) can also be used at 50 μg/mL.
11. Hybridization mix: 5X Denhardts solution, 5X SSC, 0.1% disodium pyrophosphate, 0.5% SDS, 10% sodium dextran sulfate (Pharmacia). Filter through a Millipore (Bedford, MA) 8-μm SCWP filter (omitting the SDS, which should be filtered separately). Denhardts 20X stock contains, per 100 mL, 0.4 g Ficoll (Sigma type 400), 0.4 g Polyvinylpyrrolidone, 0.4 g bovine serum albumin, BSA (Sigma fraction V)—20X SSC—*see* Section 2.9., point 4. Store at 4°C.
12. SSC washes contain 0.1% SDS and 0.1% disodium pyrophosphate. Maintain at 68°C until required.
13. Autoradiography film—use Kodak XAR-5.

3. Methods

3.1. Preparation of Chromosomal DNA from Saccharomyces cerevisiae

1. Pick a single colony from a freshly grown culture, streaked on a YPD plate, and inoculate 100 mL of YPD medium in a 500-mL flask (*see* Section 4.1., Note 1).
2. Shake for 24 h at 30–33°C, at approx 200 rpm.
3. Dilute an aliquot 1/10 in YPD, and either count the number of cells using a hemocytometer or measure the OD_{600}. Cell count should be ~1 × 10^8 cells/mL and $OD_{600} \cong 0.45$.

4. Chill the culture on ice for 15 min, and then harvest the cells by spinning at 2000*g* for 10 min at 4°C.
5. Discard the supernatant, and gently disrupt the pellet with a sterile loop before adding 50 mL of chilled 50 m*M* EDTA, pH 7.5. Make sure the cells are thoroughly dispersed.
6. Spin at 2000*g* for 5 min at 4°C.
7. Repeat steps 5 and 6.
8. Finally, discard the supernatant and take up the pellet in 3 mL of ice-cold 50 m*M* EDTA, pH 7.5 (gives a final vol of approx 3.5 mL).
9. Transfer the cells to a 20-mL universal container, with a fine-tip sterile Pastet (to disrupt any cells that are clumped), and heat to 37°C.
10. Add 6 mL of 1% low melting temperature agarose (in 0.125*M* EDTA, pH 7.5), which has been cooled to 50°C.
11. Finally, add 1.2 mL of cell wall digestion solution, which has been freshly prepared and stored on ice until required. (*see* Section 4.1., Note 5).
12. Immediately, mix thoroughly and dispense into plug molds (*see* Section 3.6.).
13. Eject the plugs into a 50-mL Falcon tube containing 25 mL of ETM solution, and incubate overnight at 37°C in a water bath.
14. Replace ETM with 20 mL 1% NDS containing 1 mg/mL proteinase K (*see* Section 3.6.).
15. Finally store plugs in 20 mL ETM at 4°C.
16. Plugs should be equilibrated for at least 1 h in gel running buffer before use.

The separation of chromosomes from two common laboratory strains of *S. cerevisiae* is shown in Fig. 1. The chromosome sizes are presented in Table 1 (*see* Section 4.1., Notes 3 and 4).

3.2. Preparation of Chromosomal DNA from Schizosaccharomyces pombe

1. Inoculate 5 mL of YPD medium from a single colony taken from a freshly grown plate (*see* Section 4.2., Note 1).
2. Shake at 30°C, in a universal container, overnight.
3. On the next day, add the overnight culture to 100 mL of YPD in a 500-mL flask. Shake at 30°C for 24 h.
4. Dilute an aliquot of the culture 1/10 in YPD, and count the number of cells in a hemocytometer. The count should be $3–5 \times 10^7$ cells/mL, giving a total yield of $3–5 \times 10^9$ cells.
5. Chill the culture on ice for 15 min.
6. Spin at 2000*g* for 10 min at 4°C.

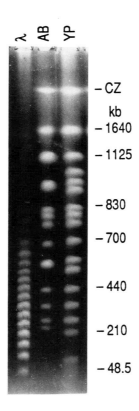

Fig. 1. The separation of chromosomes from two strains of *S. cerevisiae,* AB970 and YP148 *(4)* and concatemers of bacteriophage λ (monomer size 48.5 kb). The sizes of the yeast chromosomes are depicted in Table 1. Samples were separated in a CHEF apparatus *(23)* using a 1% medium EEO agarose gel, in 0.5X TAE, at 12°C and in an electric field of 3.8 V/cm. The following pulse time regime was employed; 120 s for 25 h, 180 s for 25 h, and 360 s for 25 h.

7. Discard the supernatant and gently disrupt the pellet with a sterile loop before adding 50 mL ice-cold 50 mM EDTA, pH 7.5.
8. Repeat steps 6, 7, and then 6.
9. Resuspend the pellet in 2 mL CPES, containing 0.6 mg (60 U) zymolyase 100T and 2.5 mg Novozym 234 *(see* Note 10).
10. Incubate at 37°C for 2 h.
11. Check for successful cell-wall digestion by mixing equal volumes of cell culture and 0.1% SDS and viewing the cells under the microscope. Cells without cell walls are lysed by SDS, and normally ≥ 50% of the cells are in this condition *(see* Note 11).

Table 1
S. cerevisiae Chromosome Sizes (kb)

Chromosome no.	AB970	YP148
XII	1095+rDNA	1095+rDNA
IV	1640	1640
XV	1130	1125
VII	1120	–
VII (part)	–	1030
XVI	955	1000
XIII	930	920
II	830	830
XIV	790	790
X	750	750
XI	690	700
V	585	600
VIII	585	550
IX	445	440
III	350	350
VI	285	270
I	240	210
VII (part)	–	90

12. Mix the cell culture (preheated to 37°C) with an equal volume of 1% low melting temperature agarose (in 0.125M EDTA, 0.9M sorbitol, pH 7.5), which has been cooled to 50°C.
13. Dispense into plug molds, and incubate the plugs in 1% NDS + proteinase K (*see* Section 3.6.).
14. Store the plugs in 1% NDS at 4°C.
15. Soak the plugs for at least an hour in gel running buffer before use.
    The electrophoretic karyotype of a *S. pombe* strain is depicted in Fig. 2, with chromosome sizes shown in Table 2.

3.3. Preparation of Chromosomal DNA from Escherichia coli

1. Inoculate 5 mL of LB from a single colony taken from a freshly grown plate (*see* Section 4.3., Note 2).
2. Incubate overnight at 37°C in a universal container.
3. On the next day, add to 100 mL LB, and shake at 37°C in a 500-mL flask.
4. Grow until OD_{600} = 0.4 (about 2–3 h).
5. Add 750 µL of chloramphenicol (*see* Note 13).
6. Continue shaking at 37°C for 1–2 h, until OD_{600} = 0.6.
7. Chill the culture on ice for 15 min.

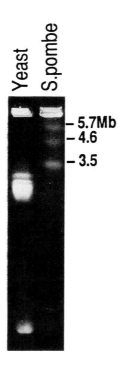

Fig. 2. Separation of *S. pombe* chromosomes by CHEF electrophoresis. The running conditions were 1% agarose gel in 0.5X TBE buffer at 12°C. A 2 V/cm electric field was applied at 60-min pulse times for 120 h. The gel illustrates the relative sizes of *S. pombe* and the largest *S. cerevisiae* chromosomes. The sizes of the *S. pombe* chromosomes are shown in Table 2. (The band at the bottom of the gel in the yeast track is mitochondrial DNA.)

8. Spin at 2000g for 10 min at 4°C.
9. Resuspend the pellet in 50 mL ice-cold TN.
10. Repeat steps 8, 9, and then 8.
11. Take up the pellet in 8 mL TN, and warm to 37°C.
12. Add an equal vol of 1% low melting temperature agarose, in TN, cooled to 50°C.
13. Dispense into plug molds (*see* Section 3.6.).
14. Incubate the plugs overnight in 20 mL EC lysis solution, at 37°C, with gentle mixing.
15. Incubate the plugs in 1% NDS + proteinase K (*see* Section 3.6.).
16. Store the plugs in 1% NDS at 4°C.

Table 2
S. pombe Chromosome Sizes (Mb)

Chromosome no.	Size
I	5.7
II	4.6
III	3.5

3.4. Preparation
of Bacteriophage Lambda Concatemers

1. Use lysogen N1323(λ)—*lop*8, *cts*I857, *Sam*7. Check fresh single colonies for lysogens by picking, say, six colonies, inoculating each into 2 mL LB in a bijoux bottle, and growing up to exponential phase at 33°C (*see* step 5). Induce at 43°C for 15 min, transfer the culture to a glass test tube, add a few drops of chloroform, vortex, and incubate at 37°C for 10 min without shaking. Lysogens should clear after a few minutes. Use a culture without chloroform as a comparison.
2. To prepare a bulk preparation, inoculate from a single colony of a lysogen into 25 mL of LB.
3. Incubate overnight at 33°C.
4. Add the overnight culture to 500 mL of prewarmed LB in a 2-L flask.
5. Shake at 33°C until $OD_{600} = 0.45$ (~3 h).
6. Induce for 15 min at 43°C.
7. Incubate for 2 h at 39°C with vigorous shaking (*see* Note 19).
8. Test for successful induction by adding a few drops of chloroform to a 2-mL aliquot of the culture (*see* step 1).
9. Pellet the cells at 4000*g* for 10 min at 4°C.
10. Gently disrupt the pellets with a sterile plastic loop, and take up in a total volume of 200 mL of ice-cold TE.
11. Spin as in step 9.
12. Take up the cells in a total vol of 23 mL of ice-cold TE, having disrupted the pellets as in step 10.
13. Add 0.5 mL chloroform, and shake gently at 37°C for 15 min.
14. Add 20 µL each of RNaseA and DNase1, and shake gently at 37°C for 15 min.
15. Spin at 8000*g* for 15 min at 4°C.
16. Heat the supernatant to 37°C, and mix with an equal vol of 1% low melting temperature agarose (in TE), cooled to 50°C, and dispense into plug molds (*see* Section 3.6.).
17. Incubate the plugs in 1% NDS + proteinase K (*see* Section 3.6.).

18. Rinse the plugs in 0.1M EDTA, pH 8.0, and incubate in the same for 48 h. at 50°C.
19. Rinse the plugs in 0.5M EDTA pH 8.0, and store in the same at 4°C.
20. Plugs should be cut in half before use and soaked for at least 1 h in gel running buffer before loading on a gel.

λ Concatemers separated by PFGE are shown in Fig. 1.

3.5. Preparation of Chromosomal DNA from Cultured Mammalian Cells

1. Harvest the cells from culture flasks, and transfer to 50-mL Falcon tubes (*see* Note 2).
2. Spin 2000g for 10 min at 4°C.
3. Discard the supernatant, and resuspend the cells in residual medium by vigorously flicking the base of the tube.
4. Add 25 mL of PBS/tube.
5. Spin as in step 2, and discard the supernatant.
6. Resuspend the cells as in step 3, and add 10 mL PBS/tube. At this point, the contents of the tubes can be combined into one or more 50-mL Falcon tubes. Transfer the contents by using a fine-tip Pastet, which helps to break up any cell clumps (*see* Note 22).
7. Count an aliquot of the cell suspension using a hemocytometer, and calculate the total cell number.
8. Repeat steps 2 and 3.
9. Resuspend the cells in a sufficient vol of PBS to give a cell density of 2×10^7 cells/mL (*see* Note 23).
10. Transfer the cells to a universal container, once again using a fine-tip Pastet.
11. Warm the cells to 37°C, and mix with an equal vol of 1% low melting temperature agarose (in PBS), which has been cooled to 50°C.
12. Dispense into plug molds (*see* Section 3.6.).
13. Incubate the plugs in 1% NDS + proteinase K (*see* Section 3.6.).
14. Store the plugs in 1% NDS at 4°C.

3.6. Preparation of Agarose Plugs

Agarose plugs can be conveniently formed, in large numbers, using a mold made from a 96-well microtiter plate *(26)* (*see* Notes 26 and 27).

1. Spray the mold with 70% ethanol and air-dry, prior to use.
2. Cover the base of the plate with a sealing strip and place on ice.
3. Pour the molten mixture of cells and agarose into a trough, and using an eight-channel micropipet, dispense 100-μL aliquots into the mold, one row after another. The trough can be tilted on end to remove the remaining liquid using a standard micropipet.

4. Allow the plugs to set, on ice, for 20 min.
5. Remove the sealing strip and, using a sterile yellow plastic micropipet tip, eject the plugs from the mold into a Falcon tube. Care must be taken not to poke holes in the plugs during ejection, and this can be avoided by running the tip down the wall of each well, making contact with the circumference of the plug, and rapidly pushing downward until the plug drops from the mold.
6. The mold can now be cleaned by soaking in 0.1*M* HCl and then thoroughly rinsed in distilled water.
7. The plugs are now incubated in a detergent + proteinase K solution, although yeast plugs require a cell-wall digestion step before reaching this stage (*see* Section 3.1., step 13): Up to 96 plugs are incubated in 20 mL of 1% NDS + 1 mg/mL proteinase K for 48 h at 50°C in a water bath. The solution is changed after 24 h. (*see* Note 29).
8. Finally, the plugs are rinsed in the storage solution and stored in the same at 4°C. Plugs generally remain in good condition for at least a year under these conditions.

3.7. Restriction Endonuclease Digestion of DNA Embedded in Agarose Plugs

1. Soak the plugs for 10 min in a large excess of sterile TE, at room temperature. Typically, up to ten plugs are immersed in 20 mL of TE.
2. Invert the tube frequently to achieve efficient mixing.
3. Immerse the plugs in 5 mL TE containing phenylmethylsulfonylfluoride (PMSF) at 40 µg/mL.
4. Incubate at 50°C for 30 min.
5. Repeat steps 3 and 4.
6. Soak the plugs for 2 h in 10 vol of 1X restriction enzyme buffer at room temperature, inverting the tube frequently to achieve efficient mixing. This preequilibriation step can be reduced to 1 h, if the PMSF treatment is performed in 1X restriction enzyme buffer rather than TE (*see* Note 30).
7. The plugs are now ready for digestion, which is performed in 1.5-mL microcentrifuge tubes—1 plug/tube.
8. Mix in each tube, on ice, 1X restriction enzyme buffer containing 0.1% Triton X-100 and 200 µg/mL BSA. Add 20 U of restriction enzyme. The final volume should be 100 µL (*see* Note 3).
9. Transfer the plug to the tube, checking that it is completely immersed in liquid and that no air bubbles are trapped around the plug.
10. Incubate overnight, in a water bath, at the recommended temperature (*see* Note 23).
11. On the next day, cool the tube on ice for 15 min and then remove the liquid with a fine-tip Pastet.

12. Add 1 mL of ice-cold TE/tube, invert once, and remove TE (*see* Note 33).
13. Add 200 µL of stop buffer/tube, and maintain on ice for 20 min (*see* Note 34).
14. The plug is now ready for loading onto the gel.

Digested genomic DNA, in agarose plugs, is shown separated by PFGE in Fig. 3, and a comprehensive list of rare cutter restriction enzymes appears in Table 3.

3.8. Resolution
of Large DNA Molecules Using the CHEF

1. Select a suitable buffer for use in the CHEF. Only two buffers are commonly used: TAE (1X or 0.5X) or TBE (0.5X).
2. Prepare a sufficient volume of the buffer to provide enough for the gel and the running buffer. This ensures that the gel and surrounding buffer are in ionic equilibrium.
3. Fill the gel tank with the correct volume of buffer, and precool to the desired temperature.
4. Meanwhile, prepare the gel, having selected the most suitable type and concentration of agarose. Dissolve the agarose by either microwaving or heating on a hotplate. Using a conical flask 2.5× the volume of the agarose solution either cover the top of the flask with perforated aluminium foil/ cling wrap (for microwaving), or preweigh the flask and contents and replenish with distilled water after the agarose has dissolved. Check that the agarose has completely dissolved by holding the flask up to the light, swirling the contents, and checking to ensure there are no translucent lumps of solid left undissolved. Some of the PFGE agaroses are supplied with special instructions for dissolving.
5. Allow the agarose to cool to hand hot (45°C) before pouring into the gel former. Before the agarose sets, remove any air bubbles with a Pastet. It is essential that gels are cast on a level surface—if in doubt, check with a spirit level (*see* Note 37).
6. If there is likely to be any delay between casting and running the gel, cover the surface with cling wrap to prevent evaporation.
7. Prior to loading, gently remove the comb, and fill the slots with running buffer. This will help to prevent the formation of air pockets when loading the sample plugs.
8. Plugs should be maneuvered into the gel slots by using sterile disposable inoculating loops and fine-tip Pastets. If the plugs require cutting, stand them on edge (supported by an inoculating loop), and slice downward with a sterile scalpel blade.

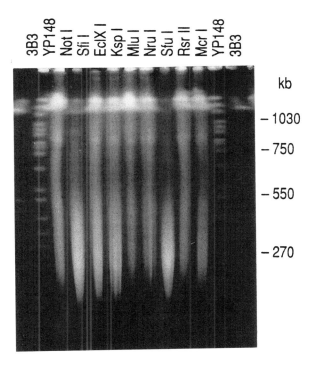

Fig. 3. Digestion of total human DNA with rare cutter restriction enzymes; 5 μg of DNA/plug were digested overnight with 20 U of restriction enzyme (Boehringer) and then separated by CHEF electrophoresis on a 1% agarose gel in 0.5X TAE buffer at 12°C. An electric field of 4.5 V/cm was applied using the following pulse time regime: 70 s for 27 h, followed by 120 s for 21 h. The gel was stained in ethidium bromide before photography. The size markers are *S. cerevisiae* YP148 and a *S. pombe* strain carrying a minichromosome of 550 kb in size. (*see* Section 4.2., Note 2).

9. Gently blot the gel to remove any buffer displaced from the wells, taking care not to disturb the plugs.
10. Seal the plugs into position by dripping cool, molten 0.5% agarose over the slots, and allow to set.
11. Load the gel into the CHEF bath, checking that it is immersed in the correct depth of buffer. Follow the manufacturer's instructions or, if using homemade equipment, aim for 7.5 mm of buffer above the gel. It is essential that the gel bath be level during the run (*see* Note 38).
12. Select an appropriate pulse time, voltage, and run time to separate the molecular-size range of interest and commence the run (*see* Note 39).

Table 3
Rare Cutter Restriction Enzymes

Enzyme	Recognition sequence[a]
*Not*1	GC/GGCCGC
*Asc*1	GG/CGCGCC
*Bss*H11	G/CGCGC
*Sse*83871	CCTGCA/GG
*Sfi*1	GGCCNNNN/NGGCC
*Rsr*11	CG/GwCCG
Sgr A1	Cr/CCGGyG
*Xma*111, *Eag*1, *Ecl*X1	C/GGCCG
*Sst*11, *Sac*11, *Ksp*1	CCGC/GG
*Mlu*1	A/CGCGT
*Pvu*1	CGAT/CG
*Nru*1	TCG/CGA
*Aat*11	GACGT/C
*Sal*1	G/TCGAC
*Nae*1	GCC/GGC
*Nar*1	GG/CGCC
*Sna B*1	TAC/GTA
*Bsi*W1, *Spl*1	C/GTACG
*Sma*1	CCC/GGG
*Xho*1	C/TCGAG
*Bse A*1, *Acc*111, *Mro*1	T/CCGGA
*Cla*1	AT/CGAT
*Sfu*1, *Asu*11	TT/CGAA
*Swa*1	ATTT/AAAT
*Pac*1	TTAAT/TAA
*Pme*1	GTTT/AAAC

[a]w = A or T, r = A or G, y = C or T, N = A, C, G, or T.

13. A visual check to ascertain which electrodes are fizzing will confirm that the machine is operating correctly. Electrodes on the sides marked E and A will fizz alternatively as the field direction changes from one pulse to the next (*see* Fig. 4).
14. At the termination of the run, remove the gel and stain in distilled water containing 1 µg/mL ethidium bromide, for 20 min, with gentle agitation.

3.9. Southern Transfer from Pulsed Field Gels

1. The large DNA molecules separated by PFGE need to be fragmented to allow efficient transfer to the hybridization membrane: Immerse the gel in 2.5X its vol of 0.25*M* HCl, and agitate gently for 20 min at room

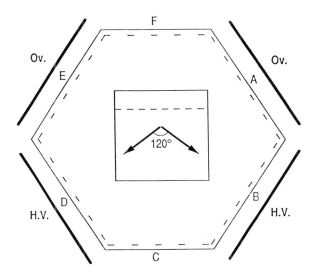

Fig. 4. Schematic diagram of the CHEF apparatus. The field switches through 120° from A -> D to E -> B and then back again. DNA migrates toward C.

    temperature. Do not exceed this time. This process leads to the partial depurination of the DNA (*see* Note 40).

2. Rinse the gel in distilled water.
3. Immerse the gel in 2.5X its volume of denaturant and agitate gently for 20 min. Repeat with fresh denaturant (*see* Note 41).
4. Repeat step 2.
5. Immerse the gel in 2.5X its volume of neutralizer and agitate gently for 40 min (*See* Note 42). Do not exceed this time.
6. Set up a device for Southern transfer by filling a plastic tray to the brim with 20X SSC. A sheet of 5 mm thick plastic rests across the top of the tray lengthwise, with a gap on each side to allow two sheets of Whatman 17Chr paper, placed on top of the plastic sheet, to dip into the buffer on both sides. This forms a wick that draws buffer up from the tray. Allow the paper to become saturated before the next stage.
7. Invert the gel, so that the base is now the top, and lay on the paper wick, checking that there are no air bubbles trapped between the gel and the paper (*see* Note 43).
8. Cover the surrounding paper with cling wrap to prevent evaporation of the buffer.
9. Lay the hybridization membrane onto the gel, following manufacturer's instructions.

10. The membrane may be gently rolled with a glass pipet to squeeze out any trapped air bubbles.
11. Mark the position of the slots, on the membrane, with a ballpoint pen, numbering the first and last tracks so that the membrane can be orientated relative to the autoradiogram.
12. Lay on two sheets of Whatman 17Chr paper, slightly larger than the gel.
13. Lay on paper towels to cover the sheets of Whatman paper, stacked to a height of 5 cm.
14. Finally, lightly compress the paper towels with a 1-kg weight, resting on a sheet of plastic or glass to distribute the weight over the whole area of the gel.
15. After 24 h, discard any wet towels and replace with dry ones.
16. After a further 24 h, remove the membrane, and wash in 2X SSC for 5 min.
17. The gel may be stained in ethidium bromide to check the efficiency of transfer.
18. Crosslink the DNA to the membrane by treating with UV light or baking, or both. Follow the manufacturer's instructions.

3.10. Hybridization of Radiolabeled Probes to Pulsed Field Gel Filters

1. Hybridization procedures using filters carrying DNA from pulsed field gels are not essentially any different from those methods used for filters from conventional gels.
2. The detection of single-copy sequences, from pulsed field gels, does seem to be more difficult than from conventional gels, and every effort must be made to optimize labeling and hybridization conditions in order to produce a clear, positive result.

3.10.1. Preparing and Labeling Probes

1. Single-copy genomic probes should be prepared by isolating the insert away from the vector sequence, by digestion with appropriate restriction enzymes and separating the products on a preparative gel, using a high-quality agarose, such as FMC Seakem GTG.
2. The insert band is excised from the gel (after staining with ethidium bromide and viewing with a midrange, 302-nm UV source). Since the DNA band may not occupy the whole depth of the gel, it is worth turning the gel slice on its side and trimming off excess agarose.
3. DNA may be extracted from the gel by centrifugation through a nitrocellulose membrane: Cut up the gel slice into small blocks, using a sterile scalpel, and load into a Spin-X tube. Spin, at room temperature, for 20 min in a microfuge, at full speed. The DNA will be in the buffer

collected in the tube. Run out a small aliquot of this on a minigel to check for successful recovery. For subsequent labeling, one should expect to see 50–100 ng in a few microliters. If the concentration is below this, the DNA should be concentrated by ethanol precipitation: Add $^1/_{10}$ volume of $3M$ sodium acetate, pH 5.5, and 2 vol of ice-cold ethanol. Invert the tube and leave at –70°C for 30 min. Spin at 4°C, in a microfuge for 10 min. Wash the pellet in half the volume of 70% cold ethanol, and dry the pellet under vacuum in a freeze-drier. Finally, take up in TE at, say, $^1/_{10}$ of the original volume. Run an aliquot on a minigel to check the concentration. Divide up the sample into aliquots, each sufficient for a single labeling experiment, and store at –20°C. (*see* Note 46).

4. Label the probe using a random prime kit (Boehringer), in a total volume of 20 µL, using 30 µCi [α^{32}P] CTP. Follow the kit instructions.

5. Check the percentage of incorporation by spotting 1 µL from the labeling reaction onto a Whatman GF/B filter circle and counting in a scintillation counter. Incorporated label can be measured by passing 20 mL 5% TCA solution through the filter and counting again. Incorporation should be at least 50%; if not, add another $^1/_2$ µL of Klenow enzyme, and incubate for 30–60 min (*see* Note 47).

6. Unincorporated label should be separated from the labeled DNA by passage through a NICK column: Rinse the column with 10 mL TNE. Add the labeling reaction mix, made up to 100 µL with TNE. Allow to run through, then rinse the column with 300 µL of TNE, and finally elute with 400 µL of TNE, collecting the eluate in a microcentrifuge tube.

7. Add sonicated salmon sperm DNA, so that the final concentration in the hybridization mix will be 100 µg/mL.

8. Pierce the lid of the tube with a pin, and denature the probe by heating at 100°C for 10 min.

9. Add directly to the hybridization mix, or store on ice until required.

3.10.2. Hybridization and Autoradiography

1. Prehybridize the filter, sealed in a polythene bag, by incubating in a shaking water bath at 68°C for at least 2 h. The bag should contain 10 mL of hybridization mix/100 cm^2 of filter. Try to exclude all air bubbles from the bag (*see* Note 48).

2. Drain out the hybridization mix from the bag, and replace with 5 mL of fresh hybridization mix, at 68°C, per 100 cm^2 of filter (*See* Note 49). Add the denatured probe, reseal the bag, and incubate overnight at 68°C, in a shaking water bath (*see* Note 50).

3. On the next day, remove the filter from the bag, rinse in 2X SSC wash, and then incubate in the same for 20 min at 68°C on a rotary platform.

4. Repeat, using if necessary progressively lower concentrations of SSC wash (e.g., 0.5X, 0.1X) until a reasonable signal:background level has been established, as monitored by a Geiger counter.

5. Drain the filter, enclose in cling wrap, and place in a film cassette fitted with an intensifying screen.

6. Place an autoradiography film that has been preexposed by a short flash of light (~1 ms) from a photographic flash gun fitted with Kodak Wratten 22A filter *(27)* next to the filter, and close the cassette. Store at -70°C for an appropriate length of time, and then develop the film. (*see* Note 51).

An autoradiograph of the digested genomic DNA, depicted in Fig. 3, hybridized with a single-copy probe is shown in Fig. 5.

4. Notes

1. *S. cerevisiae* strains are best preserved by storage in 15% glycerol at –70°C.
2. This procedure is based on the published method by Carle and Olson *(1)*.
3. Beware of contamination by wild yeasts—they may look and smell similar to *S. cerevisiae,* but give a totally different electrophoretic karotype. In particular, they tend to have a few large chromosomes (≥1 Mb) rather than the large number of smaller chromosomes characteristic of *S. cerevisiae (5)*.
4. Many *S. cerevisiae* strains exhibit chromosome length polymorphisms (CLPs), which lead to slightly differing electrophoretic karotypes *(1)*. This property can be used to advantage in the resolution of bands that comigrate.
5. The inclusion of 2-mercaptoethanol at Section 3.1., step 11, is important, because SH compounds are activators for zymolyase.
6. *Candida albicans* chromosomes, which can provide size markers in the 1–5 Mb range, are prepared by a variation of this protocol *(28)*.
7. *S. pombe* strains may be preserved in 30% glycerol + YPD at –70°C.
8. A series of *S. pombe* strains possessing a single minichromosome are available *(29)* and these provide an additional size marker of ≤1 Mb.
9. It is important to use ice-cold reagents throughout this protocol. Failure to do so results in extensive degradation of the DNA.
10. Spheroplast (cells without cell walls) formation in *S. pombe* is more difficult than in *S. cerevisiae.* Novozyme 234 is therefore added to increase the yield.
11. Spheroplasts must be maintained in an osmotically stabilized environment by including sorbitol in the medium during spheroplast formation. Spheroplasts are sensitive to hypotonic conditions and traces of detergent, so cell-wall digestion can be monitored by the addition of 0.1% SDS.

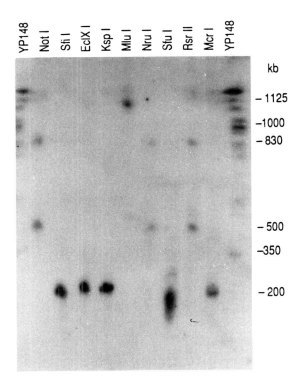

Fig. 5. Autoradiograph of the gel illustrated in Fig. 3, hybridized with a single-copy probe. Following Southern transfer onto Hybond N (Amersham), the filter was hybridized to a human chromosome 11p probe and a probe carrying the Ty-1 repetitive element from yeast. Autoradiography was for 4 d at –70°C using Kodak XAR-5 film. Note that several of the enzymes cut within CpG islands, generating fragments of ~200 kb as seen following hybridization with this specific probe.

12. This protocol gives consistently better results than procedures based on the method given in Section 3.1., where spheroplast formation takes place within the agarose plugs.
13. This protocol is based on the published method of Smith et al. *(30)*.
14. Although earlier protocols recommended the growth of *E. coli* in minimal medium, using LB is acceptable and provides for a more rapid doubling time.
15. Chloramphenicol is added to the cells in late exponential phase to synchronize replication forks. It allows the completion of rounds of replication that have already begun, but no new rounds are initiated. This may be important in bacterial chromosome mapping.

16. This protocol can be adapted for the preparation of chromosomes from other bacteria *(10)*.

17. λ has 12 base, single-stranded, complementary (cohesive) ends, which join under appropriate conditions and between a range of DNA concentrations *(31)*. λ DNA, in solution, at above 10 mg/mL will spontaneously undergo limited concatemerization. Within agarose plugs, concatemerization is probably a very efficient process, because λ DNA molecules, even at modest concentrations, are maintained in close proximity to each other, thus providing a beneficial environment for intermolecular association. The upper limit of concatemerization is probably influenced by termination resulting from damaged single-strand ends.

18. Wild-type λ has a monomer size of 48.5 kb, but concatemers can be formed based on other smaller λ genomes, e.g., λvir (42.5 kb) and λgtll (43.7 kb). Bacteriophages P2 and P4 have 19 base single-strand cohesive ends, can form concatemers, and have monomer sizes of 31.8 and 11.6 kb respectively.

19. A good yield of phage is only produced if adequate aeration is achieved at Section 3.4., step 7, so vigorous shaking is important. An incubation temperature of 39°C may be beneficial in improving the phage yield.

20. This protocol provides a rapid method for the production of λ concatemers up to ~1 Mb and does not involve the time-consuming preparation of DNA by cesium chloride density centrifugation.

21. Cells grown in culture should be harvested when just confluent; growth beyond this stage is characterized by the overproduction of mitochondrial DNA and the degradation of genomic DNA.

22. Some cells in culture readily form clumps, and it is essential that these are disrupted before plug formation. If passage through a fine-tip pastet fails to disperse the cells, then ejection from a syringe fitted with a 19-gage, or even a 21-gage needle should be considered.

23. Each plug contains 1×10^6 cells in 100 μL of agarose, and this is equivalent to about 10 μg of DNA. The plug may be cut in half if this quantity of DNA overloads the gel.

24. Methylation differences between cell lines often account for different restriction patterns, since most rare cutter enzymes are methylation-sensitive. Growth of cells in the presence of 5-azacytidine inhibits cytosine methylation *(32)* and partially overcomes this problem.

25. Genomic DNA for PFGE can also be isolated from blood *(33)*, frozen cells *(34)*, and even a single human hair *(35)*.

26. This protocol allows the rapid production of several hundred plugs at a time. The plugs are round in shape, which is beneficial for maintaining them intact during repeated manipulation.

27. The grid numbering system of microtiter plates allows different plugs to be formed within the same mold and yet preserve their identity.
28. Agarose beads allow another way to encapsulate DNA in an agarose matrix *(36)*. They are, however, more difficult to produce and more cumbersome to manipulate. Their high surface area to volume ratio, however, means that restriction enzymes can easily penetrate the beads and make contact with the DNA, thus reducing the amount of enzyme necessary for complete digestion.
29. The plugs should clear during Section 3.6., step 7, indicating that cell lysis has occurred, although those containing yeast still remain opaque.
30. Good digestion of DNA in plugs is very dependent on adequate equilibration of the plug in restriction buffer, so Section 3.7., step 6 should not be rushed.
31. The amount of restriction enzyme that needs to be added can be adjusted from experience. Some enzymes do not remain active throughout the incubation period, in which case further enzyme can be added the next day and incubation continued for a few more hours.
32. Some enzymes are unstable at the recommended incubation temperature. This may present a problem for the digestion of DNA in agarose, since by the time the enzyme has diffused into the plug, its activity has diminished. A preincubation period on ice may be beneficial, particularly since some enzymes are stabilized by their substrates. An alternative approach involves returning plugs to the plug mold, melting briefly at 68°C, cooling to the desired incubation temperature, and gently pipeting in the restriction enzyme. Following incubation, the plug may be solidified again on ice prior to loading on a gel.
33. It is important to wash the plug at Section 3.7., step 12. During extended incubation, some DNA seeps out of the plug into the surrounding buffer and would be sheared during subsequent manipulations.
34. The inclusion of tracking dye in the stop mix colors the plugs and makes loading easier. It also allows a visual check on the correct migration of the sample during early stages of electrophoresis.
35. Several methods are available for purposely creating partial digests in agarose plugs. These include adjusting the Mg concentration *(37)*, using ethidium bromide *(38)*, and varying the amount of added enzyme *(38)*. A method is also available for methylating DNA in agarose *(39)*.
36. Gels may be cast and run on glass plates, when using homemade equipment. The gel thickness should be 5 mm. The glass plate does not distort the electric field *(23)*.
37. Gel combs should be of minimal thickness to provide slots tailored to the size of the plugs, and should be positioned to give a gap of 0.5 mm between the bottom of the teeth and the gel support.

38. Manufacturers frequently recommend TBE as the running buffer and, in the case of the CHEF DR-II, the top of the gel should be 2 mm below the buffer surface. If using 0.5X TAE in the DR-II, this figure should be increased to 3 mm.

39. The behavior of CHEF pulsed field gels is influenced by five important parameters, and since they interact, the establishment of optimal run conditions has been very much an empirical process. Each of these parameters will be briefly described in the following notes, but for a more rigorous assessment, readers should consult refs. *40* and *41*.

   a. Temperature: Buffer temperature should be constant during the run. In general, the cooler the buffer, the tighter the bands and better the resolution, but the migration is slower. Temperatures between 10–15°C provide a good compromise between band tightness and migration speed.

   b. Buffer: The choice of buffer can influence the velocity of DNA migration. Using the standard medium EEO agarose, as well as the low EEO agaroses, the migration rate is faster in lower ionic strength buffers, such as 1X TAE, compared with the higher ionic strength TBE. The effect is even more pronounced if the TAE concentration is dropped to 0.5X. TBE has a higher buffering capacity than TAE and may be the buffer of choice for prolonged electrophoretic runs as well as providing better resolution when separating molecules in the megabase range.

   c. Agarose: Both the type and concentration of agarose are important factors in the speed and resolution of large DNA molecules. As the agarose concentration is decreased, the DNA migration rate increases, but resolution diminishes. Furthermore, as the agarose concentration increases, separation is achieved over a smaller size range. In general, as the EEO of the agarose is decreased, the DNA migration rate increases, and this effect is particularly pronounced in TAE buffer. Gels composed of 1% medium EEO agarose provide a good starting material for most separations, but the concentration should be decreased for the separation of megabase-sized molecules.

   d. Pulse time: The most important single variable in determining the size range of molecules separated is the pulse time—the interval between the electric field switching from one direction to another. Smaller molecules, which are capable of rapid responses to changes in field direction, are separated preferentially by short pulse times. As the pulse time is increased, progressively larger molecules are separated, but the window of good resolution changes, such that molecules at the smaller end of the range are less well resolved. Pulsed field gels run at single pulse times exhibit distinct regions of separation: Toward the top of the gel there is a region, called the compression zone (CZ), in which all molecules greater than a certain size comigrate. Below this is a region of maximum resolution in which bands are well separated, and below that is a region characterized by poorer resolution, in which mobility is linear relative to size. Thus, maximum resolution is achieved by using the minimum pulse time capable of resolving the largest molecule of interest. Multiple consecutive pulse time regimes can be used to achieve good separation over a wide size range on a single gel. An increase in linearity of size relative to mobility can be achieved using a pulse time ramp, and this approach is particularly effective if nonlinear time ramps are employed *(23)*.

e. Field strengths of up to 10 V/cm (the distance being measured between opposite electrodes) can be used to separate molecules up to about 1 Mb. The higher the voltage, the faster the run time, although lower voltages give better resolution, but over a narrower size range. Separation of molecules greater than about 1 Mb can only be achieved at reduced voltages, e.g., 2 V/cm for *S. pombe*. For separation over a given size range, or window of resolution, W, the product of the voltage gradient, V (expressed as V/cm), and pulse time, P, is roughly constant or, more accurately, according to Gunderson and Chu *(42)*:

$$W = V^{1.4} \times P \qquad (1)$$

This means in practice that, for separation in a given size range, an increase in voltage must be accompanied by an appropriate decrease in pulse time and vice versa. By solving this equation for P, it is possible to specify a pulse time for carrying out separation in the same size range, using different apparatus, as long as the voltage and distance, D, between opposite electrodes are known. Typical values for D are 33.5 cm for CHEF DR-II and 28 cm for Pulsaphor hexagon system. When the experimenter wishes to separate molecules up to a certain size limit and has no clues as to the most appropriate conditions under which to run the gel, mathematical expressions are now available that allow the various parameters to be established. An example of such a relationship (according to Smith *[43]*) is:

$$P = [R/V \times A^{(-0.5)} \times 5.25]^{(1.25)} \qquad (2)$$

where P = pulse time, R = maximum size of molecule to be resolved, A = % agarose concentration, and V = V/cm. Based on a limited amount of data, the relationship seems to hold good and provides pulse times with a reasonable degree of accuracy. As more data become available, the formula can be refined and additional variables included.

40. DNA molecules may be fragmented with UV light, in the presence of ethidium bromide, as an alternative to partial depurination. A controlled source of UV of the type used to crosslink DNA to nylon membranes, e.g., Stratalinker (Stratagene), is ideal for this technique. The makers claim that the output delivered by the machine is constant regardless of the age of the UV source. A test gel should be exposed to various doses of UV to establish the optimum exposure for efficient transfer. Remember that exposure of the gel to UV during photography should be taken into account.

41. It is important to change the denaturant halfway through step 3, Section 3.9., since the HCl present in the gel will reduce the pH of the solution.

42. It is appropriate to prepare neutralizer at pH 5.5, because the pH of the solution rises to neutrality as the denaturant is neutralized.

43. The upper layer of the gel becomes depleted of DNA during electrophoresis, so it is important to invert the gel prior to Southern transfer so that the DNA has least distance to pass through the gel before making contact with the membrane.

44. Alkali transfer is an alternative method worth considering *(44)*.

45. Vacuum blotting has been reported as an alternative approach to capillary transfer, albeit from special low EEO PFGE agarose *(42)*.

46. The probe may be labeled directly from a gel slice as an alternative to DNA extraction. In this case, the insert band must be separated on a preparative gel, using low melting temperature agarose (e.g., BRL Ultrapure). The excised gel slice is melted for 10 min at 68°C, and a small aliquot run out on a minigel to check the DNA concentration. The molten gel slice is then divided into aliquots, each sufficient for a single labeling experiment, and stored at 4°C. Follow the random prime kit instructions for labeling from gel slices, but use a total vol of 20 µL.

47. Accurate determinations of radioactive incorporation can be achieved by counting the filter in scintillation fluid. Approximate estimates can be made by Cerenkov counting, the accuracy of which depends on a number of factors, including the age of the counter. A typical SA of ~10^9 dpm/µg is usually achieved.

48. Hybridization ovens, using roller bottles, can be used as an alternative to the polythene bag method. They are intrinsically safer and use smaller volumes of reagents. Care must be taken, however, to check the temperature inside the oven with a thermometer and not always rely on the electronic temperature indicator.

49. Experienced workers have their own favorite hybridization membrane and mix. The large choice of membranes can be categorized into nitrocellulose, nylon, and nitrocellulose/nylon mixtures. The former is reputed to be more sensitive, but fragments on repeated reprobing, a property not shared by nylon membranes. The hybridization method of Church and Gilbert *(45)* gives less background, but the signal intensity is reduced.

50. Filters from pulsed field gels carrying size markers can be hybridized with radiolabeled markers at the same time as the probe or separately if crosshybridization is a problem. λ DNA can be labeled and hybridized to concatemers. *S. cerevisiae* chromosomes can be hybridized to the Ty-1 repetitive element, which is present to various extents in all yeast chromosomes. The 90- and 1030-kb chromosomes of YP148 also crosshybridize with pBR322 sequences. *S. pombe* chromosomes can be hybridized to a centomeric probe, such as pSS166, which is derived from the dg11a region *(46)*. Minichromosomes, carried by some *S. pombe* strains, tend to crosshybridize with Ty-1 and pBR322 sequences.

51. Autoradiographs should be initially developed after 1 d and then reexposed for additional periods if necessary.

52. A good, clear, positive signal, when probing pulsed field gels, is influenced by sample loading, which can make all the difference between clean sharp bands and autoradiographs with high background or no bands at all. Where problems occur with signal strength and clarity, try loading only half a sample plug.

References

1. Carle, G. F. and Olson, M. V. (1985) An electrophoretic karyotype for yeast. *Proc. Natl. Acad. Sci. USA* **82,** 3756–3760.
2. Fan, J. B., Chikashige, Y., Smith, C. L., Niwa, O., Yanagida, M., and Cantor, C. R. (1988) Construction of a Not1 restriction map of the fission yeast *Schizosaccharomyces pombe* genome. *Nucleic Acids Res.* **17,** 2801–2808.
3. Orbach, M. J., Vollrath, D., Davis. R. W., and Yanofsky, C. (1988) An electrophoretic karotype of *Neurospora crassa. Mol. Cell. Biol.* **8,** 1469–1473.
4. Link, A. J. and Olson, M. V. (1991) Physical map of the *Saccharomyces cerevisiae* genome at 110-kilobase resolution. *Genetics* **127,** 681–698.
5. Johnston, J. R. and Mortimer, R. K. (1986) Electrophoretic karyotyping of laboratory and commercial strains of *Saccharomyces* and other yeasts. *Int. J. Syst. Bacteriol.* **36,** 569–572.
6. Magee, B. B., Koltin, Y., Gorman, J. A., and Magee, P. T. (1988) Assignment of cloned genes to the seven electrophoretically separated *Candida albicans* chromosomes. *Mol. Cell. Biol.* **8,** 4721–4726.

7. Brody, H. and Carbon, J. (1989) Electrophoretic karyotype of *Aspergillus nidulans. Proc. Natl. Acad. Sci. USA* **86,** 6260–6263.
8. Howlett, B. J. (1989) An electrophoretic karyotype for *Phytophthora megasperma. Exp. Myc.* **13,** 199–202.
9. Krawiec, S. and Riley, M. (1990) Organization of the bacterial chromosome. *Microbiol. Rev.* **54,** 502–539.
10. McClelland, M., Jones, R., Patel, Y., and Nelson, M. (1987) Restriction endonucleases for pulsed field mapping of bacterial genomes. *Nucleic Acids Res.* **15,** 5985–6005.
11. Gemmill, R. M., Coyle-Morris, J. F., McPeek, F. D., Ware-Uribe, L. F., and Hecht, F. (1987) Construction of long-range restriction maps in human DNA using pulsed field gel electrophoresis. *Gene Anal. Techn.* **4,** 119–131.
12. Smith, S. B., Aldridge, P. K., and Callis, J. B. (1989) Observation of individual DNA molecules undergoing gel electrophoresis. *Science* **243,** 203–206.
13. Carle, G. F. and Olson, M. V. (1984) Separation of chromosomal DNA molecules from yeast by orthogonal-field-alternation gel electrophoresis. *Nucleic Acids Res.* **12,** 5647–5664.
14. Schwartz, D. C. and Cantor, C. R. (1984) Separation of yeast chromosome-sized DNAs by pulsed field gradient gel electrophoresis. *Cell* **37,** 67–75.
15. Chu, G., Vollrath, D., and Davis, R. W. (1986) Separation of large DNA molecules by contour-clamped homogeneous electric fields. *Science* **234,** 1582–1585.
16. Gardiner, K., Laas, W., and Patterson, D. (1986) Fractionation of large mammalian DNA restriction fragments using vertical pulsed-field gradient gel electrophoresis. *Somatic Cell Mol. Genet.* **12,** 185–195.
17. Southern, E. M., Anand, R., Brown, W. R. A., and Fletcher, D. S. (1987) A model for the separation of large DNA molecules by crossed field gel electrophoresis. *Nucleic Acids Res.* **15,** 5925–5943.
18. Serwer, P. (1987) Gel electrophoresis with discontinuous rotation of the gel. *Electrophoresis* **8,** 301–304.
19. Carle, G. F., Frank, M., and Olson, M. V. (1986) Electrophoretic separations of large DNA molecules by periodic inversion of the electric field. *Science* **232,** 65–68.
20. Ziegler, A., Geiger, K-H., Ragoussis, J., and Szalay, G. (1987) A new electrophoretic apparatus for separating very large DNA molecules. *J. Clin. Chem. Clin. Biochem.* **25,** 578–579.
21. Clark, S. M., Lai, E., Birren, B. W., and Hood, L. (1988) A novel instrument for separating large DNA molecules with pulsed homogeneous electric fields. *Science* **241,** 1203–1205.
22. Bancroft, I. and Wolk, C. P. (1988) Pulsed homogeneous orthogonal field gel electrophoresis (PHOGE). *Nucleic Acids Res.* **16,** 7405–7418.
23. Maule, J. C. and Green, D. K. (1990) Semiconductor-controlled contour-clamped homogeneous electric field apparatus. *Anal. Biochem.* **191,** 390–395.
24. Arker, W., Enquist, L., Hohn, B., Murray, N. E., and Murray, K. (1983) Experimental methods for use with lambda, in *Lambda II* (Hendrix, R. W., ed.) Cold Spring Harbor Laboratory, Cold Spring Harbor, NY, pp. 433–466.

25. Gottesman, M. M., Hicks, M. L., and Gellert, M. (1973) Genetics and function of DNA ligase in *Escherichia coli. J. Mol. Biol.* **77,** 531–547.
26. Porteous, D. J. and Maule, J. C. (1990) Casting multiple aliquots of agarose embedded cells for PFGE analysis. *Trends Genet.* **6,** 346.
27. Sambrook, J., Fritsch, E. F., and Maniatis, T. (1989). *Molecular Cloning—A Laboratory Manual,* 2nd ed. Cold Spring Harbor Laboratory, Cold Spring Harbor, NY.
28. Vollrath, D. and Davis, R. W. (1987) Resolution of DNA molecules greater than 5 megabases by contour-clamped homogeneous electric fields. *Nucleic Acids Res.* **15,** 7865–7876.
29. Niwa, O., Matsumoto, T., and Yanagida, M. (1986) Construction of a minichromosome by deletion and its mitotic and meiotic behaviour in fission yeast. *Mol. Gen. Genet.* **203,** 397–405.
30. Smith, C. L., Klco, S. R., and Cantor, C. R. (1988) Pulsed-field gel electrophoresis and the technology of large DNA molecules, in *Genome Analysis* (Davies, K. E., ed.) IRL, Oxford. pp. 41–71.
31. Mathew, M. K., Smith, C. L., and Cantor, C. R. (1988) High-resolution separation and accurate size determination in pulsed-field gel electrophoresis: DNA size standards and the effect of agarose and temperature. *Biochemistry* **27,** 9204–9210.
32. Dobkin, C., Ferrando, C., and Brown, W. T. (1987) PFGE of human DNA: 5-azacytidine improves restriction. *Nucleic Acids Res.* **15,** 3183.
33. Nguyen, C., Djabali, M., Roux, D., and Jordan, B. R. (1991) Very high molecular weight DNA for pulsed-field gel studies can be obtained routinely from conventional frozen blood aliquots. *Nucleic Acids Res.* **19,** 407.
34. Petrukhin, K. E., Broude, N. E., and Smith, C. L. (1988). A simple and efficient method for isolating high molecular weight DNA from frozen mammalian tissues. *Nucleic Acids Res.* **16,** 5698.
35. Boultwood, J., Abrahamson, G. M., and Wainscoat, J. S. (1990) Structural DNA analysis from a single hair root by standard or pulsed field gel electrophoresis. *Nucleic Acids Res.* **18,** 4628.
36. Cook, P. R. (1984) A general method for preparing intact nuclear DNA. *EMBO J.* **3,** 1834–1842.
37. Albertsen, H. M., Paslier, D. Le, Abderrahim, H., Dausset, J., Cann, H., and Cohen, D. (1989) Improved control of partial DNA restriction enzyme digest in agarose using limiting concentrations of Mg^{++}. *Nucleic Acids Res.* **17,** 808.
38. Barlow, D. P. and Lehrach, H. (1990) Partial Not1 digests, generated by low enzyme concentration or the presence of ethidium bromide, can be used to extend the range of pulsed-field gel mapping. *Technique* **2,** 79–87.
39. Wilson, W. W. and Hoffman, R. M. (1990) Methylation of intact chromosomes by bacterial methylases in agarose plugs suitable for pulsed field electrophoresis. *Anal. Biochem.* **191,** 370–375.
40. Birren, B. W., Lai, E., Clark, S. M., Hood, L., and Simon, M. I. (1988) Optimised conditions for pulsed field gel electrophoretic separations of DNA. *Nucleic Acids Res.* **16,** 7563–7582.

41. Birren, B. W., Hood, L., and Lai, E. (1989) Pulsed field gel electrophoresis studies of DNA migration made with the PACE electrophoresis system. *Electrophoresis* **10,** 302–309.
42. Gunderson, K. and Chu, G. (1991) Pulsed-field electrophoresis of megabase-sized DNA. *Mol. Cell. Biol.* **11,** 3348–3354.
43. Smith, D. R. (1990) Genomic long-range restriction mapping. *Methods* **1,** 195–203.
44. Reed, K. C. and Mann, D. A. (1985) Rapid transfer of DNA from agarose gels to nylon membranes. *Nucleic Acids Res.* **13,** 7207–7221.
45. Church, G. M. and Gilbert, W. (1984) Genomic sequencing. *Proc. Natl. Acad. Sci. USA* **81,** 1991–1995.
46. Chikashige, Y., Kinoshita, N., Nakaseko, Y., Matsumoto, T., Murakami, S., Niwa, O., and Yanagida, M. (1989) Composite motifs and repeat symmetry in *S. pombe* centomeres. *Cell* **57,** 739–751.

CHAPTER 15

Immunofluorescence Techniques Applied to Mitotic Chromosome Preparations

Peter Jeppesen

1. Introduction

Immunofluorescence has proven to be a powerful technique for the *in situ* localization of antigens at a cytological level. Whether utilized to determine the cellular distribution of known antigens using defined antibodies, to aid in the characterization of novel antigens recognized, for example, by autoimmune sera, or to screen monoclonal antibodies for their cognate antigens, the immunofluorescence method has the merit of combining high sensitivity with the ability apparently to "visualize" antigens directly.

The basic requirement for successful immunofluorescence is to be able to maintain in vivo cellular organization while retaining antigenicity and allowing access for antibodies. This requirement contains often conflicting concepts: Accessibility necessitates rendering cell membranes permeable, which in turn allows compartmentalized soluble antigens to diffuse, unless they are previously fixed; fixation can reduce or even abolish the antigenicity of some proteins. Therefore, most published immunofluorescence methods are tailored very much to suit the particular antigen(s) under study, e.g., whether or not they are diffusible, whether they can tolerate certain fixation procedures without loss of antigenicity, and so forth. The techniques to be described here are no exception and present an immunofluores-

From: *Methods in Molecular Biology, Vol. 29: Chromosome Analysis Protocols*
Edited by: J. R. Gosden Copyright ©1994 Humana Press Inc., Totowa, NJ

cence method that has been specifically designed for the localization of structural nuclear antigens. Furthermore, this chapter will concentrate on applying the method to mitotic cell preparations. However, where the method has been successfully applied to other types of antigen, with or without minor modifications to the basic techniques, this will be mentioned in the text where appropriate.

1.1. Scope of Immunofluorescence Applied to Metaphase Preparations

Immunofluorescence has been used for two main areas of study with metaphase chromosome preparations. The first is in the detection of DNA sequences hybridized *in situ,* and the second is for the localization of antigenic chromosomal proteins. Most immunofluorescence studies are *indirect,* that is, primary antibody binding is detected by a fluorescently conjugated secondary antibody, rather than by fluorescently tagging the primary antibody itself.

1.1.1. Detection of in Situ *Hybridization of DNA*

In situ hybridization of metaphase chromosomes is well established as a method for mapping the chromosomal location of DNA sequences complementary to specific nucleotide sequences contained in nucleic acid probes. The probe is first labeled in some way that can be detected following hybridization with the fixed metaphase chromosome preparation. Until relatively recently, a radioisotope, such as ^{3}H, was used to label the nucleic acid probes, either by "nick" translation or end labeling. Then, after hybridization to the metaphase chromosome preparation, the sites of hybridization were located by coating the slide containing the sample in photographic emulsion and detecting the radioactive disintegration by autoradiography. This technique requires a radioisotope with a very low energy emission and, hence, a short path length, in order that the developed silver grains remain close to the site of disintegration. The method has a number of inherent drawbacks: e.g., the inconvenience of coating slides with photographic emulsion, often long exposure times, and the residual uncertainty of the exact site of disintegration owing to the finite path length of the emitted radiation, especially when dealing with weak signals and few silver grains.

The availability of biotinylated nucleotide 5'-triphosphates for labeling of DNA probes by nick translation has meant that an alternative approach to identifying sites of hybridization can be utilized. Biotin-containing probes may be localized using fluorescently tagged antibiotin, avidin, or streptavidin, or alternatively, in order to amplify the signal, by first binding (strept)avidin and then detecting the complex with fluorescently tagged anti(strept)avidin. In both cases, the sites of hybridization are observed directly by fluorescence microscopy. (Although the use of fluorescently tagged avidin or streptavidin to localize biotinylated probes is not strictly immunofluorescence, in practice, the techniques involved are so similar that they may be conveniently considered together under the same heading.) A recent modification of the *in situ* hybridization technique is to use short, unlabeled, synthetic oligonucleotides for the initial hybridization, which then act as primers for extension by DNA polymerase with biotinylated deoxynucleolide 5'-triphosphates (*Pr*imed in s*itu* or PRINS). The sites of biotin incorporation are then localized as above. Fluorescence microscopy *in situ* hybridization techniques are addressed in detail in Chapters 18, 25, and 26 of this volume.

The advantages of immunofluorescence over autoradiography to detect *in situ* hybridization are self-evident: The results are immediately apparent on viewing the chromosomes in the fluorescence microscope, and the fluorescence exactly corresponds to the sites of hybridization. Given that the manipulations involved are straightforward and the sensitivity of the method high, it is not surprising that immunofluorescence has rapidly established itself as the method of choice for the detection of *in situ* hybridization.

1.1.2. Localization of Protein Antigens

Approximately half the metaphase chromosome mass is composed of protein, of which histones account for the major fraction. Histones may exist with a wide range of posttranscriptional modifications to their primary amino acid sequences *(1)*, whose functions are only beginning to be investigated. Immunofluorescence can be used to monitor variation in modification states along the chromosome, and even detect subtle differences in histone and/or nucleosome conformation *(2)*. These studies will eventually assist in understanding how histone modification is related to gene function.

Among the nonhistone proteins are the so-called scaffold proteins, responsible for organizing DNA into the looped domains, which are believed to form the fundamental higher order structure of mammalian chromosomes throughout the cell cycle *(3)*. Toward the end of G2 and during prophase, transcriptional activity is progressively shut down, with simultaneous condensation of the chromatin into individually distinguishable chromosomes. By metaphase, transcription is virtually abolished, and chromosome compaction is at its greatest. It is not clear at present what drives this process, but there is evidence that the comparably condensed organization of heterochromatin is controlled by DNA-binding nonhistone proteins (discussed in ref. *2*), and it is tempting to speculate that similar proteins are involved in mitotic chromosome condensation and may be constituents of the metaphase chromosome. Nonhistone proteins are also components of the kinetochore, the specialized structure located at the primary constriction or centromere in metaphase chromosomes that is responsible for interaction with the mitotic spindle, enabling chromosome division and segregation to take place. A number of centromere-specific proteins have been identified, some of which may be localized in the kinetochore *(4,5)*. In addition to these known or inferred proteins, metaphase chromosomes are likely to contain many other nonhistone proteins of as yet unknown or only surmised functions.

Compared with total histones, nonhistone chromosomal proteins are in minor to extremely low yields. Individual modified histone species may also not be very abundant. It is their scarcity, together with a lack of functional assays, which has, until relatively recently, largely impeded progress in understanding the roles played by these minor protein constituents of the chromosome. Antibodies have provided a number of new approaches to analyzing chromosomal proteins.

If antibodies already exist or can be raised to them, possible candidate chromosomal proteins can have their presence verified by protein blotting with nuclear extracts and their chromosomal localization determined by immunofluorescence. Probably the first example of this approach was the demonstration that topoisomerase II is a major constituent of the chromosome scaffold *(6)*. Another immunological approach is the use of sera from patients with certain autoimmune conditions who spontaneously produce autoantibodies to nuclear constituents, for reasons that are not yet understood *(7)*. However, the antibodies provide potentially powerful probes for dissecting nuclear substructure, and recognizing autoantigens that may be previously unknown or that are poorly immunogenic in experimental animals. Thus, autoantibodies from CREST patients *(8)* have been crucial in beginning to unravel the complexities of centromere and kinetochore structure.

In both of these examples, immunofluorescence has played important roles: in the first case, showing directly the localization of topoisomerase II along the scaffold axis, and in the second, initially demonstrating the nature of the autoantibodies present in CREST sera, and subsequently aiding in the analysis of the centromere epitopes recognized *(9)*. The importance of immunofluorescence is unlikely to diminish in the near future, as the renewed interest in the structure of the eukaryotic chromosome that these pioneering studies have engendered leads to the discovery of new antigenic determinants and antibody probes.

1.2. Special Requirements for Immunofluorescence of Metaphase Preparations

In order to correlate immunofluorescence data with structure and organization of mammalian chromosomes, it is necessary to conserve features of interest during reaction with antibodies. Conservation of subcellular structure is normally achieved by some form of fixation, usually maintaining, as far as possible, the in vivo state, but for certain applications, modifying this in some way to allow easier interpretation of the results. This latter approach has traditionally been employed in the study of metaphase chromosomes. The identification of individual chromosomes and chromosomal substructure is facilitated if the microtubular mitotic spindle is disrupted and chromosomes are prepared so as to be spread out with minimal overlapping. For conventional metaphase chromosome staining studies, for example, karyotyping and banding, this state is commonly attained by using a drug, such as colchicine or vinblastine, or cold treatment, to disrupt the spindle, followed by hypotonic swelling to disperse the chromosomes, and finally fixation with methanol:acetic acid (3:1). When mechanisms of chromosome motility and segregation are under study, it is, of course, not desirable to disrupt the mitotic apparatus in this way.

For fluorescence *in situ* hybridization and PRINS techniques, where DNA is the target molecule in the metaphase chromosome, methanol:acetic acid fixation has been successfully used. Not only does the method give good spreading of chromosomes, but by disrupting the native nucleosome structure of chromatin and extracting a large fraction of the histones, the DNA is in an easily accessible state for subsequent hybridization procedures. However, the use of methanol:acetic acid fixation is not, in general, suitable for the localization of protein antigens.

1.2.1. Limitations of Methanol:Acetic Acid (3:1) for Immunofluorescence

The antigenicity of many proteins is significantly reduced and, in some cases, completely abolished by fixation in methanol:acetic acid, presumably through denaturation of the native polypeptide conformation. Even when sufficient antigenicity is retained for immunofluorescence following methanol:acetic acid fixation, there is the further problem of extracting basic proteins, such as histones, by exposure to acidic conditions. An example of the difficulties in interpretation that this might lead to is provided by anticentromere labeling with CREST sera. The two major human centromeric antigens recognized by most CREST sera are CENP-A, a 17-kDa histone-like protein found in approximately equal amounts at all centromeres *(10,11),* and CENP-B, an 80-kDa protein varying considerably in abundance at different centromeres *(10).* When a nonacidic fixative is used to prepare chromosomes, as described below, immunofluorescence at the centromeres appears relatively uniform, a result of the combined anti-CENP-A and anti-CENP-B activities. In contrast, if brief methanol:acetic acid fixation is used to prepare spreads, although labeling of centromeres is still observed, the intensity of immunofluorescence varies significantly from centromere to centromere (unpublished observation of the author). Knowing the properties of the antigens concerned, this observation can be readily understood: the basic CENP-A is largely extracted by acid during fixation, leaving CENP-B, with its variable distribution between centromeres, to be immunolabeled. Clearly, the use of methanol:acetic acid fixative should be avoided when screening novel or uncharacterized antibody activities, since its effects cannot be predicted.

1.2.2. Nonextracting Fixatives

Alternative fixatives avoiding methanol:acetic acid include organic solvents, such as methanol and acetone, and the protein crosslinking agents formaldehyde and glutaraldehyde. Unfortunately, none of these provides a one-step fixing and spreading procedure, as is the case for methanol:acetic acid. The cells must first be prepared in some way so as to give a spread on a microscope slide in which the features of interest are retained and that can subsequently be fixed for preservation of the sample. There are a number of possible ways of obtaining the initial spreads. Tissue culture cells that grow by adhesion to a surface may be grown directly on glass slides or cover slips. Detached cells or suspension cultures may be transferred to slides or cover slips by a variety of means. These include: making smears from concentrated cell suspensions, allowing cells to settle under gravity from a drop of more dilute suspension, or sedimenting cells out of suspension by centrifugation.

Once the cells are attached to the slide, they need to be treated to enable antibodies to gain access to nuclear components, and at the same time ensuring that the structure and morphology of the organelles under study are maintained in as near their in vivo states as possible. The fixatives methanol and acetone dissolve the lipid cell membrane, thus allowing access for antibodies, but the resulting nuclear morphology is not as good as using methanol:acetic acid. In particular, metaphase chromosomes are much more swollen with a less well-defined appearance, making further identification of individual chromosomes difficult. In contrast, formaldehyde and glutaraldehyde give quite good morphology of chromosomes, but by crosslinking the protein components of the cell membrane, can lead to reduced accessibility for antibodies. An additional drawback is that many proteins exhibit loss or reduction of antigenicity after exposure to aldehyde fixatives, especially glutaraldehyde. Limited fixation with formaldehyde has, however, been used successfully for the localization of structural antigens *(8)*.

1.2.3. Cytocentrifugation to Obtain Metaphase Spreads

The most important factor in achieving good chromosome preparations for immunofluorescence, avoiding the use of methanol:acetic acid, is the technique adopted for making the initial metaphase spreads on microscope slides or cover glasses, irrespective of subsequent fixation procedures. The author has experimented with numerous methods of obtaining cell spreads, few of which even approach the results routinely achieved by conventional methanol:acetic acid. The most generally applicable technique is cytocentrifugation of cell suspensions onto microscope slides. Two main strategies exist for cytocentrifugation: Either the supernatant solution is retained above the sedimenting cells during centrifugation and is subsequently removed, or the cells are sedimented onto the slide through an aperture in a porous card that absorbs the supernatant solution during centrifugation, resulting in a "dry" cell preparation. The latter technique has been found to give the best results for preparation of metaphase spreads. In conjunction with a prior hypotonic treatment, the resulting chromosomes are reasonably well dispersed over a somewhat greater area than is achieved by "wet" cytocentrifugation—the swollen cells appear to be "flattened" more by the dry technique. Also, cell adhesion through subsequent manipulations is better, the brief air-drying presumably helping to anchor the cells to the slide.

Perhaps surprisingly, the majority of nuclei and chromosomes retain good morphology following this procedure, although a small fraction of cells with disrupted outer membranes do show evidence of internal disintegration, presumably through the effects on the cell contents of exposure to a high-salt concentration during drying. When the membrane remains intact, however, either it prevents the cell interior from drying out, or the other soluble components of the cytoplasm (e.g., proteins, carbohydrates, and so on) help protect labile structures from the effects of drying. It has been found empirically that the fraction of cells ruptured during cytocentrifugation is relatively high if the cells are sparse, but decreases as the cell density on the slide is increased, and reaches a minimum as the cells approach a monolayer in the final preparation. It appears that cells in contact are able to provide each other with mutual mechanical support during centrifugation. In practice, the aim is to cover 50–70% of the slide surface with cells in the sample area.

Following cytocentrifugation, as pointed out in the previous section, the cells require permeabilizing in order that antibodies can reach their target antigens. For soluble and other labile antigens, a brief (5-min) treatment with cold (–20°C) methanol serves both to permeabilize cells and to fix the antigens without significant loss of antigenicity. However, for better morphology when studying mitotic chromosomes, the following method has been developed, in which nonionic detergent is used to permeabilize cell membranes and chromosomes remain unfixed until after the antibody reactions are completed.

1.2.4. An Immunofluorescence Method
Avoiding Prior Fixation

A method has previously been described for the isolation of mammalian metaphase chromosomes under "physiological" conditions *(12),* in which chromosome structure was stabilized in an isotonic salts solution based on potassium chloride and including 0.1% Triton X-100 ("potassium chromosome medium" or "KCM"). When cytocentrifuged metaphase cell spreads prepared as described above are treated with KCM, the lipid membrane is dissolved allowing access to antibodies, whereas at the same time, metaphase chromosomes remain condensed and retain good morphology when viewed by phase optics microscopy. Slides can be stored in KCM at room temperature for several hours with no apparent deterioration. It was also previously shown that KCM provided a good medium in which to carry out antibody reactions for immunofluorescence *(13).* Using the procedures to be described in detail in the remainder of this chapter, it is therefore possible to label immunofluorescently metaphases derived from cultured mammalian cells, avoiding the many problems associated with using fixatives and retaining, as far as can be judged, the native chromosome structure.

2. Materials

2.1. Tissue Culture Media and Reagents

Media and reagents for cell culture are standard formulations obtainable from a number of tissue culture suppliers. The culture media for the cell types used in the illustrations to this chapter were:

1. Dulbecco's Modified Eagle's Medium (DMEM) supplemented with 10% (v/v) fetal bovine (calf) serum (FCS).
2. RPMI 1640 medium supplemented with 10% (v/v) FCS.

Other tissue culture reagents used were:

1. Trypsin-EDTA solution (TE): 0.05% (w/v) trypsin and 0.02% (w/v) EDTA in buffered saline.
2. Ficoll-plaque (Pharmacia, Uppsala, Sweden).
3. Phytohemagglutinin (PHA) solution (Gibco-BRL, Gaithersburg, MD).

2.2. Solutions for Chromosome Preparation

Analytical reagent (AR) grade chemicals should be used if available; otherwise, substitute general laboratory reagent grade (*see also* Note 1).

1. Colcemid stock solution (100X): 10 µg/mL Colcemid (Fluka, Buchs, Switzerland) in water, filter sterilized.
2. Hypotonic solution: 75 mM KCl.
3. "Potassium chromosome medium" (KCM): 120 mM KCl, 20 mM NaCl, 10 mM Tris-HCl, pH 8.0, 0.5 mM EDTA, and 0.1% (v/v) Triton X-100.
4. Dulbecco's phosphate-buffered saline (PBS): 0.2 g/L KCl, 8.0 g/L NaCl, 0.2 g/L KH_2PO_4, and 1.15 g/L Na_2HPO_4.
5. Formaldehyde solution: 40% (w/v), diluted (1:10) just before use to 4% formaldehyde in KCM (or PBS).
6. Hoechst "33258" or DAPI (4',6-diamidino-2-phenylindole), both obtained from the Sigma (St. Louis, MO). Stock solutions: 50 µg/mL in water.

2.3. Antibodies and Sera

The choice of antibodies and sera for immunofluorescence of metaphase chromosome preparations is clearly dictated by the nature of the study (*see also* Note 7). The following lists the antibodies used for the illustrations to this chapter.

2.3.1. Primary Antibodies

Autoimmune anticentromere sera were gifts from George Nuki at the Rheumatic Diseases Unit, Western General Hospital, Edinburgh, UK. Mouse monoclonal antibody HBC-7 (subclone B11-1B8) against histone H2B, and rabbit sera R15/0 and R5/12, against histone H4 nonacetylated and acetylated at Lys-12, respectively, were gifts from Bryan Turner at the Department of Anatomy, University of Birmingham Medical School, UK. For use, antibodies were diluted 1:100 for whole sera and 1:20 for HBC-7 hybridoma supernatant, in KCM containing 10% (v/v) normal goat serum (NGS).

2.3.2. Secondary Antibodies

Fluorescein isothiocyanate (FITC) and tetramethylrhodamine isothiocyanate (TRITC) conjugated, affinity-isolated goat antihuman, antimouse, and antirabbit immunoglobulins were obtained from

Sigma. They were used diluted 1:20 in KCM containing 10% (v/v) NGS.

2.4. Cytocentrifugation

There are a number of different models of cytocentrifuge available on the market. The author has no reason to believe that any one is more suitable for the procedures described here than another. Different designs of cytocentrifuge use different volumes of cell suspension for centrifugation onto different sample areas on the slide. The optimum cell density for a particular machine is estimated from the principles outlined in Section 1.2.3. For the results illustrating this chapter, an Ames Cyto-Tek cytocentrifuge (Bayer Diagnostics UK Ltd., Basingstoke, UK) was used, employing 1-mL disposable sample chambers. The author also has experience with the use of the Shandon Cytospin and Sakura Autosmear machines, both of which give similar results to the Cyto-Tek.

2.5. Fluorescence Microscopy

The fluorescence micrographs shown here were taken by epi-illumination on a Leitz Ortholux-2 microscope using filter sets A, I 2/3, and N 2 to detect Hoechst 33258, FITC, and TRITC/rhodamine/Texas red fluorescence, respectively. When using other models of fluorescence microscope, it is important to use narrow band filter sets where possible, to avoid spillover of signal from one channel to another. When counterstaining for DNA with Hoechst 33258 or DAPI, the UV fluorescence signal can be very strong, and without a narrow-band FITC filter, the signal spilling over from the UV fluorescence channel can completely swamp the FITC signal. With the Leitz filters specified here, a very strong FITC signal can be observed as green fluorescence in the UV channel, but this is not usually a problem. A strong TRITC/rhodamine/Texas red signal can also be detected in the FITC channel as a weak orange fluorescence, which can be a problem when recording FITC + TRITC double-labeling results in monochrome.

To minimize fading, slides were mounted for fluorescence microscopy in antifade AF3 PBS (Citifluor Ltd., Connaught Building, London EC1V 0HB, UK):glycerol (1:1). Other additives to reduce fading of fluorescence, such as *p*-phenylene diamine *(14)* or *n*-propylgallate *(15),* are probably equally effective, but have not been tested by the author.

3. Methods

3.1. Cell Culture

Monolayer or suspension cultures of established cell lines are grown by standard tissue culture procedures. For the examples illustrating this chapter, Don Chinese hamster fibroblasts (ATCC no. CCL 16), mouse L929 fibroblasts (ATCC no. CCL 1), and mouse C127 cells (derived from a mouse mammary tumor, ATCC no. CRL1616) were grown as monolayer cultures in DMEM containing 10% FCS. For culture conditions to induce undercondensation of heterochromatin, *see* Note 2.

3.1.1. Monolayer Cultures

1. Split subpassage confluent cultures at a ratio of 1:5. After 24 h, add Colcemid (final concentration 0.1 µg/mL) to approx 10^6 total cells (10 mL culture), and continue incubation for 1 h. (The quantities in parentheses represent a typical preparation). Harvest as follows:
2. Remove and save on ice the supernatant culture medium, while incubating the cell layer with TE (4 mL) at 37°C to detach the cells.
3. Dilute TE cell suspension with an equal vol of saved, cold, culture medium, and centrifuge at 1000 rpm for 10 min at 4°C. Discard the supernatant, and gently resuspend and wash the cell pellet with the remaining saved culture medium. (Further trypsin action is prevented by the serum contained in the medium.)
4. Centrifuge cells again (1000 rpm, 10 min, 4°C), and remove all but approx 0.1 mL of supernatant; gently resuspend cell pellet in this, and add 5 mL of cold KCl hypotonic solution, initially dropwise, maintaining a homogeneous suspension of cells.
5. Incubate at 37°C for 10 min, and then finally cool and keep the hypotonic cell suspension on ice.

3.1.2. Suspension Cultures

1. Dilute late exponential phase (or early stationary phase) cells 1:5 with fresh growth medium. After 24 h, add Colcemid (final concentration 0.1 µg/mL) to approx 10^6 total cells (10 mL culture), and continue incubation for 1 h.
2. Collect cells by centrifugation at 1000 rpm for 10 min at 4°C, and remove all but approx 0.1 mL of supernatant; continue as detailed in steps 4 and 5, Section 3.1.1.

3.1.3. Blood Lymphocytes

For preparation of metaphases by cytocentrifugation from lymphocyte cultures, it is important to remove red blood cells at the outset:

1. Dilute 20 mL of defibrinated blood with 10 mL of RPMI 1640 medium, and layer onto 7.5 mL of Ficoll-paque. Separate lymphocytes by centrifugation at 2600 rpm for 20 min, and then wash twice with RPMI medium, centrifuging the lymphocytes at 1000 rpm for 12 min at each washing and carefully resuspending each time in 20 mL RPMI.
2. Establish 5–10 mL lymphocyte cultures (approx 10^6 cells/mL) in RPMI supplemented with 10% FCS, and stimulate with PHA at a 1:100 dilution of the stock solution.
3. After 72 h growth at 37°C, accumulate metaphases by adding colcemid to a final concentration of 0.1 µg/mL 1–2 h before collecting cells and swelling in hypotonic as described above for suspension cultures, from step 2, Section 3.1.2.

3.2. Preparation of Metaphase Spreads

The suggested quantities apply to the Cyto-Tek centrifuge fitted with 1-mL disposable chambers. For an explanation, and to use other cytocentrifuges, *see* Note 3.

1. With a hemocytometer or other cell-counting device, determine the cell density of the hypotonic KCl suspension. Dilute with further 75 mM KCl if necessary to obtain $1–2 \times 10^5$ cells/mL.
2. Use the appropriate volume per slide (0.5–1.0 mL) to contain approx 10^5 cells, and centrifuge for 10 min at 2000 rpm onto clean slides.
3. After removing slides from the cytocentrifuge, allow any visible moisture to dry briefly, and then immerse in a Coplin jar containing KCM at room temperature for at least 10 min before carrying out the first antibody incubation (*see also* Notes 4 and 5).

3.3. Antibody Reactions

After permeabilizing the cells by immersion in KCM, they must not be allowed to dry at any stage until finally fixed with formaldehyde. Therefore, if several slides are being processed, steps 1 and 2 below should be carried out on one slide at a time before starting on the next slide.

1. Remove slide from KCM and allow to drain briefly. Then with a tissue, carefully wipe and dry the back of the slide and the edges of the slide around the sample area, leaving the cells with an approx 5-mm wet margin all around.
2. With the slide horizontal, carefully apply 40 µL of first antibody dilution to the sample area, and cover with an approx 1-cm square of Parafilm or other laboratory film. Then, keeping slide horizontal, transfer it to a humid chamber (e.g., a sealed plastic sandwich box containing wetted tissues) maintained at room temperature (*see* Note 6).

3. After the primary antibody incubation of 1–2 h, remove slide from the humid chamber, and carefully remove Parafilm square by lifting from a corner with forceps. Then, gently rinse off the antibody with a few milliliters of KCM directed from a Pasteur pipet, holding the slide at an angle to form a ramp down which the solution flows. Transfer the slide to a Coplin jar containing KCM.
4. After 5 min, transfer slides to a second Coplin jar containing KCM for a further 5-min wash. Then repeat steps 1 and 2 for the second antibody.
5. After 30-min secondary antibody incubation, rinse off and transfer to KCM as described in step 3. After 5 min, transfer to fresh KCM for a further 5-min wash.
6. Finally, fix slides in a Coplin jar containing KCM + 4% formaldehyde for 15 min at room temperature, transfer to distilled water for 5 min, drain, and allow to dry.

3.4. Fluorescence Microscopy

For ease of observation, slides are counterstained for DNA.

1. Immerse slides for 10 min in a Coplin jar of Hoechst 33258 or DAPI at 0.5 µg/mL in water. Wash 5 min in water, drain, and dry.
2. Mount cover glasses on a small volume of antifade/glycerol, blot excess mountant with filter paper, and seal around the edges with rubber solution (*see* Note 8).

3.5. Illustrations of the Method

The following specific examples of immunofluorescence applied to metaphase chromosomes, drawn from a variety of cell types and antibodies, serve to illustrate some of the results that have been obtained in this laboratory using the techniques described in this chapter.

3.5.1. Autoimmune Sera

It is well established that many CREST patients possess anticentromere autoantibodies (ACAs) in their sera *(8)*. When ACA sera are studied in more detail, however, a number have been shown to contain additional autoantibodies (e.g., ref. *13*), including some that recognize other chromosomal antigens. Figure 1a shows a metaphase spread from the mouse L929 cell line, immunofluorescently labeled with a CREST serum that exclusively recognizes centromeres, whereas Fig. 1c shows a similar metaphase labeled with a serum (EP) that recognizes mouse pericentromeric heterochromatin in addition to true centromeres. Heterochromatin labeling in Fig. 1c is so strong

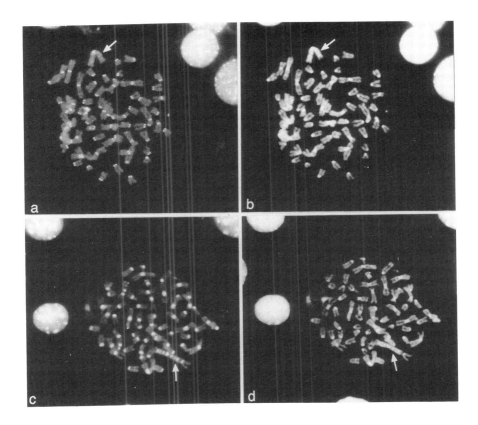

Fig. 1. Immunofluorescent labeling of mouse pericentromeric heterochromatin by a CREST anticentromere serum. **a.** FITC immunofluorescence of a mouse L929 metaphase cell, using a CREST serum that exclusively recognizes centromeres. **b.** Hoechst 33258 fluorescence of same cell shown in a. **c.** FITC immunofluorescence of a similar L929 metaphase cell using CREST serum EP, which labels the pericentromeric heterochromatin in addition to centromeres. **d.** Hoechst 33258 fluorescence of same cell shown in c. The octacentric marker chromosome is indicated by arrows in both cells.

that it obscures the typical ACA "double-dot" immunofluorescence pattern seen in Fig. 1a, and is particularly striking in the case of an "octacentric" fusion marker chromosome (arrowed), where the fluorescence of each block of residual centric heterochromatin is clearly evident. This autoantibody activity appears similar to that described previously elsewhere *(16)*.

When the same serum EP is used to label human metaphase chromosomes prepared from normal cultures, it produces a typical double-dot centromere fluorescence pattern. However, if the human lymphocytes are cultured in the presence of 5-azacytidine or DAPI prior to preparing spreads, the major heterochromatic domains are caused to decondense (*see* Chapter 9) and are now immunofluorescently labeled by serum EP (Fig. 2a). It seems that decondensation is required to make the heterochromatin antigen accessible for antibody binding in human chromosomes, but this is not required in mouse chromosomes. In Chinese hamster where there are no large blocks of heterochromatin, serum EP labels centromeres and, in addition, gives a banded appearance to the chromosomes (Fig. 2c). In this case, the antigen, which we believe to be closely related to those localized in mouse and human heterochromatins (L. Nicol and P. Jeppesen, in preparation), appears to be distributed nonuniformly along the chromosome arms, perhaps at sites containing smaller blocks of heterochromatin-like structure.

3.5.2. Antihistone Antibodies

Immunofluorescence of metaphase chromosomes using antibodies raised against whole histone fractions normally leads to homogeneous labeling, reflecting the constancy of the chromatin nucleosome subunit structure, which comprises all of the histones in stoichiometric amounts. When antibodies recognizing defined histone epitopes or modifications are used, however, nonuniform labeling of the chromosomes may be seen, indicating variations in chromatin conformation and/or modification state at different positions in the chromosomes.

3.5.2.1. MONOCLONAL ANTIBODY AGAINST HISTONE H2B

Mouse monoclonal antibody HBC-7 recognizes the N-terminal region of histone H2B (*17*). Figure 3a shows a mouse L929 metaphase immunofluorescently labeled using HBC-7. Comparing Fig. 3a with the Hoechst 33258 fluorescence of the same spread shown in Fig. 3b, which distinguishes heterochromatin as more brightly fluorescent than euchromatin, it can be seen that binding of HBC-7 to heterochromatin is completely absent. This is evidenced by an unlabeled "hole" at the centromeres of the acrocentric chromosomes, but is even more clearly apparent in the dicentric fusion chromosomes and the octacentric marker chromosome (arrowed) present in this cell line.

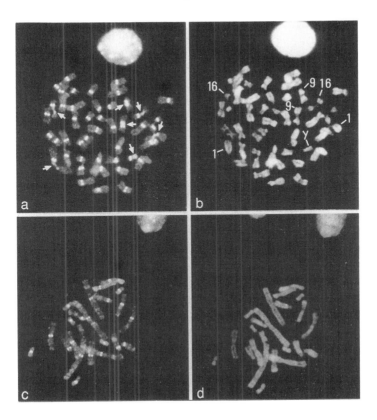

Fig. 2. Different patterns of immunofluorescence in human and Chinese hamster metaphase chromosomes using CREST anticentromere serum EP. **a.** FITC immunofluorescence of a metaphase cell prepared from a human lymphocyte culture grown in the presence of 5-azacytidine to induce decondensation of the major heterochromatic domains. In addition to typical "double-dot" centromere fluorescence, the decondensed heterochromatin also shows bright fluorescence, indicated by arrows. **b.** Hoechst 33258 fluorescence of same cell shown in a, identifying chromosomes with decondensed heterochromatic domains. **c.** FITC immunofluorescence of a metaphase cell prepared from Chinese hamster (Don) cell line, showing banding pattern along chromosome arms in addition to bright centromere fluorescence. **d.** Hoechst 33258 fluorescence of same cell shown in c.

Paradoxically, the opposite result is obtained when HBC-7 is used to label human metaphase chromosomes. In Fig. 4a–c, the same human lymphocyte metaphase is illustrated by Hoechst 33258 fluorescence, immunofluorescence using HBC-7, and after staining by the methyl green/DAPI C-banding procedure, which causes heterochromatin to

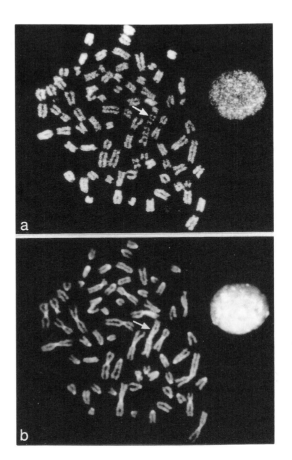

Fig. 3. Lack of immunofluorescent labeling of mouse pericentromeric heterochromatin by mouse monoclonal antibody HBC-7 against histone H2B. **a.** FITC immunofluorescence of a mouse L929 metaphase cell, showing uniform fluorescence of euchromatin, but complete lack of labeling of pericentromeric heterochromatin, clearly demonstrated by the dark bands present on the octacentric marker chromosome (indicated by arrow). **b.** Hoechst 33258 fluorescence of same cell shown in a.

fluoresce more brightly *(18),* respectively. The chromosomes containing major heterochromatic domains are identified in Fig. 4c, and, as shown in Fig. 4b, these domains are also immunofluorescently labeled by HBC-7, mostly at a higher level than euchromatin. If the heterochromatin is induced to decondense as described above, however, the enhanced immunofluorescence with HBC-7 is abolished, as shown in Fig. 4e. In this example, the heterochromatin of one chromosome 9 has undergone decondensation and lost its bright appearance with HBC-7, whereas the other chromosome 9 is normally condensed and has retained a brightly immunofluorescent heterochromatin domain.

Immunofluorescence using monoclonal antibody HBC-7 has shown that the N-terminal region of histone H2B has different properties when found in heterochromatin compared with euchromatin, and that these heterochromatin specific properties are not the same in mouse and human. It is not yet possible to define the differences more precisely. They could be:

1. Differences in accessibility resulting from altered conformations of the nucleosome in mouse and human heterochromatins;
2. In the case of mouse heterochromatin, masking of the epitope by heterochromatin-specific protein; or
3. A heterochromatin-specific modification to histone H2B resulting in a loss of antigenicity.

3.5.2.2. RABBIT ANTISERUM TO ACETYLATED HISTONE H4

The variation in chromatin structure leading to differential heterochromatin immunofluorescence with monoclonal antibody HBC-7, as described above, is not yet understood. However, R5/12, a rabbit antiserum that specifically recognizes histone H4 when acetylated at position Lys-12 *(19)*, gives precise information on the distribution of one type of histone modification, namely, acetylation. Acetylation and deacetylation of histones are rapidly cycling processes whose exact relationship with transcription is not clear, although it is known that actively transcribing chromatin is maintained in a hyperacetylated state *(1)*. R5/12 has been shown to be a good indicator of hyperacetylation in histone H4 *(19)*, and the use of this antibody in immunofluorescence experiments has enabled patterns of H4 acetylation on chromosomes to be studied *in situ.*

When human lymphocyte metaphase preparations are immunofluorescently labeled with R5/12, as shown in Fig. 5a, the majority of metaphases are very weakly stained compared with interphase nuclei present in the same sample. This is consistent with the low level of transcription, and hence acetylation, to be expected during mitosis.

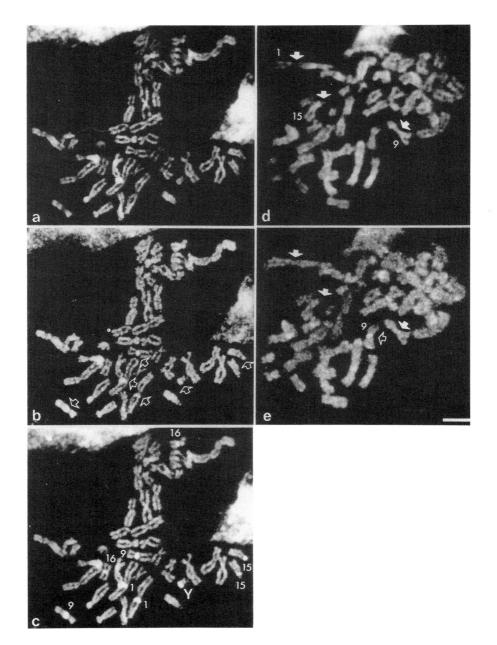

However, occasionally, metaphases that are presumed to have been labeled soon after entering metaphase arrest, and have therefore not undergone significant deacetylation, are more brightly fluorescent (an example is shown in the center of Fig. 5a). If such a spread is inspected in more detail (Fig. 5c), the distribution of fluorescence has the appearance of a banding pattern resembling R-bands. It is widely believed that genes are concentrated in R-bands, and the finding that an increased level of histone acetylation is also found in R-bands is consistent with the association of acetylation and transcription, and suggests that the pattern of immunofluorescence seen reflects the transcriptional activity of different regions of the genome just prior to mitosis. Of particular interest in this respect is the observation that the major heterochromatic domains, which are transcriptionally inactive, are unlabeled, and thus appear to contain underacetylated histone H4 (some examples are identified in Fig. 5c). Figure 5d,f illustrates the more uniform immunofluorescence obtained in both interphase and mitotic chromatin when using an antibody that recognizes total histone H4, where there is no evidence for any unlabeled regions.

The association of histone acetylation with transcriptionally active chromatin is dramatically demonstrated in Fig. 6, where serum R5/12 was used to label immunofluorescently a metaphase prepared from the female mouse cell line C127. In addition to the "R-like" banding

---

Fig. 4. *(previous page)* Enhanced immunofluorescence of human heterochromatic domains using mouse monoclonal antibody HBC-7 against histone H2B. **a.** Hoechst 33258 fluorescence of a metaphase cell from a normal human lymphocyte culture. **b.** FITC immunofluorescence of the same cell shown in a, indicating bright fluorescence of heterochromatic domains. **c.** UV fluorescence of metaphase depicted in a and b following C-banding with methyl green/DAPI. Chromosomes containing the major heterochromatic domains revealed by this procedure are identified. **d.** Hoechst 33258 fluorescence of a metaphase cell from a human lymphocyte culture grown in the presence of DAPI to induce undercondensation of the heterochromatic domains. Three "stretched" centromeres are arrowed and the chromosomes identified. **e.** FITC immunofluorescence of the same metaphase shown in d. The solid arrows point to undercondensed heterochromatic domains that have lost their bright fluorescence. The unfilled arrow indicates a chromosome 9 heterochromatic domain that has not undergone decondensation and that retains its bright fluorescence. Bar represents 5 µm. (Reproduced from ref. 2, with the permission of Springer–Verlag.)

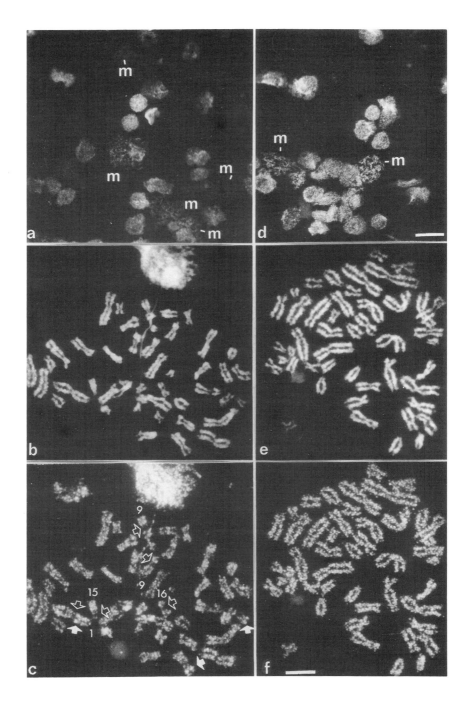

noted above for human lymphocytes, comparison of immunofluorescence (Fig. 6a) with Hoechst 33258 fluorescence (Fig. 6b) reveals
one chromosome that is almost completely unlabeled by the antibody
(arrowed in Fig. 6a). This is the inactive X chromosome, identified
by its characteristically bright Hoechst 33258 fluorescence and curved
appearance (large arrow, Fig. 6b). X inactivation, therefore, also appears
to be associated with underacetylation of histone H4.

As found with the major human heterochromatic domains, mouse
pericentromeric heterochromatin is also unlabeled by R5/12. This is
clearly seen by comparing the bright C-bands in Fig. 6b with the corresponding "holes" in the immunofluorescence patterns shown in Fig. 6a.
Three tiny marker chromosome fragments in this cell line (small arrows,
Fig. 6b) are absent from the R5/12 immunofluorescence picture (Fig. 6a)
and, therefore, appear to be entirely composed of heterochromatin.

3.5.3. Double Labeling

3.5.3.1. DOUBLE ANTIBODY

Where two antibodies are derived from different species, they may
be used to label their respective antigens simultaneously by indirect
immunofluorescence, using secondary antibodies tagged with differ-

---

Fig. 5. *(previous page)* Histone H4 acetylation in human metaphase chromosomes detected by immunofluorescence using rabbit antiserum R5/12. **a.** Low magnification photomicrograph of cells from a human lymphocyte culture showing
variation in intensity of FITC immunofluorescence exhibited by different cells with
R5/12 In general, metaphases (m) show weaker fluorescence than interphase nuclei,
although the metaphase in the center of the field is as intensely labeled as the weaker
nuclei. **b.** Hoechst 33258 fluorescence of a metaphase cell. **c.** FITC immunofluorescence of same cell shown in b, revealing distribution of histone H4 acetylation
at position Lys-12. Unfilled arrows indicate the lack of labeling at centromeres of
chromosomes containing major heterochromatic domains (identified). The solid
arrows point to typical examples of chromosomes exhibiting bright punctate fluorescence patterns repeated on both chromatids. **d.** Low magnification photomicrograph of cells from a human lymphocyte culture to show similar intensities of
immunofluorescence of metaphases (m) and nuclei using rabbit serum R15/0, which
recognizes total histone H4. **e.** Hoechst 33258 fluorescence of metaphase cell from
a similar culture as in d. **f.** FITC immunofluorescence of same metaphase shown in
e, demonstrating uniform binding of serum R15/0 to total histone H4. Bars represent 30 μm (a,d) and 5 μm (b,c,e,f). (Reproduced from ref. 2, with the permission
of Springer–Verlag.)

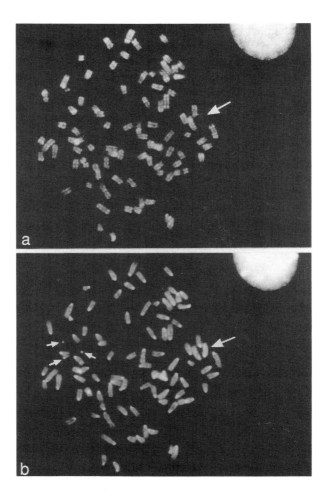

Fig. 6. Histone H4 acetylation in mouse C127 metaphase chromosomes detected by immunofluorescence using rabbit serum R5/12, revealing underacetylation of inactive X chromosome. **a.** FITC immunofluorescence of metaphase cell, showing "R-like" banding pattern and nonfluorescence of centric heterochromatin. The low level of fluorescence of the inactive X chromosome is indicated by the arrow. **b.** Hoechst 33258 fluorescence of same cell shown in a. The characteristic bright fluorescence and curved appearance of the inactive X chromosome, corresponding to the underlabeled chromosome in a, is indicated by the large arrow. Three chromosome fragments, apparently containing only centric heterochromatin, are indicated by the small arrows. These fragments exhibit no immunofluorescence and are not visible in a.

ent fluorochromes. Figure 7 illustrates this in the case of a mouse L929 metaphase simultaneously labeled with rabbit antiacetylated histone H4 serum R5/12 (Section 3.5.2.2.) and human CREST autoimmune serum EP (Section 3.5.1.). The primary antibody reaction mixture contained both R5/12 and EP, and binding was detected by TRITC-antirabbit IgG and FITC-antihuman IgG, respectively, both contained in the secondary reaction mixture. TRITC fluorescence is shown in Fig. 7a, FITC fluorescence in Fig. 7b, and Hoechst 33258 fluorescence in Fig. 7c, each recorded in successive exposures under appropriate filter conditions. This particular example demonstrates the negligible crosscontamination inherent in the method, since human serum EP labels the pericentromeric heterochromatin strongly (Fig. 7b), which is unlabeled by rabbit serum R5/12 (Fig. 7a). The complementary labeling patterns are particularly striking in the octacentric marker chromosome arrowed in Fig. 7a–c.

3.5.3.2. COMBINED ANTIBODY AND PRINS

The immunofluorescence technique can also be followed by *in situ* DNA hybridization or PRINS (*See* Chapter 18) (Section 1.1.1) in order to determine where protein antigens are located in relation to specific DNA sequences. This approach has been useful in mapping the distribution of different human satellite DNA sequences in relation to the centromere identified by CREST anticentromere sera *(20)*. Figure 8 shows a metaphase prepared from a human lymphocyte culture grown in the presence of 5-azacytidine to induce heterochromatin decondensation. After labeling centromeres by immunofluorescence using a CREST serum, the sample was subsequently subjected to the PRINS technique using an oligonucleotide primer derived from the satellite 3 DNA sequence *(20)*. The metaphase includes a chromosome 9, in which the centric heterochromatin has undergone decondensation, leading to a stretched appearance when viewed by Hoechst 33258 fluorescence (arrow in Fig. 8c). It can be seen in Fig. 8a that there is a strong Texas red fluorescence signal from the PRINS reaction coincident with the stretched region of chromosome 9 (arrow), localizing the satellite 3 sequences to the decondensed heterochromatin. FITC immunofluorescence in Fig. 8b defines the position of the centromere in this chromosome by its characteristic "double-dot" appearance.

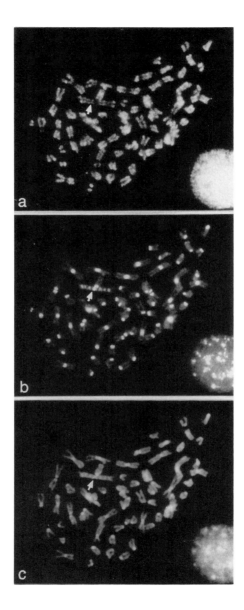

Fig. 7. Double labeling of mouse L929 metaphase chromosomes with rabbit
serum R5/12 and CREST anticentromere serum EP. **a.** TRITC immunofluorescence localizing binding of antiserum R5/12 showing distribution of histone H4
acetylation. **b.** FITC immunofluorescence of same cell shown in a, localizing bind-

Because of slight overspill of the strong Texas red signal into the FITC channel, both satellite 3 hybridization and anticentromere staining can be observed simultaneously in Fig. 8b, clearly showing the physical separation of the two.

In contrast, Fig. 9 shows the result of a similar experiment, but using an α-satellite-derived oligonucleotide for the primer reaction *(20)*. In this case, the PRINS signal also has a "double-dot" appearance (Fig. 9a) that is coincident with the CREST anticentromere immunofluorescence (Fig. 9b), demonstrating that α-satellite DNA sequences are very tightly linked to the centromere. It is also clear from observation of the stretched chromosome (arrowed) that the α-satellite sequences do not undergo decondensation and form a separate domain from the satellite 3 DNA sequences localized in Fig. 8.

4. Notes

1. Since antibody incubations are carried out on unfixed cell preparations over a period of hours at room temperature, it is important to minimize possible degradation occurring as a result of contamination of solutions by nucleases and proteases. A major source of contamination is through the growth of microorganisms in nonsterile solutions, and to prevent this, KCl, KCM, and PBS solutions should be freshly prepared from sterile stocks, or, if stored, should be sterilized by autoclaving immediately after preparation and then refrigerated.

2. In some of the examples illustrating this chapter, metaphase chromosomes exhibiting decondensed heterochromatin are shown. To induce decondensation of heterochromatin in spreads, add either (a) 0.37 μ*M* 5-azacytidine for 5 h, or (b) 100 μg/mL DAPI for 16–18 h before addition of colcemid (*2; see also* Chapter 9).

3. The optimum spreading of metaphases when cytocentrifuged cells cover 50–70% of the sample area of the slide was discussed in Section 1.2.3. The Cyto-Tek centrifuge takes 0.5–1 mL of cell suspension and has a 6-mm square aperture in the filter card. For most cell types, the optimum is achieved by centrifuging approx 10^5 cells into this area. The density of the hypotonic cell suspension is adjusted to give a minimum sample vol of 0.5 mL/slide. For other models of cytocentrifuge, the

ing of CREST serum EP autoantibodies. **c.** Hoechst 33258 fluorescence of same cell shown in a and b. The pericentromeric heterochromatin, which is strongly labeled by CREST serum EP in b, is completely unlabeled by rabbit serum R5/12 in a. These opposite labeling patterns are most clearly evident in the octacentric marker chromosome, indicated by an arrow in each panel.

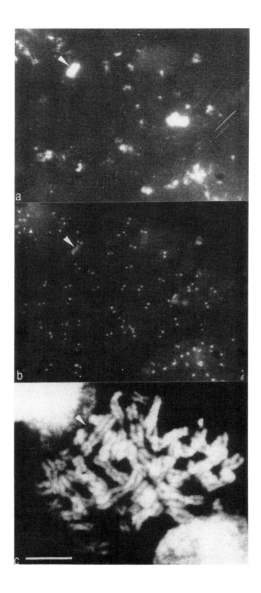

Fig. 8. Mapping of human satellite 3 in relation to the centromere in chromosome 9, using CREST anticentromere serum to locate the centromere, followed by PRINS *in situ* hybridization with a satellite 3-derived oligonucleotide primer. **a.** Texas red fluorescence showing localization of satellite 3 sequences as determined by PRINS using oligonucleotide 266 *(20)* in a metaphase cell prepared from a human lympho-

required cell densities should initially be estimated proportionately, taking into account the area of the aperture and the minimum recommended sample volume, and then adjusted in the light of experience to obtain the best results. Glass microscope slides should be clean: If not purchased prewashed, then acid or detergent used to clean them should be removed by thoroughly rinsing with distilled water. Then the slides should be allowed to dry. To remove dust and so forth, slides are wiped with ethanol just prior to use.

4. For antigens suspected of being soluble or labile, slides may be mildly prefixed by immersing for 5 min in 100% MeOH at –20°C after centrifugation and then transferred to KCM. It has occasionally been observed that the intensity of subsequent immunofluorescence for certain antigens is increased by MeOH pretreatment. This may be owing to improved accessibility in the somewhat more swollen chromatin that results from this procedure or to a more favorable conformation of the antigen following exposure to MeOH.

5. With minor modifications, the immunofluorescence technique described here can also be applied to the localization of cytoplasmic antigens. In order to preserve cytoplasmic organization, the hypotonic KCl treatment may be omitted and the cells suspended instead in PBS for cytocentrifugation, after which a brief (5-min) pretreatment with 100% MeOH at –20°C is used, as described above for the preservation of soluble or labile antigens. Most cytoplasmic antigens can then be detected following the procedures described for nuclear and metaphase preparations, using KCM as the antibody dilution medium. However, for some cytoplasmic antigens, it has been found that antibody dilutions made into PBS (including 10% NGS) produce higher levels of immunofluorescence, possibly at the expense of a slightly higher background.

6. For low background levels with indirect immunofluorescence, primary antibodies are diluted into KCM, including 10% of normal serum from the species in which the secondary antibody was raised (goat in the examples shown here), which reduces by competition nonspecific anti-

---

cyte culture grown in the presence of 5-azacytidine to induce decondensation of the heterochromatic domains. **b.** FITC immunofluorescence of same cell shown in a, with positions of centromeres defined by CREST autoantibodies. **c.** Hoechst 33258 fluorescence of same cell shown in a and b. Bar represents 10 µm. The same chromosome 9 containing a decondensed heterochromatic domain is indicated in each panel. (The fluorescence of the decondensed region in b is owing to overspill into the FITC channel of the very strong Texas red signal in a, which serves to show the physical separation of the "double-dot" centromere fluorescence and the satellite 3 sequences.) (Reproduced from ref. *20,* with the permission of Springer–Verlag.)

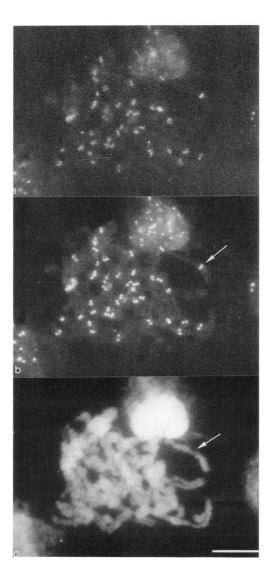

Fig. 9. Mapping of human alphoid satellite in relation to the centromere, using CREST anticentromere serum followed by PRINS *in situ* hybridization with an alphoid oligonucleotide primer. **a.** Texas red fluorescence showing localization of alphoid sequences as determined by PRINS using oligonucleotide 405 *(20)* in a metaphase cell prepared from a human lymphocyte culture grown in the presence

body binding. Failing this, normal serum from a noncrossreacting species may be substituted. It has been found that using a normal serum as competitor produces lower levels of background fluorescence than, for example, nonfat milk or bovine serum albumin, also commonly used as competitors for immunofluorescence. The same medium is used for secondary antibodies. The serum in the medium also helps to stabilize purified antibody dilutions, e.g., secondary antibodies and affinity purified antibodies. Whole sera are usually diluted 1:100. Affinity-purified antibodies and hybridoma supernatants require less dilution, from 1:5–1:20, and fluorescently conjugated secondary antibodies are also normally diluted in the range 1:5–1:20. The antibody dilutions can be covered by glass cover slips instead of Parafilm during incubation, but these are sometimes difficult to remove by gentle rinsing, particularly if the solution has dried slightly around the edges. Parafilm is simply removed by lifting off with forceps.

7. Instead of fluorescent tagging, secondary antibodies can be conjugated to biotin, which is in turn detected by a third "layer." This may be fluorescently labeled antibiotin, avidin, streptavidin, or ExtrAvidin™ (Sigma). Introducing an extra layer leads to amplification, which may be an advantage when the original signal is weak. However, any low-level nonspecific background binding of primary antibody also produces an amplified signal and, in the author's experience, this can often outweigh the advantage of amplifying the specific signal. Procedures for detecting biotinylated probes at high sensitivity are dealt with elsewhere in this volume (Chapters 18 and 26) and will not be duplicated here.

8. Slides mounted in the medium described in Section 2.5. can be stored refrigerated in the dark for several days. For longer periods, slides should be stored unmounted in the dark, desiccated, and refrigerated.

E. Merck (Darmstadt) produces a special grade of glycerol for use in mounting media for fluorescence microscopy. It is standard practice in a number of groups in this laboratory to use Merck glycerol for mount-

---

of 5-azacytidine to induce decondensation of the heterochromatic domains. **b.** FITC immunofluorescence of same cell shown in a with positions of centromeres defined by CREST autoantibodies. **c.** Hoechst 33258 fluorescence of same cell shown in a and b. Bar represents 10 μm. The PRINS labeling produces a "double-dot" fluorescence pattern in a that can be superimposed on the CREST immunofluorescence shown in b, demonstrating the colocalization of alphoid sequences and CREST antigens. The arrows in b and c indicate a decondensed heterochromatic domain that is clearly distinct from the alphoid domain, which does not undergo decondensation. (Reproduced from ref. *20,* with the permission of Springer–Verlag.)

ing conventional fluorescence metaphase preparations (i.e., those fixed with methanol:acetic acid [3:1]). However, it has been found that for immunofluorescence using the technique described here, mounting slides in Merck glycerol leads to a noticeable autofluorescence in the specimen after a few hours, visible in both the FITC and rhodamine channels. The level of autofluorescence progressively increases, and after a day or two, it can completely swamp out weak immunofluorescence signals. The mechanism responsible for this effect is not understood, but seems to be dependent on formaldehyde fixation, and is accentuated by the use of antifade in the mounting medium. The problem is completely avoided by the use of analytical-grade glycerol in the mountant.

References

1. Wu, R. S., Panusz, H. T., Hatch, C. L., and Bonner, W. M. (1986) Histones and their modifications. *CRC Crit. Rev. Biochem.* **20,** 201–263.
2. Jeppesen, P., Mitchell, A., Turner, B., and Perry, P. (1992) Antibodies to defined histone epitopes reveal variations in chromatin conformation and underacetylation of centric heterochromatin in human metaphase chromosomes. *Chromosoma* **101,** 322–332.
3. Jeppesen, P. and Bower, D. J. (1986) Towards understanding the structure of eukaryotic chromosomes, in *Cytogenetics: Basic and Applied Aspects* (Obe, G. and Basler, A., eds.) Springer-Verlag, Berlin, pp. 1–29.
4. Cooke, C. A., Bernat, R. L., and Earnshaw, W. C. (1990) CENP-B: a major human centromere protein located beneath the kinetochore. *J. Cell Biol.* **110,** 1475–1488.
5. Compton, D. A., Yen, T. J., and Cleveland, D. W. (1991) Identification of novel centromere/kinetochore-associated proteins using monoclonal antibodies generated against human mitotic chromosome scaffolds. *J. Cell Biol.* **112,** 1083–1097.
6. Earnshaw, W. C., Halligan, B., Cooke, C. A., Heck, M. M. S., and Lin, L. F. (1985) Topoisomerase II is a structural component of mitotic chromosome scaffolds. *J. Cell Biol.* **100,** 1707–1715.
7. Tan, E. M. (1982) Autoantibodies to nuclear antigens (ANA): their immunobiology and medicine. *Adv. Immunol.* **33,** 167–240.
8. Moroi, Y., Peebles, C., Fritzler, M. J., Steigerwald, J., and Tan, E. M. (1980) Autoantibody to centromere (kinetochore) in scleroderma sera. *Proc. Natl. Acad. Sci. USA* **77,** 1627–1631.
9. Earnshaw, W. C., Sullivan, K. F., Machlin, P. S., Cook, C. A., Kaiser, D. A., Pollard, T. D., Rothfield, N. F., and Cleveland, D. W. (1987) Molecular cloning of cDNA for CENP-B, the major human centromere autoantigen. *J. Cell Biol.* **104,** 817–829.
10. Earnshaw, W. C. and Rothfield, N. (1985) Identification of a family of human centromere proteins using autoimmune sera from patients with scleroderma. *Chromosoma* **91,** 313–321.

11. Palmer, D. K., O'Day, K., Wener, M. H., Andrews, B. S., and Margolis, R. L. (1987) A 17-kD centromere protein (CENP-A) copurifies with nucleosome core particles and with histones. *J. Cell Biol.* **104,** 805–815.
12. Gooderham, K. and Jeppesen, P. (1983) Chinese hamster metaphase chromosomes isolated under physiological conditions: a partial characterization of associated non-histone proteins and protein cores. *Exp. Cell Res.* **144,** 1–14.
13. Jeppesen, P. and Nicol, L. (1986) Non-kinetochore directed autoantibodies in scleroderma/CREST: identification of an activity recognizing a metaphase chromosome core nonhistone protein. *Mol. Biol. Med.* **3,** 369–384.
14. Johnson, G. D. and Nogueira Araujo, G. M. de C. (1981) A simple method of reducing the fading of immunofluorescence during microscopy. *J. Immunol. Meth.* **43,** 349–350.
15. Giloh, H. and Sedat, J. W. (1982) Fluorescence microscopy: reduced photobleaching of rhodamine and fluorescein protein conjugates by n-propylgallate. *Science* **217,** 1252–1255.
16. Haaf, T., Dominguez-Steglich, M., and Schmid, M. (1990) Immunocytogenetics: IV. Human autoantibodies to heterochromatin-associated proteins. *Cytogenet. Cell Genet.* **53,** 40–51.
17. Whitfield, G. F., Fellows, G., and Turner, B. M. (1986) Characterization of monoclonal antibodies to histone 2B. Localization of epitopes and analysis of binding to chromatin. *Eur. J. Biochem.* **157,** 513–521.
18. Donlon, T. A. and Magenis, R. E. (1983) Methyl green is a substitute for distamycin A in the formation of distamycin A/DAPI C-bands. *Hum. Genet.* **65,** 144–146.
19. Turner, B. M. and Fellows, G. (1989) Specific antibodies reveal ordered and cell-cycle-related use of histone-H4 acetylation sites in mammalian cells. *Eur. J. Biochem.* **179,** 131–139.
20. Mitchell, A., Jeppesen, P., Hanratty, D., and Gosden, J. (1992) The organization of repetitive DNA sequences on human chromosomes with respect to the kinetochore analyzed using a combination of oligonucleotide primers and CREST anti-centromere serum. *Chromosoma* **101,** 333–341.

CHAPTER 16

Immunocytochemical Techniques Applied to Meiotic Chromosomes

Christa Heyting, Axel J. J. Dietrich, J. Hans de Jong, and Edgar Hartsuiker

1. Introduction

During the prophase of the first meiotic division, homologous chromosomes align, pair, recombine, and segregate. These processes are accompanied by the appearance of meiosis-specific structures. Chromosome alignment is accompanied by the formation of axial elements along each chromosome (1); in meiocytes of some species, fibers appear to pull the axial elements of homologous chromosomes together (2). Alignment is followed by a process called synapsis: The axes of homologous chromosomes are closely apposed, and a tripartite structure, called the synaptonemal complex (SC), is formed. It consists of the axial elements of the homologs, connected by transversal filaments, and a central element that is formed on the transversal filaments between the axes (1).

The SC disassembles during diplotene/diakinesis, when chiasmata (resulting from homologous reciprocal exchanges between nonsister chromatids) have been formed. During zygotene and pachytene, electron-dense structures appear on the SCs, the so-called recombination nodules (RNs) (3). In various species, early and late RNs can be discriminated on the basis of their morphology (reviewed in ref. 4). The distribution and number of late nodules correlate with those of chiasmata, and late nodules are, therefore, supposed to have a function in recip-

From: Methods in Molecular Biology, Vol. 29: Chromosome Analysis Protocols
Edited by: J. R. Gosden Copyright ©1994 Humana Press Inc., Totowa, NJ

rocal exchange *(4)*. The significance of the early nodules is still a matter of debate. It has been suggested *(4)* that the early nodules are involved in homology search, and that they can leave gene conversion events without reciprocal exchange as "footprints" of their activity. Thus, when chromosomes have to fulfill meiosis-specific functions, they associate with meiosis-specific structures. Those structures provide just as many good reasons to analyze meiotic chromosomes immunocytochemically: Virtually nothing is known about the composition of these structures, the regulation of their (dis)assembly, and the way in which they perform their presumed functions. One of the strategies to fill these gaps in our knowledge is to isolate the structures, elicit specific antibodies, and use these to identify components to study the assembly and disassembly, and to isolate and characterize genes encoding specific components. In the next paragraphs, we will describe protocols for the isolation of SCs from pollen mother cells (PMCs) of the tomato and for the immunocytochemical staining of SCs with anti-SC antisera.

A method to isolate SCs from rat spermatocytes has been described earlier *(5)*. The procedure involves the purification of spermatocytes, lysis in Triton X-100, EDTA and DTT, digestion of the lysed nuclei with DNase II, and centrifugation through $1.5M$ sucrose. Sixty to eighty percent of the resulting preparation consists of SCs. Most of the substructures of SCs that can be discerned in sections or surface-spread spermatocytes are also present in isolated SCs. These SC preparations have been very useful for the identification and characterization of the major components of SCs *(5–10)*. However, the lateral elements of isolated SCs of the rat appear less dense than in sections, the central element is fragmented or absent, and RNs are very rare *(5)*. Furthermore, zygotene SCs are underrepresented, and (unpaired) axial elements of zygotene SCs from rat spermatocytes are virtually absent in these SC preparations. In an attempt to isolate more complete SCs for immunizations, we turned to the tomato. In hypotonic burst preparations of zygotene up to and including diplotene PMCs of the tomato, SCs show up relatively intact, with complete central elements and abundant early as well as late RNs (depending on the stage). These SCs look particularly useful for the identification and characterization of components of RNs.

Of the procedures required for the immunocytochemical analysis of meiotic prophase chromosomes, the preparative procedures are the most characteristic. These procedures will therefore be described in detail in the next paragraphs. The procedures for immunization and immunocytochemical staining are more or less standard, although several adaptations to the specific properties of meiotic prophase cells are required. Of these procedures, only these adaptions will be discussed.

2. Materials

2.1. Plants

We used the cherry-tomato cv Evita, grown in the greenhouse, as the source of material.

2.2. Solutions

1. 10 mL Acetocarmine solution: 1% carmine in 45% (v/v) acetic acid in distilled water.
2. 10 mL PMC isolation medium: $0.7M$ mannitol, 2% polyvinylpyrrolidone (PVP) (mol-wt average 10,000, Sigma [St. Louis, MO]), $0.1M$ PIPES (Merck no. 10220), 0.56 mM KH_2PO_4, 0.3% potassium dextran sulfate (Calbiochem). Adjust the pH to 5.1 with KOH and filter through a 0.2-μm filter. The solution has to be made fresh; mannitol and PVP are added as solids; the other components are added from stock solutions.
3. 10 mL Lysis mix: 8 mM Tris-HCl, 10 mM EDTA, 1 mM dithiothreitol (DTT), 2% (v/v) Triton X-100, 1 mM phenylmethylsulfonylfluoride (PMSF), pH 7.0; PMSF is added from a $1M$ stock solution in dimethylsulfoxide (DMSO) immediately before use. Filter the solution through a 0.2-μm filter as soon as the PMSF has dissolved. DTT is added immediately before use from a $0.5M$ stock solution.
4. 8 mM Tris-HCl, 1 mM PMSF, pH 7.0, 20 mL buffer A: The PMSF is added immediately (*see* as described for Solution 3) before use. Filter the solution through a 0.2-μm filter as soon as the PMSF has dissolved.
5. DNase II solution: Dissolve 12,000 U of DNase II (Sigma cat. no. D5275) in 1 mL of buffer A. Aliquot in portions of 60 μL, freeze in liquid N_2, and store at −20°C.
6. Cytohelicase solution: Reconstitute 10 mL of freeze-dried cytohelicase (JBF Biotechnics, France) with distilled water, and desalt this solution on a Sephadex G50 column at 4°C in the dark; elute with distilled water. Pool the protein-containing fractions, and freeze-dry again. To obtain the cytohelicase solution, dissolve 100 mg of freeze-dried desalted

cytohelicase in 1 mL 50% (v/v) glycerol in distilled water, and store at
–20°C. The solution is stable for months. NB: Cytohelicase is light-
sensitive: Perform incubations in cytohelicase in the dark.

7. 1.5*M* Sucrose in buffer A, 10 mL. Filter through 0.2 µm.
8. 2.4*M* Sucrose in buffer A, 10 mL. Filter through 0.2 µm.
9. Aprotinine solution: Dissolve 2 mg of aprotinine (Boehringer, [India-
napolis, IN] cat. no. 9815) in 1 mL of buffer A. Aliquot in portions of
100 µL, freeze in liquid N$_2$, and store at –20°C.
10. Trypsin inhibitor solution: Dissolve 10 mg of trypsin inhibitor (Sigma)
in 1 mL of buffer A. Aliquot in portions of 100 µL, freeze in liquid N$_2$,
and store at –20°C.
11. Paraformaldehyde (PFA) (4% w/v): Add 2 g of PFA (Merck [Rahway,
NJ] no. 4005) to 40 mL of distilled water, heat to 70°C while stirring,
and add dropwise 1*N* NaOH until the solution becomes clear. Add 5
mL of 0.1*M* sodium phosphate buffer, pH 7.0, cool to 20°C, and adjust
the pH to 7.3 with NaOH and the vol to 50 mL. Filter through a 0.2-µm
filter, and cool the solution to 4°C. This solution has to be made fresh.
12. 1*M* PMSF in DMSO; store at –20°C.
13. 0.1% β-mercaptoethanol in distilled water, freshly made.
14. 1*M* Sucrose in buffer A, filtered through a 0.2 µm filter.

2.3. Equipment

1. Forceps with fine tips (e.g., Balzers, Lichtenstein) and scalpel no. 11
with holder.
2. Dissection microscope with measuring eye piece.
3. Phase-contrast microscope.
4. Beckman high-speed centrifuge J 2.21 with rotors JS 13 or JS 13.1 and
JA 20 (or equivalents).

3. Methods
3.1. Preparation of Antigens
3.1.1. Outline of the Protocol for the Isolation of SCs from Tomato Anthers

Figure 1 shows the outline of a procedure to isolate SCs from PMCs
of the tomato. In principle, the procedure is similar to the method
described for the isolation of SCs from rat spermatocytes *(5)*. First,
cells in meiotic prophase are purified; then they are lysed, the SCs are
liberated from the chromatin by digestion with DNase II, and then
they are purified by centrifugation through sucrose. However, as will
become clear below, many details of the protocol had to be adapted
to the tomato as source of material.

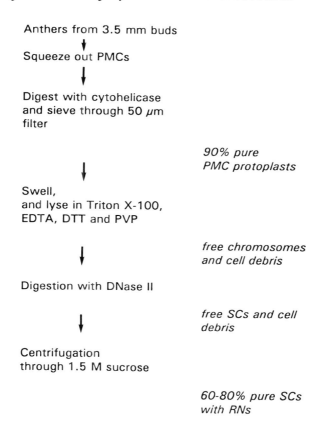

Fig. 1. Outline of the procedure for the isolation of SCs from pollen mother cells of the tomato.

3.1.2. Selection of Buds and Preparation of Anthers

1. Pick about ten 3–4 mm long buds, and measure them precisely, using the dissection microscope with measuring eye piece.
2. Prepare the anthers from the buds as follows: Keep the tip of the sepals between the forceps, and cut the bud across where its diameter is greatest. Thus, the anthers are left intact in the tip of the bud, the part of the petals that is grown together is cut off, and the ovary is cut into two halves.
3. Using a scalpel, lift the upper half of the ovary out of the tip of the bud. Press gently with the blunt side of the scalpel on the tip of the bud, so that the anthers come out. If the petals also come out, push them back with the blunt side of the scalpel while pushing the anthers out.
4. Cut a piece of about 1 mm from the middle of an anther, and put it onto a microscope slide into a drop of solution 1.

5. Squeeze the contents out of the piece of anther by pressure on the coverslip.
6. Examine the contents with a phase-contrast microscope (100× objective). The appearance of aceto-carmine-treated PMCs in meiotic prophase can be found in ref. *2*.
7. Determine the range of bud sizes within which almost all buds contain PMCs in meiotic prophase (we find mostly between 3.2 and 3.6 mm).
8. Collect as many buds of approximately the right size as possible in 0.1% β-mercaptoethanol (buffer A).
9. Select the buds of the right size under the dissection microscope; prepare the anthers from these buds (steps 2 and 3), and collect them in solution 13 on ice.
10. Rinse the anthers twice with distilled water.

3.1.3. Isolation and Lysis
*of Pollen Mother Cells (*See *Note 1)*

The following protocol applies to anthers from 75–200 buds of the right size:

1. Transfer the anthers to a microscope slide, and drain all adhering water with filter paper.
2. Add three drops of isolation medium, and cut all anthers across with a scalpel.
3. Put a second slide onto the anthers, and squeeze the PMCs out by manual pressure. Most of the anthers release their contents as coherent "sausages" consisting of PMCs. This can be observed through the dissection microscope.
4. Transfer PMCs and debris to a small Petri dish, rinse adhering PMCs off the slides into the Petri dish using 1.5 mL of isolation medium, and adjust the vol to 2 mL with isolation medium.
5. Add 25 µL of cytohelican solution, and incubate for 30 min in the dark on a shaker at 20°C. The walls of the PMCs are now digested by the cytohelicase. (*See* Note 2).
6. Disperse the PMCs by pipeting the suspension several times through a fine plastic pipet tip (e.g., Stratagene, La Jolla, CA); this takes about 15 min.
7. Sieve the suspension through a nylon mesh (50-µm pore size) prewetted with isolation medium, and wash the nylon mesh with 2.5 mL of isolation medium. The sieved fluid contains PMCs with partially digested walls. Transfer the PMCs to a plastic 50-mL tube (e.g., Greiner [Solingen, Germany] cat. no. 227261).
8. Mix the suspension well, and take a sample for counting and inspection of the purity of the suspension. We obtain about 4500 cells/anther, of which about 77% is in meiotic prophase. (*See* Note 1)

9. Add 4 mL of buffer A, cap the tube, and mix by quietly turning the tube upside down two to three times.
10. Allow the PMCs to swell for 1 min.
11. Using a plastic 10-mL pipet, blow 9 mL of lysis mix into the suspension, and mix rapidly by pipeting the suspension once with the 10-mL pipet. (The PMCs lyse almost instantaneously, whereas their nuclei fall apart into separate chromosomes. The nuclei of other cell types or stages do not fall apart.) (*See* Notes 3 and 4).
12. Divide the lysate over 18 1.5-mL plastic reaction vessels (1 mL/tube), and pipet in each tube 250 µL of solution 14 underneath the lysate.
13. Centrifuge for 5 min at 2300*g*.
14. Remove the lysate plus 0.5 mm of the 1*M* sucrose cushion. (*See* Note 5).

3.1.4. Digestion of Meiotic Prophase Chromosomes by DNase II

1. Mix each sucrose cushion with 800 µL of buffer A, and add 1.5 µL of each of the solutions 5, 9, 10, and 12/tube.
2. Incubate for 45 min at 20°C on a shaker.
3. After 20 min, add fresh DNase II (1.5 µL of solution 5/tube).
4. During the DNase II digestion, prepare two sucrose step gradients as described in Section 3.1.5., step 3, and make DFA solution (2.2.11.).

3.1.5. Purification of SCs

1. After the DNase II digestion, collect the contents of the ten 1.5-mL tubes in one conical tube, and centrifuge for 1 min at 60*g*.
2. Load the supernatant except the lower 1.0 mL onto the two sucrose step gradients.
3. To make the step gradients, pipet into each of two 15-mL siliconized Corex glass tubes 2 mL of Fluorinert FC77 (3M; St. Paul, MN) and 3 mL of 1.5*M* sucrose. Insert a layer of 400 µL of 2.4*M* sucrose–buffer A between the Fluorinert and the 1.5*M* sucrose layer.
4. Load the DNase II-digestion mixture onto the step gradients.
5. Centrifuge for 50 min at 13,000 rpm in a Beckman JS13.1 rotor at 20°C. The SCs are now in the 2.4*M* sucrose and on the Fluorinert-2.4*M* sucrose interface. (This is just visible as some fine dust on the interface.)
6. Remove the supernatant plus 1 mL of the 1.5*M* sucrose layer. Dry the wall of the tube carefully with paper towels, and remove the remainder of the 1.5*M* sucrose layer.
7. Collect the 2.4*M* sucrose layer; avoid mixing the 2.4*M* sucrose with the Fluorinert. Wash the Fluorinert surface twice with 800 µL of buffer A, and mix these well with the 2.4*M* sucrose, to obtain the final SC suspension.

8. Mix a sample of 100 µL of the SC suspension with 100 µL of PFA solution, and put it on ice for 15 min. Put droplets of 30 µL of this mixture onto an agar filter for ultrastructural analysis *(5)*.

3.2. Analysis of Isolated SCs

Isolated SCs can be analyzed ultrastructurally by means of the agar filtration technique. For this purpose, the final SC suspension is mixed with an equal vol of 4% PFA and incubated on ice for 15 min. Subsequently, droplets of 30 µL of fixed SCs are put onto agar filters. Agar filters are perforated collodion films on dry agar plates (*see* refs. *9* and *11* for the preparation of agar filters). After the SC-suspension has been put onto the filter, the fluid is sucked through the holes into the dry agar before the droplets can evaporate. Therefore, the SCs do not aggregate, but spread evenly on the filter. Agar filters can be stained with uranylacetate and mounted on grids *(5)*.

Figure 2 shows an example of an isolated SC from the tomato after fixation in PFA, agar filtration, and staining with uranylacetate. The preparations of isolated SCs from the tomato differ in several aspects from those of rat SCs:

1. Isolated zygotene SCs of the tomato are not rare;
2. The central element is still intact in isolated tomato SCs; and
3. Recombination nodules are abundant on isolated tomato SCs. It still has to be sorted out which of these differences are owing to differences between the isolation procedures and which to differences between the SCs.

We estimate that about 25% of the SCs from pachytene PMCs are recovered. The recovery of SCs from other stages cannot be estimated, because these SCs tend to clump together.

3.3. Preparation of Anti-SC Antibodies

Anti-SC antibodies can be obtained by standard immunization protocols *(6)*. We have obtained good monoclonal as well as polyclonal antibodies against rats' SCs by immunization according to the following protocol: one injection with 5×10^8 SCs, followed by four injections with 2.5×10^8 SCs; the interval between the injections was 2 wk. Prior to injection, the SCs were pelletted, washed twice with PBS, resuspended in 150 µL of PBS, and sonicated until the pellet had fallen apart. Subsequently, the antigen was mixed by sonication with 150 µL of complete (first injection) or incomplete Freund's adjuvant, and injected ip (mice) or sc and im (rabbits). Native SCs appear to

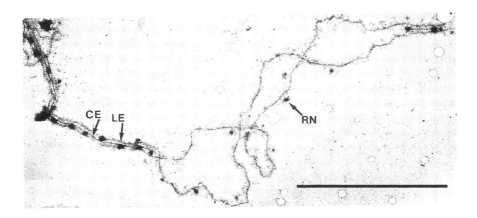

Fig. 2. Agar filtrate of an isolated zygotene SC from the tomato. RN, recombination nodule; CE, central element; LE, laberal element. Bar represents 4 μm.

be more immunogenic than SCs or SC proteins that have been treated with SDS (unpublished observations). For the preparation of monoclonal antibodies, the spleen cells of the immunized mouse are isolated 75 h after the last injection of antigen. We have not yet sorted out whether smaller amounts of SCs per injection are sufficient to elicit antibodies. Also, we have not yet tried to elicit antibodies against tomato SCs.

3.4. Immunocytochemical Analysis of Meiotic Prophase Chromosomes

Meiotic prophase chromosomes have been analyzed immunocytochemically in surface-spread spermatocytes *(6,10),* agar filtrates of lysed spermatocytes *(6),* frozen sections of the testes of rats *(7)* and mice (Dietrich and Heyting, unpublished), and ovaries of mice *(12).* In addition, using a crossreacting polyclonal antirat SC antiserum, we have performed immunocytochemical staining of SCs of the tomato in hypotonic burst *(13)* preparation of PMCs and frozen sections of anthers. (*see* Section 3.4.2.)

3.4.1. Localization in Tissue Sections

We have attempted to analyze meiotic prophase chromosomes immunocytochemically in sections of frozen as well as paraffin-embedded testes of the rat and in frozen sections of anthers of the tomato. We never obtained any signal on sections from paraffin-embedded tissue.

With the rat testis, a strong signal and a reasonable conservation of morphological detail could be obtained with frozen sections that were fixed postsectioning for 45 min at –20°C in acetone *(7)*. A weaker signal and a better conservation of morphology were obtained with frozen sections, fixed for 30 min at 4°C in 1% PFA and 10 mM sodium phosphate buffer, pH 7.3. Glutaraldehyde fixation abolished the antigenicity of all antigens analyzed so far.

For visualization of antibody binding to sections of the testes, we prefer indirect immunofluorescence above the indirect immunoperoxidase technique, because the acetone-fixed sections are damaged considerably during exposure to DAB and H_2O_2. Immunofluorescence staining also has the advantage that it can be used for the analysis of the three-dimensional distribution of antigen within the meiotic prophase nucleus by means of confocal laser scanning microscopy (CSLM) *(see* Fig. 3).

We have also tried to perform immunocytochemical staining of frozen sections of tomato anthers, using a crossreacting polyclonal antiserum elicited against rat SCs, but without much success: Using the indirect peroxidase technique, we could obtain a signal on the SCs in frozen sections of anthers, fixed postsectioning with acetone at –20°C, but the sections were damaged by the exposure to H_2O_2. Indirect immunofluorescence staining with goat-antirabbit FITC conjugate as second antibody had the disadvantage that the anther cells show autofluorescence at the same wavelengths as FITC. It is possible that use of TRITC instead of FITC will provide better results, but we have not yet tested this.

In conclusion, any treatment that may cause crosslinking (e.g., glutaraldehyde fixation) or aggregation (e.g., embedding in paraffin) will reduce or abolish the antigenicity of meiotic prophase chromosomes. If such treatments are avoided, immunocytochemical analysis of meiotic prophase chromosomes in tissue sections may be performed by otherwise standard procedures.

3.4.2. Localization of Antigens in Meiotic Preparations, Obtained by Lysis, Surface Spreading, or Hypotonic Bursting

For the analysis of complete prophase chromosome complements, we have performed immunocytochemical staining of surface-spread spermatocytes *(6,10)*, agar filtrates of lysed spermatocytes *(6,8)*, and preparations obtained by hypotonic bursting *(13)* of PMCs of the tomato.

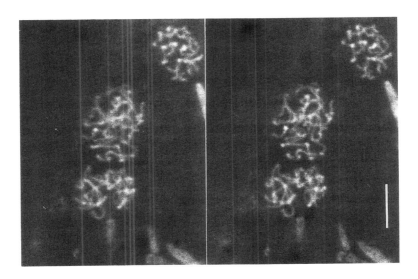

Fig. 3. CSLM analysis of the distribution of an SC antigen in late pachytene spermatocytes in a frozen section of the rat testis. The section was stained by the indirect immunofluorescence technique, with mouse monoclonal antibody II52F10, which recognizes two components of the lateral elements of SCs (of 30 and 33 kDa ref. 6), as first antibody, and goat antimouse FITC conjugate as second antibody. The pictures were taken with a Bio-Rad (Richmond, CA) MRC 600 CSLM equipment with an Argon ion laser, in combination with a Nikon microscope with a 100× objective. Bar represents 10 μm.

For light microscopical analysis, the indirect immunoperoxidase or immunofluorescence staining of agar filtrates of lysed spermatocytes is the most easy and reliable technique. The immunocytochemical incubations can be performed according to standard procedures *(6,9)*.

Unfortunately, agar filtration of lysed PMCs cannot be used for the analysis of whole chromosome complements, because on lysis of PMCs, the chromosomes are not kept together, but float apart immediately. However, preparations obtained by hypotonic bursting *(13)* can also be used for immunocytochemical analysis, as is shown in Fig. 4. Indirect immunoperoxidase staining can be applied to these preparations according to standard procedures *(6,9)*.

Ultrastructural immunocytochemical analysis of whole chromosome complements has been performed by immunogold labeling of agar filtrates of lysed spermatocytes *(6)* and surface-spread spermatocytes *(10)*. *Surface spreading* provides the highest labeling inten-

Heyting et al.

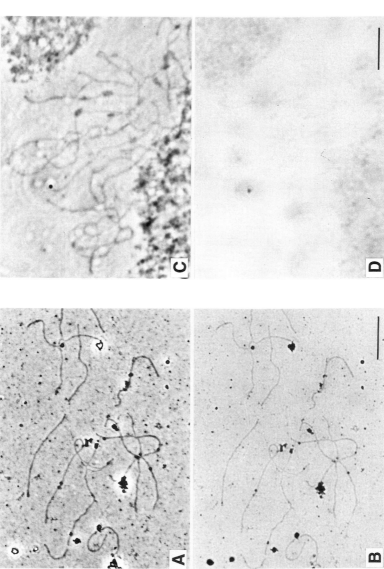

Fig. 4. Immunocytochemical staining of PMCs of the tomato. PMCs were isolated and subjected to the hypotonic burst technique of Stack (*13*). Subsequently, they were incubated with a crossreacting polyclonal antiserum, elicited in a rabbit by immunization with rat SCs, and subjected to indirect immunoperoxidase staining according to standard procedures (*6*). The antiserum also recognizes tomato SCs. **A** and **B**, incubated in immune serum, diluted 1:100; **C** and **D**, incubated in the same dilution preimmune serum. **A** and **C**, phase contrast; **B** and **D**, bright field illumination. Bar represents 10 μm.

sity and best conservation of ultrastructural detail; *agar filtration* allows a higher yield of cells. Immunogold labeling of preparations obtained by the hypotonic burst technique has not yet been attempted. In both types of preparations, access of the antibodies to their targets is enhanced by incubation in DNase I *(9,10)*.

In conclusion, the bottleneck for the immunocytochemical analysis of meiotic prophase chromosomes is the preparation of specific antibodies. Once these have been obtained, there are no obvious obstacles for the immunocytochemical analysis of meiotic prophase chromosomes, provided that conditions are avoided that may hamper access of the antibodies to their target.

4. Notes

1. An essential step in the procedure for the isolation of SCs from the tomato is the purification of PMCs. As has been discussed earlier for the isolation of SCs from the rat *(5,9),* the conditions for cell lysis and enzymatic digestion of chromatin are such that the nuclear matrix falls apart, whereas the SCs remain intact. However, the nuclear lamina is also resistant against these treatments *(14);* fortunately, the lamina is absent from spermatocytes and, apparently, also from PMCs. The purification of PMCs therefore serves to avoid contamination of the SC preparation with nuclear laminae from other cell types. The above described procedure to isolate PMCs yields about 5000 cells/anther, of which about 77% is PMC in meiotic prophase. Most of the contaminating cells or their nuclei are removed by the low speed centrifugation step after the DNase II digestion. The isolation procedure of tomato SCs is derived from an earlier described procedure for the isolation of SCs from the rat *(5).*

    For the tomato, it had to be adapted in several respects as explained in Notes 2–5.

2. Digestion of the cell wall with cytohelicase: This also serves as an extra purification step of the PMCs; other cell types than PMCs are relatively insensitive to cytohelicase. These cells will not lyse in the lysis mixture, and are removed by the low-speed centrifugation step after the DNase II digestion.

3. Shorter exposure to lysis mix: Tomato SCs fall apart after prolonged exposure to the lysis mix.

4. Presence of cytohelicase and PVP during lysis: If these components are omitted during lysis, the tomato SCs will fall apart. Probably the SCs are stabilized by PVP and one or more components of the cytohelicase solution *(15).*

5. Pelletting of the meiotic prophase chromosomes into 1*M* sucrose: In contrast to rat spermatocytes, PMCs do not yield coherent swollen nuclear matrices after exposure to lysis mix, but free meiotic prophase chromosomes (unpublished observations). After centrifugation, these will stick together in a very compact pellet, which is not easily attacked by DNase II.

To avoid such large compact pellets, we perform the cell lysis in several small instead of one large tube; furthermore, to separate the meiotic prophase chromosomes from the lysis mix, we centrifuge them into 1*M* sucrose.

Acknowledgments

We thank J. van Eden and A. C. G. Vink for expert technical assistance.

References

1. von Wettstein, D., Rasmussen, S. W., and Holm, P. B. (1984) The synaptonemal complex in genetic segregation. *Annu. Rev. Genet.* **18,** 331–413.
2. Stack, S. and Anderson, L. K. (1986) Two-dimensional spreads of synaptonemal complexes from solanaceous plants. II. Synapsis in Lycopersicon esculentum (tomato). *Amer. J. Bot.* **73,** 264–281.
3. Carpenter, A. (1975) Electron microscopy of meiosis in Drosophila melanogaster females: II: The recombination nodule: a recombination-associated structure at pachytene? *Proc. Natl. Acad. Sci. USA* **72,** 3186–3189.
4. Carpenter, A. T. C. (1987) Gene conversions, recombination nodules, meiotic recombination and chiasmata. *BioEssays* **6,** 232–236.
5. Heyting, C., Dietrich, A. J. J., Redeker, E. J. W., and Vink, A. C. G. (1985) Structure and composition of synaptonemal complexes, isolated from rat spermatocytes. *Eur. J. Cell Biol.* **36,** 307–314.
6. Heyting, C., Moens, P. B., van Raamsdonk, W., Dietrich, A. J. J., Vink, A. C. G., and Redeker, E. J. W. (1987) Identification of two major components of the lateral elements of synaptonemal complexes. *Eur. J. Cell Biol.* **43,** 148–154.
7. Heyting, C., Dettmers, R. J., Dietrich, A. J. J., Redeker, E. J. W., and Vink, A. C. G. (1988) Two major components of synaptonemal complexes are specific for meiotic prophase nuclei. *Chromosoma* **96,** 325–332.
8. Heyting, C., Dietrich, A. J. J., Moens, P. B., Dettmers, R. J., Offenberg, H. H., Redeker, E. J. W., and Vink, A. C. G. (1989) Synaptonemal complex proteins. *Genome* **31,** 81–87.
9. Heyting, C. and Dietrich, A. J. J. (1991) Meiotic chromosome preparation and labeling. *Meth. Cell Biol.* **35,** 177–202.
10. Moens, P. B., Heyting, C., Dietrich, A. J. J., van Raamsdonk, W., and Chen, Q. (1987) Synaptonemal complex antigen location and conservation. *J. Cell Biol.* **105,** 93–103.
11. Fukami, A. and Adachi, K. (1965) A new method of preparation of a self-perforated microplastic grid and its application. *J. Electron Microsc.* **14,** 112–118.

12. Dietrich, A. J. J., Kok, E., Offenberg, H. H., Heyting, C., Deboer, P., and Vink, A. C. G. (1992) The sequential appearance of components of the synaptoneural complex during meiosis of the female rat. *Genome* **35,** 492–497.
13. Stack, S. (1982) Two-dimensional spreads of synaptonemal complexes from Solanaceous plants. I. The technique. *Stain Technol.* **57,** 265–272.
14. Galcheva-Gargova, A., Petrov, P., and Dessev, G. (1982) Effects of chromatin decondensation on the intra nuclear matrix. *Eur. J. Cell Biol.* **28,** 155–159.
15. de Jong, J. H. and van Eden, J. (1988) The effect of bovine serum albumin and cytohelicase on surface-spread synaptonemal complexes of Rye (*Secale cereale*). *Stain Technol.* **63,** 213–220.

CHAPTER 17

Immortalized Cell Lines

Their Creation and Use in Gene Mapping

Veronica van Heyningen

1. Introduction

Unequivocal physical ordering of genes and genetic markers along chromosomes has been an essential component of gene mapping for much longer than the span of the current genome mapping effort. Human geneticists contemplate mapping a gene as soon as its presence can be identified either directly at the DNA level or through its product (RNA, protein, or even an abnormal disease state). Unlike the situation in the mouse, physical rather than genetic mapping is the method of first choice. Accurate chromosomal localization is usually a multistep process starting first with assignment to one of the 23 chromosomes, and progressing to increasingly refined subregional localization. Somatic cell hybrids and *in situ* hybridization (*see* Chapter 25) have been the techniques most often used.

In situ hybridization, which requires the availability of a cloned DNA probe, allows us to jump directly to the second stage, but the accuracy of subregional assignment afforded by this technique is limited. Very frequently when unequivocal order for relatively close markers is required, preexisting or induced chromosomal breakpoints are used for mapping, although the development of multicolor fluorescent *in situ* hybridization has made possible the ordering of close markers by this method (*see* Chapter 25). Because of the very high efficiency of nonradioactive *in situ* hybridization (in normal diploid

From: *Methods in Molecular Biology, Vol. 29: Chromosome Analysis Protocols*
Edited by: J. R. Gosden Copyright ©1994 Humana Press Inc., Totowa, NJ

cells, both chromosome homologs are labeled with >90% frequency and all four chromatids carry signal in ~75% [J. A. Fantes, unpublished data]), it is now possible to carry out deletion mapping without the need for difficult DNA dosage analysis by Southern blotting or for laborious somatic cell hybrid segregation of deleted chromosomes. This technology will surely become part of the routine repertoire of clinical cytogenetics. It has already been used to demonstrate submicroscopic deletions. However, in many instances, reassessment of patients with new markers has only been possible because Epstein-Barr virus (EBV)-transformed cell lines were available.

In a number of cases, the chief aim is the mapping and isolation of an actual, usually disease-associated, cytogenetic (translocation or deletion) breakpoint. This approach has been an essential component of most of the successes in positional gene cloning (the genes for retinoblastoma, Duchenne muscular dystrophy, Wilms' tumor, neurofibromatosis, familial polyposis, and so forth), most of which were identified as deletion-associated abnormalities. It has also been fundamental to understanding the molecular biology underlying many other tumor-associated cytogenetic rearrangements, particularly in the field of hematological malignancies (*see* Chapter 24). *In situ* hybridization on mitotic chromosome spreads (*see* Chapters 5 and 25) is now the method of choice for the initial definition of the breakpoint(s) with available flanking markers, but in most cases, to clone the actual breakpoint will require the generation of many new markers (e.g., Chapters 20–23) for the region. These will probably include a variety of different types of DNA clones (small phage or plasmid inserts, PCR products, cosmids, and perhaps YAC clones) that require different mapping techniques.

When a particular breakpoint is to be used repeatedly for mapping purposes, it is more or less essential to "immortalize" the breakpoint by setting up a permanent cell line bearing the chromosome of interest. For constitutional cytogenetic changes, setting up an EBV-transformed lymphoblastoid cell line (LCL) from peripheral blood B lymphocytes is the easiest way to achieve this. The technique can only be used for human and primate samples. Among the advantages of this route is that the cell lines almost invariably have exactly the same karyotype as the donor cells—indeed when mosaicism is present in the lymphocyte lineage, it is possible to produce independent cell lines from each component. Only on prolonged culture, usually combined with neglect, are karyotypic changes observed. Assiduous cryopreservation at early stages after transformation will avoid such problems. Other viral transformations, e.g., SV40 or adenovirus, (or constructs derived from these) can be used to immortalize fibroblasts or other cell types, but the process is almost always accompanied by severe karyotypic changes.

If the karyoptypic alteration that needs to be investigated is not constitutional, but arises in somatic cells, for example in association with malignancy, then the preservation of the altered chromosome can be achieved by long term-direct culture or by fusion with an appropriate rodent cell line. Permanent cell lines have been established from a wide variety of cancers, as witnessed by the American and European cell culture collections (*see* Note 1). However, not all malignant cells are amenable to in vitro culture. For these, immortalization by fusion is described below.

When *in situ* hybridization is not the mapping technique of choice, it is frequently necessary to segregate specific rearranged chromosomes from their normal homologs on a rodent cell background in somatic cell hybrids. A large number of breakpoint hybrids have now been produced and accumulated by groups interested in different chromosomes. In many cases, panels covering a whole chromosome with well-spaced breakpoints have been assembled for quick mapping of new markers by Southern blotting or PCR. Some of these panels are now being made available through the Coriell Institute (*see* Note 1).

Selectable markers encoded by the chromosome of interest are essential for efficient hybrid cell production. Classical biochemical selection systems are still the easiest, most efficient, and most widely used. Appropriate mutant rodent cell lines are readily available as fusion partners. The best known systems are: HAT (hypoxanthine, aminopterin, thymidine) selection for the enzymes HPRT (hypoxanthine guanine phosphoribosyl transferase) and TK (thymidine kinase chromosome) on chromosomes X and 17, respectively *(1),* and a related system for the selection of APRT (adenosine phosphoribosyl transferase) on chromosome 16 *(1).* Other rodent cell mutants have been developed to allow selection of a number of different chromosomes. For example, hamster cell lines carrying genes encoding temperature-sensitive aminoacyl t-RNA synthetases have been described for chromosome

5 *(2)*. Working predominantly, but not exclusively, with chromosome 11, we have found selection and screening for human cell-surface marker expression a very useful technique for the isolation of hybrid cells bearing abnormal or fragmented chromosome 11. Although the immunomagnetic bead selection that we favor is transient, the subcloned selected hybrids become increasingly stabilized *(3)*. Immunofluorescent screening, using a fluorescence-activated cell sorter (FACS), is quantitative, so the proportion of cell-surface marker-positive cells gives a clear measure of selection efficacy. There are a number of cell-surface markers encoded on different chromosomes that are widely expressed in different cell types and could be used in the same way (*see* the reports of the International Workshops on Human Gene Mapping published in *Cytogenetics and Cell Genetics*).

If naturally occurring breakpoints are not available in a region of interest, it is possible to produce them by random breakage, usually using X-irradiation *(1)* or CMGT (*see* Chapter 20). The most widely used method recently has been through the lethal, but low-dose X-irradiation of single-chromosome hybrids (somatic cell hybrids carrying a single intact human chromosome), followed immediately by rescue of random chromosome fragments through fusion with another selectable rodent cell line. Human chromosome fragments of interest can then be identified (*see* Chapter 26) and propagated relatively stably as a refined mapping or cloning resource *(4,5)*.

This chapter describes the techniques for:

1. Setting up EBV-transformed permanent cell lines;
2. Cell fusion to produce rodent–human somatic cell hybrids;
3. Cell-surface antigen selection and screening methods to ensure retention of the chromosome of interest; and
4. Preparation of DNA from small cell pellets for marker analysis by molecular techniques.

2. Materials

2.1. EBV Transformation of Lymphocytes

General cell culture facilities include: filtered air-flow hood for tissue culture; bench-top centrifuge with calibrated rev counter and buckets to permit spinning of Universal tubes, as well as 5-mL Nunc (Roskilde, Denmark) tubes; good inverted microscope for looking at cells in culture at various magnifications.

1. Heparinized or EDTA blood sample (*see* Note 2).

2. Lymphoprep (Nycomed, Birmingham, UK).
3. Culture media:
    Serum-free medium: RPMI 1640 alone.
    RPMI-FCS: RPMI + 10% v/v fetal calf serum.
    RPMI-heparin: RPMI + FCS with 10 U/mL mucus heparin added.
4. Sterile 30-mL Universal tubes without label and sterile 5-mL tubes (Nunc) with lids (for small volumes of blood).
5. $0.17M$ NH_4Cl in double-distilled water, sterilized through 0.2-μm filter.
6. EBV stocks—prepared in advance (*see* Section 3.1.1.).
7. Feeder cells—prepared in advance (*see* Section 3.1.2.).
8. Pastets—sterile plastic Pasteur pipets (Alpha Laboratories, Eastleigh, Hampshire, UK).
9. Ninety six-well sterile tissue culture plates, 24-well tissue culture plates, 25-cm^2 tissue culture flasks (Falcon, Nunc, and so on).
10. Plastic insulating tape (1 cm wide).
11. Sterile cotton dental swabs, alcohol, and forceps—for drying plate lid when necessary.
12. Humidified cell culture incubator (37°C).
13. Freezing mix: FCS + 10% (v/v) sterilely handled DMSO (DMSO is so toxic—**Handle in fume hood**—that it is considered sterile when carefully removed from original bottle).
14. Freezing vials (1.8-mL Nunc cryotubes).
15. –70°C Freezer.
16. Freezing box: polystyrene-lined sandwich box with slots cut to hold cryotubes.
17. Liquid nitrogen tank for cell storage.

2.2. Cell Fusion

1. Fast-growing parental cells.
2. Culture medium: All additions are sterile solutions:
    Serum-free, RPMI-FCS—as in Section 2.1.
    RPMI-etc.: RPMI 1640-FCS + 1 mM oxaloacetate + 0.45 mM pyruvate (OAA + PYR diluted from combined 100X aqueous stock solution) + 0.2 IU/mL insulin (from clinical stock 100 IU/mL) + 1.25 mM MOPS buffer (from 100X aqueous stock) (Sigma, St. Louis, MO).
    RPMI-HAT: RPMI-etc. + HAT selective components (final concentrations: $10^{-4}M$ hypoxanthine, $2 \times 10^{-6}M$ aminopterin, $10^{-5}M$ thymidine; after dilution of 50X stock) (*see* Note 3).
    RPMI-HAT-OUA: RPMI-HAT with added ouabain—**Care: toxic!**—(final concentration $3 \times 10^{-5}M$ after dilution of 100X stock) (*see* Note 3).
    RPMI-TG: RPMI-etc. + $3 \times 10^{-5}M$ thioguanine (2-amino 6-mercaptopurine) (diluted from 50X aqueous stock).

3. Polyethylene glycol (PEG) (35% w/v) 1450 (Sigma): Sterile PEG can be prepared in advance and then stored at room temperature in solidi-fied state for dissolving when required. PEG 1450 is weighed out into *glass* Universals in 0.7-g aliquots. Capped Universals containing the PEG flakes are sterilized by autoclaving. Before use, the solidified sterile PEG is melted in the microwave oven (watch, 2–3 min on low setting). Serum-free medium (65% v/w) is added to the molten PEG. Have ready a syringe containing 1.3 mL for fast addition. Liquified PEG should dissolve immediately. If phenol red in medium suggests acidic solu-tion, add a few (2–5) µL of sterile 2*M* Tris base until PEG solution color suggests a pH around 7.8.
4. Trypsin/EDTA solution, T/E: Sterile trypsin stock solution is 0.25% w/v in calcium and magnesium-free Dulbecco's buffered saline. Sterile EDTA stock is 1 m*M* Na$_2$EDTA. Working solution is a 1:1 mixture of these.
5. Tissue culture plasticware as for cell transformation.
6. Cells for fusion in suitable growth state—healthy and free of myco-plasma. Rodent parent cells: HGPRT⁻ mouse myeloma cells, Sp2/0 *(6);* HGPRT⁻ RAG cells *(7);* HGPRT⁻ and TK⁻ Chinese hamster cells, WG3H *(8)* and A3, respectively *(8)*. Sp2/0 and RAG cells can be obtained from ECACC and ATCC (*see* Note 1). Human parent cells: EBV LCL in log phase; normal or leukemic cells from peripheral blood or bone marrow; other malignant tissue, disrupted to single-cell state.

2.3. Cell-Surface Marker Screening and Selection

1. Monoclonal antibody culture supernatant for coating beads. This must be sterilely collected, but one can get away with having azide in there even for selection if coated beads are thoroughly washed free of azide.
2. Negative control monoclonal antibody: Myeloma protein of appropri-ate immunoglobulin class and subclass, e.g., MOPC 21 IgG1, brought from Sigma. If purified immunoglobulin is used, then it should be diluted to 5–10 mL for coating.
3. Magnetic bead separator for Eppendorf tubes (Dynal, Wirral, UK).
4. Sterile Eppendorf tubes.
5. Dynabeads M450 sheep antimouse Ig-conjugated stock at 4 × 10⁸ or 30 mg beads/mL (Dynal). Store carefully at 4°C. These must never be allowed to dry out.
6. Sterile PBS/BSA: PBS with 1% bovine serum albumin added.
7. End-over-end rotary mixer.
8. FITC-conjugated F(ab')$_2$ fragment of goat or sheep antimouse IgG, used at the dilution recommended by the manufacturer. (We use Sigma F 2883).

9. PBS with 1% formaldehyde added (1:40 dilution of "formalin").
10. Fluorescence-activated cell sorter: (Ours is a Becton Dickinson [Oxford, UK] FACScan).

2.4. DNA Preparation from Small Pellets for Marker Analysis

1. Cell pellets containing $5–50 \times 10^6$ cells.
2. Sarstedt straight-sided, round-bottom polypropylene tubes, 4- and 13-mL sizes.
3. Lysis buffer 0.5% SDS, 150 mM NaCl, 100 mM Tris-HCl (pH 8.0), 100 mM EDTA (SDS is freshly added from 10% w/v stock just before use).
4. Boiled RNase, 10 mg/mL stock, stored at –20°C.
5. Pronase, 5 mg/mL stock, stored at –20°C.
6. Water-saturated phenol.
7. Chloroform.
8. Chloroform:isoamyl alcohol, 24:1.
9. Ammonium acetate (7.5M).
10. TE buffer 10 mM Tris-HCl, pH 7.5, 1 mM EDTA.
11. Glass Pasteur pipets.

3. Methods

3.1. EBV Transformation of Lymphocytes

3.1.1. Virus Preparation

This is done in advance as aliquoted bulk preparations. Virus stocks prepared in this way will last for years as frozen stocks in liquid nitrogen.

1. The EBV-producing marmoset cell line B95.8 (*see* Note 1) is grown under prescribed conditions for potentially hazardous virus-producing cells. It is grown as any other established lymphoblastoid cell line in RPMI-FCS to whatever volume of virus preparation it is desired to preserve (we usually produce 100 mL at a time). The cells are grown to saturation density ($5–10 \times 10^5$ cells/mL) in an appropriate number of flasks and left undisturbed (unfed) in a 37°C incubator for 14 d.
2. After 2 wk, spin the culture at 1200 rpm (300g).
3. Collect the supernatant containing the virus particles. Filter through a 0.2-µm sterile filter to remove all live cells and cell debris. (This is essential to ensure that "transformation" is not just a regrowth of B95.8.).
4. The filtered virus preparation is aliquoted directly, without addition of any cryoprotectant, into sterile freezing vials and stored in liquid nitrogen until required.

5. Freshly thawed virus is used each time lymphocyte transformation is attempted. Unused virus is discarded (following autoclaving or hypochlorite treatment to inactivate).
6. New virus preparations should be checked for the ability to transform at high frequency peripheral lymphocytes from unimportant test bloods.

3.1.2. Feeder Cells

Activated mouse peritoneal macrophages collected by sterile peritoneal lavage make excellent feeder cells and phagocytic debris-removers for newly transforming human LCLs (*see* Note 4).

1. Four days prior to peritoneal lavage, mice are injected ip with 0.8 mL 10% of normal strength fluid thioglycollate medium (Difco, Detroit, MI). This means 10% of recommended concentration for bacterial culture, i.e., we use 0.3 g/100 mL.
2. To collect macrophages, the mouse is killed by gentle cervical dislocation (do not stretch mouse too much so that bleeding into the peritoneal cavity is avoided).
3. Ice-cold phosphate buffered saline (Dulbecco A) (8 mL) is carefully injected, using 23-gage needle, into the peritoneal cavity.
4. Leave for 5 min, and then gently turn body to ensure cells are suspended in the lavage fluid.
5. Spray the abdomen with disinfectant (e.g., Hibitane).
6. Insert a new wide bore, 18–19 gage needle, keeping both the beveled needle and the plastic syringe end sterile (i.e., touch only the middle of the needle shaft) so that the lavage fluid can be allowed to drip sterilely, through what is normally the syringe end of the needle, into a Universal tube. (Care must be taken not to puncture the gut since it contains bacteria and so on, and we need sterile cells). Keep collecting tubes on ice to prevent cell loss by adherence to the tube.
7. Spin cells at 2000 rpm (900g) for 10 min at 4°C. Resuspend in fresh PBS, and count nucleated cells by diluting 50 µL of cell suspension in 450 µL of crystal violet solution (0.5% w/v solution of crystal violet in 2% v/v acetic acid), which will lyse any contaminating red cells and stain nuclei to make them visible. Correct for dilution factor when calculating total cell yield.
8. While counting, pellet the cells by centrifugation at 1200 rpm.
9. Resuspend pelleted cells in freezing mix at 2×10^6 or 10×10^6 cells/vial. (Some vials at each concentration are useful for different purposes.)
10. Freeze at controlled rate as for any other cells (*see* Section 3.1.3., no. 8).

11. When required for use as feeder cells, thaw quickly, resuspend in 10 mL RPMI-FCS, and spin immediately at 1200 rpm (300g) to prevent cell loss by adherence.
12. Plate out resuspended cells as required (2×10^6 cells/96-well plate).

3.1.3. Isolation and Transformation of Peripheral Blood Lymphocytes

All procedures are carried out under sterile conditions.

1. Dilute the heparinized or EDTA blood with an equal vol of RPMI + heparin.
2. Load this carefully on top of a cushion of 12 mL Lymphoprep in Universal tube(s) if volume of blood sample is 5 mL or more. Use 1–3 5-mL narrower tubes containing 2.5 mL Lymphoprep for better separation if blood volume is <5 mL. Spin at 3000 rpm (1500g) for 15 min (*see* Note 5).
3. With a Pastet, carefully remove white cells from the interface between the Lymphoprep and the medium above. (The yield should be 2–5 × 10^6 nucleated cells/original mL of blood. It is not necessary to make cell counts once the technique is familiar.) Resuspend in 15 mL RPMI + FCS, and spin at 1500 rpm (500g) for 8 min.
4. Resuspend cells in original blood volume of RPMI + FCS.
5. Use 1 mL of resuspended lymphocytes in a separate Universal, and add two to three drops of freshly thawed EBV. Leave for 15–20 min to allow virus to adsorb to cells at high density of both virus and cells.
6. Dilute with 10–20 mL RPMI + FCS (volume depending on whether there is already medium over feeders in the wells) and plate evenly into 80–96 0.2 mL wells, which may already contain mouse macrophage feeder cells. Wells should be relatively full so that evaporation does not leave medium too hypertonic. We like to tape the plate lid onto the plate with 1 cm insulating tape, partly to make it easier to handle.
7. Any unused peripheral blood lymphocytes are pelleted by spinning and cryopreserved in freezing mix at 3–5 mL blood equivalents (6–20 × 10^6 cells/ mL/vial). Frozen lymphocytes can be transformed nearly as successfully as fresh ones (*see* Note 2).
8. Cryopreservation of live cells is by controlled rate freezing. We achieve this by placing the vials in the freezing box into the –70°C freezer overnight and then transferring quickly to the liquid nitrogen tank. (Cells must not get above the critical temperature of –50°C at any stage after freezing.)

9. Transforming cells are fed every 2–3 d by replacing half to two-thirds of the old medium with fresh RPMI + FCS using sterile Pastets to remove and add medium. Great care must be taken to avoid cell–cell cross contamination. We use 1 Pastet/8-well vertical column to remove culture supernatant to be replaced with fresh medium. Novices should transform each individual cell line on a separate plate.
10. Transforming cells will be seen to clump and to look refractile, but "hairy" with villous projections. They will often be found at the edges of wells.
11. When 0.2-mL wells look thick with cells, their content is transferred to 2-mL wells, 2 × 2 mL wells, and eventually to 25-cm² flasks.
12. Transformed cells are cryopreserved at high density (2–5 × 10⁶ cells, equivalent to at least half the contents of a well-grown 10-mL culture, in 1 mL freezing mix, per vial). Plenty of vials (at least 6/cell line) should be put away soon after transformation when cells are growing well and likely to be karyotypically unaltered.
13. If clonal transformation is desired for some reason (e.g., because of suspected mosaicism), contents of individual 0.2-mL wells should be kept separate, and more vials should be preserved.
14. In general, it is a good idea to prepare chromosomes or freeze away cell pellets for DNA or RNA preparation soon after transformation when cells are healthy and vigorous, although in principle this state should be attainable again at any time with careful husbanding of frozen stocks.
15. Nomenclature of cell lines is a matter of individual preference. We like to give five letter names that can be pronounced and remind us of the patient's name. We tend to keep the last three letters pertaining to the family name, the same for each member of a family (e.g., ROSMI, JOSMI, PASMI—Rosemary, John, and Paul Smith). Record keeping of patient data, liquid nitrogen maps, and vials, as well as detailed cell culture histories are also of enormous importance.

3.2. Cell Fusion

This is the method we use most frequently for all types of cells. Most of our fusions involve selection in HAT for HGPRT, since the chromosomes of interest to us usually carry no particular routinely selectable biochemical marker. The rodent parent cell lines that we use are therefore thioguanine resistant. There is some evidence that fusion between cells of similar ontogenic origin produces a higher frequency of hybrid cells. We tend to fuse LCL or peripheral leukocytes with Sp2/0 myeloma cells, unless an attached hybrid cell is required for some reason, such as cell-surface marker expression. For other fusions, we use RAG or WG3H as the mouse or hamster parent line. If malignant cells from freshly collected tissue are to be used, the tissue needs to be disaggregated to a single-cell suspension for fusion.

1. Thioguanine-resistant rodent parent cells are taken out of liquid nitrogen and put into culture at least 2 wk before the scheduled fusion. Cells should be fast-growing and in log phase at time of harvesting for fusion. If there is any doubt about thioguanine resistance, the cells should be cultured in the presence of thioguanine for three passages, before returning to RPMI-etc. HGPRT$^-$ status should be checked by demonstrating 100% cell death in RPMI-HAT.

2. If the human parental line is an EBV LCL, it should be growing vigorously and at log phase for fusion. Normally 5–10-fold excess of human cells is used in fusions with Sp2/0, RAG, or WG3H. We routinely aim at 10^7 human:1–2 × 10^6 mouse cells. Hamster fusions are generally more efficient, and a three-to fivefold reduction in total numbers is possible, ratios remain 10:1, human:hamster. Similarly, I would try a 10:1 ratio with freshly dissociated malignant cells.

3. Parent cells that grow attached to the substratum have to be harvested by trypsinization. For each 25-cm^2 flask, discard the culture medium, gently rinse cells with 2.5 mL trypsin, and add about 2 mL fresh trypsin to loosen cells. When cells have rounded up and detached, gently pipet into RPMI-FCS to stop trypsin action with excess protein.

4. Centrifuge the harvested cells at 1200 rpm (300g), and wash pellet well with serum-free medium three times before fusion.

5. Other parental cells are collected by centrifugation and also washed three times in serum-free medium.

6. Parental cells in serum-free medium are added together in a Universal tube at the appropriate ratio (10:1 peripheral leukocyte to rodent cell, 5:1 for LCL).

7. The cells are spun together at 1200 rpm (300g) for 5 min.

8. All media are removed from the pellet using a narrow-tip Pastet. Pellet is tapped loose.

9. Freshly made up 35% PEG 1450 (0.5 mL) is added, the stop watch is started, and the cells are mixed by agitation.

10. Centrifuge cell suspension gently at 700 rpm (100g) for 5 min.

11. Eight minutes after PEG addition, add 5 mL serum-free medium, gently layering it on top of the still present PEG, without disturbing the pellet. Then swirl to resuspend gently over 3–4 min, to give a single-cell suspension.

12. Centrifuge at 1200 rpm for 5 min.
13. Remove supernatant carefully. Add 5 mL RPMI-HAT slowly without disturbing the pellet. Leave for 5–7 min, and then swirl gently to resuspend.
14. Make up to required volume with RPMI-HAT for dispensing into flasks or plates. We usually plate a 1–2 × 10^6 rodent cell fusion into 4 × 96 wells or 10 × 25 cm^2 flasks. The wells may already contain feeder cells, or feeders may be plated as a mixture with the freshly fused cells. (Remember that when feeder cells are required for cells under HAT selection, the macrophages can be plated directly in HAT since normal cells survive.) Attached cells (L-cells, RAG, and WG3H or A3) are normally seeded into flasks for subsequent colony picking.
15. Plated cells are incubated in the humidified CO_2 incubator, and the medium is changed (about $3/4$ is removed and replaced) every 2–3 d.
16. At the first medium change, RPMI-HAT-OUA is used to kill off the human parental cells. This double selection is repeated for at least three further media changes.
17. Hybrid cell clones are picked from 0.2-mL wells with the aid of individual sterile Pastets and transferred into 2-mL wells on 24-well plates. Monolayer cell clones are usually not too firmly attached for picking with a sterile disposable bacterial loop from a well drained flask. These are also deposited into 2-mL wells. In both cases, selection in RPMI-HAT continues until the first cells are frozen away.
18. As the cells multiply, they are subbed up into 25-cm^2 flasks from which two to four ampules are frozen before significant analysis is carried out. T/E treatment may be necessary to harvest cells from flasks.
19. Analysis for chromosome-specific markers begins around the time of first freezing.
20. Cryopreservation of cells, carried out as described for EBV-transformed cells, requires care and attention to naming, labeling, storage, and record keeping.
21. Cells are harvested for marker analysis in different ways for different analyses (*see* Note 6).
22. As soon as markers of interest are shown to be present, subcloning for stabilization begins. Different cell types are subcloned in different ways (*see* Note 7).
23. Subclones are analyzed in the same way as primary clones. The aim of subcloning is to stabilize the hybrid cell bearing the chromosome of interest and to ensure that this is present at high frequency (*see* Note 8).

3.3. Cell-Surface Marker Selection and Screening

3.3.1. Immunomagnetic Bead Selection for Cells in Suspension

The most efficient separation and simplest experimental protocol is achieved by precoating the beads with the monoclonal antibody chosen to recognize the human cell-surface markers. For the chromosome on which we have done the most work, chromosome 11 *(3)*, four or five different cell-surface antigen systems have been defined. They are encoded by genes at different positions along both chromosome arms. They are widely expressed in different proliferating cell types (i.e., most are expressed on Sp2/0, RAG, and WG3H backgrounds). However, one of the four is expressed only on adherent, fibroblastic cells. We have been able to select specifically for deleted chromosome 11 homologs and for the two halves of translocation chromosomes, so providing us with excellent material for mapping by many different techniques.

1. Wash 1 mg (33 μL = 1.3×10^7) of stock beads (which must always be stored carefully without drying out) three times in sterile PBS/BSA. Each time, they are "pelleted" using the powerful magnetic Eppendorf tube rack.
2. Incubate the washed beads in 1 mL of sterile hybridoma culture supernatant (1–10 μg/mL Ig) for 10 min with end-over-end rotation at room temperature. Occasionally, it may be advantageous to coat the beads with a mixture of more than one antibody directed to different epitopes of the same antigen or sometimes to different antigens. In these cases, use a 1:1 mixture of the antibodies.
3. Pellet the coated beads with the magnet and discard the spent antibody. Wash the beads three times with PBS/BSA. All excess antibody must be removed, since it would interfere with efficient cell selection. Coated beads can be stored in PBS/BSA for several days, certainly for up to a week.
4. Harvest the hybrid cells for antibody selection. Wash with sterile PBS/BSA. Cells from even one near-confluent 2-mL well (1.5 cm² growth area—yielding perhaps $2-5 \times 10^4$ cells depending on cell density and cell size) are often sufficient for selection. For the next stage, it is necessary to have some idea of cell numbers, but with experience of different cell types, exact counting is not required.

5. Transfer washed cells in fresh PBS/BSA to a sterile Eppendorf tube, and add 1–2 coated beads/cell. Incubate for 30 min at room temperature with end-over-end rotation. Cells in the presence of beads must be treated gently to avoid mechanical damage.
6. After adsorption, the beads are pelleted, the supernatant is discarded (**unless clones resulting from negative selection are desired**), and the beads hopefully with some cell-surface marker-positive cells attached are gently washed three times in sterile serum-free medium. The gently resuspended cells are transferred to 2-mL wells.

3.3.2. Selection of Colonies of Attached Cells

When RAG or WG3H hybrids are being selected, it is much more efficient to pick whole positive colonies. The bead selection can also be carried out in a 25-cm^2 culture flask on cells growing as independent clones.

1. The beads are used merely as visual markers for positive cells. A suspension of about 10^4 coated beads in 1 mL of PBS/BSA is added to the rinsed cells. The flask is incubated at room temperature for 30 min.
2. Positive clones are revealed when the flask, without washing away excess beads, is gently rocked, and any clusterings of beads over cell colonies are investigated under the microscope.
3. Marked colonies are then picked into fresh medium using a sterile disposable bacterial loop to scrape off cells from the gently drained flask.

This procedure is nondestructive and can be repeated with the same flask at a later date to select slower-growing and possibly more stable cells. Attached beads on the picked cells in both types of selection are found eventually to dissociate from the cell, and the cells continue to divide to produce a new selected colony.

3.3.3. Quantitative FACS Analysis for Cell-Surface Marker Expression

1. All cells have to be in suspension for analysis by FACS, so harvest attached cells by trypsinization to produce a single-cell suspension without clumps, which might clog the flow system. Loosely attached Sp2/0 hybrids are also harvested into 5-mL sterile Nunc tubes; 1–2 × 10^5 cells/assay are sufficient for modern FACS. **Do not forget to run a negative control antibody for each cell line.** If several antigens, encoded in different regions of the chromosome of interest, are available for analysis, hybrids should be checked for all of them at some point, since chromosome breakage may occur. We have picked up problems early in this

way, and we could be relatively certain that the clones we chose finally were likely to carry the "native" chromosome.

2. Wash pelleted cells in PBS/BSA, and repellet (1200 rpm for 5 min at 4°C).
3. Resuspend pellet in 200 μL of hybridoma culture supernatant, and incubate on ice for 30–60 min.
4. Wash away excess antibody with three washes in 2.5 mL PBS/BSA. Pellet at 1200 rpm for 5 min at 4°C between washes.
5. During this incubation period, make up a sufficient volume of FITC antimouse Ig for the next stage; 120 μL/tube are needed of a 1:40 dilution in PBS/BSA. This is centrifuged for 15 min in a cooled microcentrifuge to remove any antibody complexes that might increase the background.
6. Resuspend washed pellets in the diluted second antibody, leave on ice for 30 min.
7. Wash away unbound antibody thoroughly (3 × 2.5 mL PBS/BSA, 1200 rpm for 5 min at 4°C).
8. Resuspend the final pellet thoroughly in PBS with 1% formaldehyde.
9. Cells are now ready for FACS analysis, which is carried out according to the manufacturer's instructions, with gating and appropriate scatter values for each cell type (*see* Note 9).
10. If necessary, cells can be kept in the fixed state for 2–3 d at 4°C, in the dark (foil-covered) to prevent FITC fading, before FACS analysis needs to be delayed.

Examples of the type of data to be obtained are shown in Seawright et al. *(3),* although the exact format shown is from a Becton Dickinson FACS IV. Although we have not encountered this problem with any of the antigen systems we have used, there may be occasions when 100% positivity never seems achievable, however, many times a hybrid is subcloned. There may be cases where antigen expression varies with the cell cycle, for example, and so there may always be a proportion of negative cells. This can only be ascertained by comparing FACS results with cytogenetic analysis (*see* Chapter 5). It may then be possible to adjust conditions to maximize expression.

3.4. DNA Preparation from Frozen Cell Pellets

3.4.1. Preparation of Cell Pellets for Freezing

1. Harvest cells when still in log phase of growth, but near confluence. They should be adequately, but not overtrypsinized (stop trypsin action efficiently, e.g., with RPMI-FCS).
2. Wash twice with large volumes of PBS.

3. Count cells if you are not highly experienced in gaging pellet size. Variation in cell size means that different sized pellets may be produced from the same cell numbers.

4. Suspend the requisite number of cells in 1 mL PBS/Eppendorf tube. After spinning for 2 min in a microcentrifuge, the supernatant is thoroughly removed with a narrow-tip plastic Pastet.

5. Pellets are stored at –40°C until required. It is more efficient to prepare several DNA samples simultaneously.

3.4.2. Preparation of DNA

1. Thaw frozen cells quickly; suspend in a minimum volume to transfer quickly and efficiently to a Sarstedt tube (4 mL for 5×10^6 cells; 13 mL for 5×10^7 cells).

2. Quickly add appropriate volume of lysis buffer (1 mL for 5×10^6 cells; 5 mL for 5×10^7 cells), whirlimixing all the time.

3. Add 10 μL RNase/mL of lysate. Incubate at 37°C for 1 h.

4. Add 50 μL Pronase/mL of lysate. Incubate at 37°C for 4 h with occasional vortexing, or at 37°C for 1 h and 10 min at 56°C, or at 37°C overnight—whichever is most convenient.

5. Extract lysate with an equal volume of water-saturated phenol, mix for 5 min, spin at 2500–3000 rpm (1200–1800g) for 10 min to separate phases, and remove the upper aqueous layer to clean a tube for further extraction.

6. Extract lysate with an equal volume of phenol chloroform, mix for 5 min, spin at 2500–3000 rpm for 10 min, and remove the upper aqueous layer to a clean tube for further extraction.

7. Extract with chloroform isoamyl alcohol, mix for 5 min, spin at 2500–3000 rpm for 10 min, remove the upper aqueous layer to a clean tube for further extraction.

8. Add $^1/_2$ volume of 7.5M ammonium acetate, and then add $2^1/_2$ vol of absolute alcohol. Rock tubes back and forth, and when the DNA precipitates, it will be visible as a mass of white fibers.

9. Spool out this high-mol-wt DNA using a glass Pasteur pipet with a flame-sealed end.

10. Air-dry the DNA, and then wash it still on the tip of the Pasteur pipet in an Eppendorf tubeful of 66% ethanol and 0.8M ammonium acetate (diluted from 7.5M stock). Allow DNA to air-dry.

11. To dissolve the spooled DNA, cut off the sealed end of the pipet with the DNA on, using a diamond-tipped cutter. Place this carefully into a fresh Eppendorf tube containing TE buffer. The ideal final concentra-

tion of the DNA is 1 mg/mL. It will take overnight in the cold room for the DNA to dissolve. The theoretical yield from 5×10^7 cells is 300 µg.

12. Estimate DNA concentration by measuring absorbance, at 260 and 280 nm, of a 1 in 200 dilution (400 µL needed for a narrow cuvet). A 1 mg/mL solution of DNA gives an absorbance of 20 at 260 nm.

The description of techniques used to analyze the human DNA content of cell hybrids is beyond the scope of this chapter (*see* Chapters 20, 23, and 25).

4. Notes

1. American Type Culture Collection (ATCC)
12301 Parklawn Drive
Rockville, MD 20852
TEL: (1) 301-881-260
FAX: (1) 301-231-5826

   Coriell Institute for Medical Research
401 Haddon Avenue
Camden, NJ 08103
TEL: (1) 609-757-4848
FAX (1) 609-964-0254

   European Collection of Animal Cell Cultures (ECACC)
PHLS Centre for Applied Microbiology and Research
Porton Down
Salisbury
Wiltshire SP4 0JG
TEL: (44) 980 610391
FAX: (44) 980 611315

   These organizations also have important, increasing collections of cell lines, many with well-defined cytogenetic breakpoints, in some instances associated with specific disease states. See their catalogs for safety recommendations for the handling of a large variety of malignant and transformed cells. EBV-producing cell lines can be obtained from ECACC (no. 85011419); ATCC (CRL 1612); Coriell Institute (GM 07404).

2. Blood collected preferably not more than 48 h prior to processing is needed for successful transformation. Normal heparin or EDTA tubes are suitable for collection, but we now believe that EDTA blood transforms rather more quickly and at higher efficiency (on a per cell basis).

However, we have a >95% success rate either way, if no other problems are present. Problems include badly mixed, clotted samples, old samples, and contamination. If cryopreserved lymphocytes are available, transformation can be tried again at a later date. This is also useful if there are karyotypic alterations and no unaltered cell lines frozen away.

3. Hypoxanthine, thioguanine, and aminopterin are all difficult to dissolve. They should dissolve in half the final volume of dilute alkali (0.1M NaOH). pH is then adjusted to 8.0 with 1M HCl. Thymidine should dissolve in distilled water and can be added to HA after pH adjustment. The solution is then made up to required volume. Stocks are filter-sterilized and stored at −20°C in aliquots. Ouabain dissolves easily in distilled water. It is a highly toxic cardiac glycoside and should be treated with great care.

4. In the UK, Home Office licenses are required to carry out the thioglycollate injection part of this procedure.

5. Recently, we have experimented successfully with selective red cell lysis using ammonium chloride solution, which should leave the white cells intact. Take about 1 mL heparinized or EDTA blood. Spin it in a Universal at 2000 rpm. Remove the serum carefully, add 3 mL of ice-cold 0.17M NH$_4$Cl, and leave for 10 min on ice. Add 15 mL RPMI + FCS and spin at 1200 rpm (330g). Resuspend in 1 mL RPMI + FCS, and transform as usual.

6. For cell-surface marker analysis, freshly harvested viable cells are required; *see* Section 3.3. For DNA preparation or enzyme analysis, frozen cell pellets work well. Independent clones can be collected and screened in batches for convenience. (It must, however, be remembered that early rodent–human hybrids are very unstable, and subcloning should be initiated as soon as possible on clones of interest.) We harvest healthy, not over-confluent cells by collecting a cell suspension, following trypsinization, if required, and pelleting from the spent culture medium by centrifugation at 1200 rpm (330g). The cells are washed in a large volume of PBS, pelleted as before, and resuspended at an appropriate density so that a 1-mL suspension will provide enough cells for DNA preparation, lysis for enzyme assay, and so forth. In general, 75% of the contents of a 25-cm^2 flask will be sufficient for screening purposes, although making DNA from small cell pellets is a skilled task, especially if Southern blotting quality and quantity is required. Analysis by PCR is much easier and quicker and should be the method of choice.

7. We tend to release the hybrids from general selection at the time of cloning, unless the selection is maintaining the chromosome of inter-

est. Otherwise, if selection was only to ensure hybrid cell formation and to help kill off parental cells, this is the stage to stop using it. HAT selection has to be released with care, adding HT without aminopterin, until the latter is diluted out by growth and new enzyme synthesis from the dihydrofolate reductase to which it is tightly bound as competitive inhibitor.

Subcloning of attached cell is by plating very dilute single-cell suspension cultures into 25-cm^2 flasks (no more than 100 cells/flask). Unattached cells are cloned by limiting dilution into wells; this should be carried out by 1 in 10 serial dilution with no greater than 1:50 dilution for the final step, which should give about 1 cell/well. We use bijoux tubes and sterile micropipets to effect this. Remember to keep the cells in even suspension, both when making dilutions and when plating out.

If cloning efficiency is found to be too low, then the theoretical cell number per well has to be increased until clones are seen at reasonable frequency. (Poison distribution tells us that we should have single-cell clones if only 37% of wells have any colony growth in them at all.)

8. FACS analysis for human cell-surface marker expression is quantitative; enzyme analysis by electrophoretic separation and Southern blotting with cross-species hybridizing probes are semiquantitative measures of human chromosome content *(3)*.

9. If the signal for a particular antigen–antibody combination is very weak, it is usually because the number of molecules displayed on the cell surface is low. Signal-to-noise ratio can sometimes be improved by using a stronger, but more labile, fluorochrome. We have used phycoerythrin-conjugated antibody from Serotec (Oxford, UK) in such cases.

References

1. Shay, J. W., ed. (1982) *Techniques in Somatic Cell Genetics.* Plenum, New York.
2. Wasmuth, J. J. and Carlock, L. R. (1986) Chromosomal localization of human gene for histidyl tRNA synthetase: clustering of genes encoding aminoacyl tRNA synthetases on human chromosome 5. *Somatic Cell Mol. Genet.* **12,** 513–517.
3. Seawright, A., Fletcher, J. M., Fantes, J. A., Morrison, H., Porteous, D. J., Li S. S-L., Hastie, N. D., and van Heyningen, V. (1988) Analysis of WAGR deletions and related translocations with gene-specific DNA probes, using FACS-selected cell hybrids. *Somatic Cell Mol. Genet.* **14,** 21–30.
4. Cox, D. R., Burmeister, M., Price, E. R., Kim, S., and Myers, R. M. (1990) Radiation hybrid mapping: a somatic cell genetic method for constructing high resolution maps of mammalian chromosomes. *Science* **250,** 245–250.

5. Richard, C. W., Withers, D. A., Meeker, T. C., Maurer, S., Evans, G. A., Myers, R. M., and Cox, D. R. (1991) A radiation map of the proximal long arm of human chromosome 11 containing the multiple endocrine neoplasia type I (MEN1) and bcl-1 disease loci. *Am. J. Hum. Genet.* **49,** 1189–1196.
6. Shulman, M., Wilde, C. D., and Kohler, G. (1978) A better cell line for making hybridomas secreting specific antibodies. *Nature* **276,** 269–270.
7. Klebe, R. J., Chen, T-R., and Ruddle, F. H. (1970) Controlled production of proliferating somatic cell hybrids. *J. Cell Biol.* **45,** 74–82.
8. Westerveld, A., Visser, R. P. L. S., Meera Khan, P., and Bootsma, D. (1971) Loss of human genetic markers in man-Chinese hamster somatic cell hybrids. *Nature New Biol.* **234,** 20–24.

CHAPTER 18

Oligonucleotide Primed
in Situ DNA Synthesis (PRINS)

An Alternative to in Situ *Hybridization
for Gene Mapping and the Investigation
of Genome Organization*

John R. Gosden and Diane Lawson

1. Introduction

The technique of *in situ* hybridization has come of age, it being more than 21 years since the first descriptions of the procedure were published *(1)*. In that time, the capabilities of the method have expanded enormously. In the early years, the sensitivity (minimum size of target capable of being detected) was restricted to highly repeated DNA sequences, such as satellite DNAs, and detection was exclusively by autoradiography of radioisotopic label (e.g., ref. 2). In time, it became possible to map unique sequences (e.g., ref. *3*), but this was a tedious procedure involving the analysis of grain distribution over large numbers of metaphase spreads, in order to distinguish specific hybridization signal from background grains.

In 1980, Bauman et al. *(4)* described a method of *in situ* hybridization using a fluorochrome bound directly to a DNA probe, and this was followed over the next few years by a plethora of reports describing nonisotopic ways of modifying DNA, while still allowing it to be hybridized *in situ*. These methods generally involve making the DNA specifically antigenic, and include incorporating biotin into the DNA enzymically *(5)*, treating the DNA with acetylaminofluorene *(6)*,

From: *Methods in Molecular Biology, Vol. 29: Chromosome Analysis Protocols*
Edited by: J. R. Gosden Copyright ©1994 Humana Press Inc., Totowa, NJ

mercurating the DNA and coupling sulfhydryl-hapten ligands *(7)*, and incorporating digoxigenin into the DNA enzymically *(8)*. Of these, the two that have been most widely applied have been the enzymic labeling of DNA with biotin or digoxigenin (*see* refs. *9* and *10* and Chapters 25 and 26).

Nonisotopic *in situ* hybridization has reached its most sophisticated level in the elegant experiments using multiple labels described by Nederlof et al. *(11)*, but the limitations of the technology lie largely in the sensitivity of the technique—what is the smallest target that can be detected? For most cases, this seems to be in the range of 2.5–5 kilobases (kb). Although occasional reports appear describing the mapping of smaller probes (e.g., *12*), these are the exception rather than the rule, so that mapping DNA markers for which only smaller probes are available requires a fundamentally different approach. Such a method was described by Koch et al. *(13)*, with the first use of oligonucleotide primed *in situ* synthesis (PRINS).

In the PRINS method, an unlabeled oligonucleotide is annealed, under stringent conditions, to the DNA of denatured chromosomes. A DNA polymerase then extends the primer by synthesizing a copy of the complementary strand of the DNA duplex, incorporating biotin or digoxigenin-tagged nucleotides. The biotin or digoxigenin are then detected immunocytochemically, and the location of these reporter molecules indicates the site of annealing of the initial primer. Although this approach was first used to detect tandem repeated DNA sequences, the sensitivity has been improved to the point where it is used to detect very low copy repeats, e.g., the human β-satellite, which has only 25 copies of a 68 bp sequence on chromosome 9 *(14)*, and is potentially capable of detecting single-copy sequences, if the oligonucleotide primer and the annealing and extension conditions can be optimized. The selection of appropriate oligonucleotide primers is critical, and we find the OLIGO program *(15,16)* invaluable for this.

2. Materials

2.1. Primed in Situ *Synthesis*

1. 2'-Deoxyadenosine 5'-triphosphate (dATP): 100 m*M* solution (Pharmacia, Brussels, Belgium).
2. 2'-Deoxycytidine 5'-triphosphate (dCTP): 100 m*M* solution (Pharmacia).
3. 2'-Deoxy-guanosine 5'-triphosphate (dGTP): 100 m*M* solution (Pharmacia).
4. 2'-Deoxythymidine 5'-triphosphate (dTTP), 100 m*M* solution (Pharmacia).

5. 5-(n-[n-Biotinyl-ε-aminocapryl]-3-aminoallyl)-2'-deoxyuridine 5'-tri-phosphate (Bio-11-dUTP) (Sigma, St. Louis, MO).
6. Biotin-16-2'-deoxyuridine-5'-triphosphate (Bio-16-dUTP) (Boehringer, Mannheim, Germany).
7. Digoxigenin-11-deoxyuridine-5'-triphosphate (DIG-11-dUTP) (Sigma) (*see* Note 3).
8. Fluorescein-12-dUTP (Boehringer) (*see* Note 3).
9. Oligonucleotide primer (*see* Table 1) at 250 ng/μL.
10. *Taq*1 DNA polymerase (either Boehringer *Taq*1 or Ampli*Taq* [Perkin-Elmer, Norwalk, CT] cloned enzyme) (*see* Note 4).
11. Formamide (Analar).
12. 20X SSC: 3.0M NaCl, 0.30M trisodium citrate, pH 7.5.
13. Taq buffer (10X): 500 mM KCl, 100 mM Tris-HCl, pH 8.3, 15 mM $MgCl_2$, 0.1% BSA.
14. Twin-frost glass microscope slides and 20 × 40 coverslips, soaked in absolute ethanol to which concentrated HCl has been added at the rate of 1 mL/100 mL. The slides and coverslips are removed from the acid/alcohol and polished with clean muslin shortly before dropping the chromosome preparations. These are referred to as clean slides and coverslips.
15. Water bath at 70°C.
16. Water bath at 60°C.
17. Water bath (or incubator) at 50°C.

2.2. Detection

1. Dried skimmed milk powder.
2. Avidin DCS-fluorescein isothiocyanate (Av-FITC) (Vector Labs, Burlingame, CA).
3. Avidin DCS-Texas Red (Av-TR) (Vector Labs).
4. Biotinylated goat antiavidin (Bio-anti Av) (Vector Labs).
5. Antidigoxigenin-fluorescein isothiocyanate (anti-DIG-FITC) (Boehringer).
6. Propidium iodide (PI).
7. 4',6-diamidino-2-phenylindole·2 HCl (DAPI).
8. Spermidine *bis*-acridine (CMA_2S) (*see* separate protocol).
9. Citifluor AF3 (Citifluor).
10. Citifluor AF10 (Citifluor).
11. Glycerol for fluorescence microscopy (Merck, Poole, Dorset, UK).
12. Blocking buffer; 4X SSC (diluted from stock 20X SSC), 0.05% Triton X-100, 5% skimmed milk powder.
13. Wash buffer; 4X SSC, 0.05% Triton X-100.
14. Water bath (or incubator) at 45°C.
15. Water bath (or incubator) at 37°C.

Table 1
Sequences of Oligonucleotide Primers Used in PRINS

Name	Origin	Sequence
211 (22-mer)	Alu, 5' end of consensus	CCCAAAGTGCTGGGATTACAGG
450 (19-mer)	Alu, lacking 3 bases from 211	AAAGTGCTGGGATTACAGG
451 (26-mer)	Alu, 3' end of consensus	GTGAGCCGAGATCGCGCCACTGCACT
339 (16-mer)	Alphoid, consensus	TCAGAAACTTCTTTGT
340 (16-mer)	Alphoid, adjacent to 339	GAATGCTTCTGTCTAG
405 (30-mer)	Alphoid	AAAGAAGCTTTCTGAGAAACTGCTTAGTGT
266 (30-mer)	Core sequence from satellite III	[CCATT]$_6$
267 (35-mer)	Diverged satellite III	AATGGGATGGAGTGGAATCAACCCAATGGAATGG
B18 (31-mer)	Core sequence from satellite II	CGTTTGATTCCATTTGATGTTGATTCCATTC
435 (26-mer)	β-sat repeat (ref. *14*)	AGTGCAGAGATATGTCACAATGCCCC
527 (35-mer)	β-sat repeat	TCCAAAGCCCATGTAGGCCGAGCCAAGACAAGAGT
394 (24-mer)	Trypanosoma telomere-specific repeat	[TTAGGG]$_4$
395 (24-mer)	Tetrahymena telomere-specific repeat	[TTGGGG]$_4$

16. Microscope equipped for UV fluorescence (e.g., Leitz Ortholux II with Ploemopak filter/dichroic mirror system).

2.3. Spermidine Bis-Acridine Preparation

1. Dichloromethoxyacridine (Sigma).
2. Phenol.
3. Sodium hydroxide.
4. Spermidine or spermidine trihydrochloride (Sigma).
5. Ether.
6. An oil bath with thermostatic heating control.
7. A mechanical stirrer with glass paddle.

3. Methods
3.1. Primed in Situ Synthesis

1. You will need metaphase or prometaphase chromosomes, freshly prepared as described in Chapters 1, 2, and 5, and spread on acid/alcohol cleaned slides (*see* Note 1).
2. The concentration of the appropriate oligonucleotide that produces a satisfactory signal can only be obtained by experiment. As a starting point, for most repeated sequences, using primers of 16–30 bases, we use 250 ng/slide in a total of 25–50 μL (*see* Note 2).
3. The reaction mix is made up as follows: Dilute 100 mM dATP, dGTP, and dCTP 1:10 with distilled water. Dilute 100 mM dTTP 1:100. In a microcentrifuge tube, put 1 μL of each of the diluted nucleotide triphosphates, plus one of the following: 2 μL of 1 mM Bio-11-dUTP, 2 μL of 1 mM Bio-16-dUTP, 2 μL of 1 mM DlG-11-dUTP or 2 μL of 1 mM Fluorescein-12-dUTP (*see* Note 3), 5 μL of 10X buffer, 250 ng of oligonucleotide, and distilled water to 50 μL.
4. Denature the chromosomal DNA by incubating the slides in 70% formamide; 2X SSC for 2 min at 70°C, and passing through a cold (–20°C) ethanol series (70, 90, 100%). Air-dry. Add 1 U *Taq*1 DNA polymerase (*see* Note 4) to the reaction mix, mix by hand, and prewarm at the selected annealing temperature. Transfer to the slide, which has been preheated to the annealing temperature for 5 min. (Note: The optimum annealing temperature can only be determined empirically for each oligonucleotide primer; *see* Note 5.) Spread with a preheated acid/alcohol cleaned coverslip, seal with Tip-Top rubber solution, and continue to heat at the selected annealing temperature for 5 min to allow the primer to anneal to the chromosomal DNA. Transfer to a water bath or incubator at 70°C, placing the slides in a humid chamber (i.e., a plastic box with filter paper soaked in 4X SSC, 0.05% Triton X-100). Incubate for 30 min.

5. Stop the reaction by transferring slides (after removal of rubber solution seal) to 50 mL of 500 m*M* NaCl, 50 m*M* EDTA in a Coplin jar at 70°C for 5 min. The coverslip falls off at this stage. Finally, transfer to 4X SSC, 0.05% Triton X-100 at room temperature. Slides may be held at this stage overnight if convenient.

3.2. Detection

It is important that the slides are not allowed to become dry at any time during this process.

1. Prepare blocking buffer: The milk powder dissolves more readily if the solution is healed to 45°C in the water bath for a few minutes.
2. Put 40 µL blocking buffer on an acid/alcohol cleaned coverslip. Shake surplus fluid from the slide, and pick up the coverslip by inverting the slide over it. Ensure the blocking buffer spreads without bubbles, and leave at room temperature for 5 min.
3a. For reactions using Bio-dUTP: Dilute Av-FITC 1:500 in blocking buffer, mix well, and spin in microcentrifuge for 5 min. This precipitates any aggregates that form on storage and can produce high background. Gently remove coverslip, shake off surplus fluid, and put 40 µL of diluted Av-FITC on *the same* coverslip. Replace coverslip (taking care not to leave any air bubbles) and incubate in a humid chamber for 30 min at 37°C (*see* Note 6).
3b. For reactions using DIG-dUTP: Dilute anti-DIG-FITC 1:100 with blocking buffer, and treat as in step 3a.
3c. Fluorescein-12-dUTP needs no additional reporter, and is simply mounted in Citifluor AF3:Glycerol 1:1 (*see* Section 3.2.5.) after Section 3.1., step 5.
4. Remove coverslip and wash 3 × 2 min in 2X SSC, 0.05% Triton X-100 at 45°C.
5. Mount slides in Citifluor AF3:Glycerol 1:1, containing 3 µg/mL propidium iodide.
6. Examine slides under a fluorescent microscope equipped with suitable filters and dichroic mirrors for FITC and propidium iodide (e.g., Leitz Ortholux II with N2 and I2/3 Ploemopak filters).
7. As an alternative, use Av-Texas Red to detect the biotin (diluted as above), and counterstain with either DAPI (5 µg/mL in McIlvaine's buffer) or CMA_2S, as follows: Weigh out 5 mg CMA_2S. Put into screw-topped tube with 1–2 mL methanol. Use a vortex mixer to dissolve as much as possible (there will probably be some material remaining undis-

solved). Pipet off fluid, and make up to 100 mL with 10 m*M* phosphate buffer, pH 6.5. Stain slides for 10 min, rinse in same buffer, and mount in Citifluor AF10:Glycerol or the same buffer mixed 1:1 with glycerol. Examine as above.

The results, using some of the oligonucleotides in Table 1, are shown in Fig. 1.

3.3. Preparation of Spermidine Bis-Acridine (CMA₂S)

Due caution must be exercised in carrying out this preparative technique because of the dangerous nature of the constituents. It should only be carried out in an efficient fume cabinet under careful supervision.

1. Melt 60 g of phenol at 100°C in a glass beaker in the oil bath, and dissolve 4 g of NaOH in it.
2. Add 14 g of dichloromethoxyacridine while stirring. Keep at 100°C for 1.5 h stirring continuously, then pour into 500 mL of 2*N* NaOH, stir, and cool overnight.
3. Filter precipitate, wash with distilled water, break down any lumps, and dry. This intermediate is **phenoxyacridine**, and can be stored dry at 4°C almost indefinitely.
4. Dissolve 8.68 g phenoxyacridine in 27.6 g melted phenol at 80°C in a glass beaker.
5. Add 2.0 g spermidine.
6. Raise temperature to 120°C and continue heating while stirring for 1 h.

Alternatively, steps 4–6 can be replaced by the following (*see* Note 7).

4. Dissolve 7.44 g of phenoxyacridine in 23.6 g melted phenol at 80°C in a glass beaker.
5. Add 3 g spermidine trihydrochloride.
6. Raise temperature to 120°C, and continue heating while stirring for 1 h. Thereafter, complete preparation as in steps 7–9.
7. Cool and pour into 500 mL of ether.
8. Wash the precipitate with ether, and redissolve in hot methanol.
9. Cool, and add ether to precipitate. Filter through Buchner funnel with filter paper, wash with ether, and dry. The precipitate is spermidine *bis-*acridine.
10. Store at 4°C in an air-tight container.

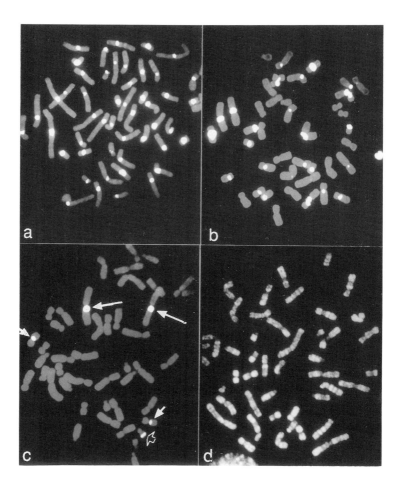

Fig. 1. Results of PRINS using four single primers. **a.** 339 Labeled with Bio-16-dUTP; 339 is an oligonucleotide derived from the consensus alphoid DNA sequence, and clearly labels all the human centromeres. **b.** 267 Labeled with DIG dUTP; 267 is derived from the satellite III DNA sequence, and gives the strongest signals on chromosomes 9 and the Y, with slightly weaker signals on chromosomes 1, the D and G group, and 20. **c.** B18 Labeled with Fluorescein-12-dUTP. B18 is an oligonucleotide derived from the satellite II DNA sequence, and, with FLU as the detector, labels only chromosomes 1 (large arrow), 16 (small arrow), and the Y (arrowhead). **d.** 450 Labeled with Bio-16-dUTP; 450 is derived from the *Alu* consensus sequence, near the 5' terminus. *Alu* sequences are known to be enriched in the R-bands of human chromosomes, and this PRINS reaction produces a distinct R-band pattern.

4. Notes

1. The age of the slides is critical. For the best results, they should be made no earlier than 1 wk before the experiment is to be performed. Cell suspensions with good quality metaphases can be stored in methanol:acetic acid (3:1) at −20°C for up to 2 mo, and fresh slides made by centrifuging to collect a pellet, resuspending in fresh methanol:acetic acid, and dropping the suspension as described in Chapter 1 onto cleaned slides. Optimum results are obtained by treating the prepared slides immediately with further fixation steps: Incubate 1 h in methanol:acetic acid (3:1), dry, and incubate 10 min in acetone, followed by air-drying.

2. The amount of oligonucleotide primer to be used in the reaction is primarily dependent on the kinetics of annealing of the primer sequence, which is, in turn, dependent on the frequency with which the primer sequence occurs in the target genome. For low-copy or unique sequences, high concentrations of primer may be necessary, in order to drive the kinetics of the annealing stage toward completion. Up to 12 µg of primer have been used in a single reaction *(17,18)*.

3. The choice of label is to some extent dependent on the sequence to be detected. For highly repeated sequences, Bio-11-dUTP is perfectly adequate and the cheapest label. For low-copy sequences, Bio-16-dUTP provides better sensitivity. Many workers have found DIG-11-dUTP to be as sensitive as or more sensitive than Bio-16-dUTP, but in our experience, although the sensitivity is certainly comparable, backgrounds tend to be higher. However, for very low-copy or unique sequences, where Bio-16-dUTP does not produce an adequate signal, DIG-11-dUTP is worth trying. A third possibility is the recently introduced Fluorescein-12-dUTP (Boehringer). Preliminary results indicate that, used in the same concentration as DIG-11-dUTP, it gives very strong signals and, of course, requires no additional detection since it contains its own reporter.

4. *Taq* I DNA polymerases show great variability in their behavior in the PRINS reaction. Of all the *Taq* I enzymes we have tested, only that made by Boehringer and the cloned enzyme produced by Perkin-Elmer Cetus (Ampli*Taq*) give clean results, free from background.

5. The optimum annealing temperature is only determined empirically. Although the OLIGO program *(18)* can give an indication of the optimum for filter hybridization, this is not necessarily the best for chromosomes. We usually try a series from 50–70°C, in 5°C steps. GC-rich primers are likely to give better results at the upper end of this scale, but there are frequently surprises. As in anything involving chromosomes, the parameter that is least controllable is the chromosome preparation!

6. It may be necessary to amplify the signal obtained with either biotin or digoxigenin label, where this is still not detectable with a single layer of reporter fluorochrome. For biotin, this is readily done by adding an incubation with biotinylated antiavidin (1:100) in the standard blocking buffer, washing as normal, adding a second incubation with avidin-FITC, washing, and mounting as described above (Section 3.2., steps 4 and 5). Digoxigenin may be amplified with a single additional incubation with FITC-antisheep IgG.

7. The original protocol for making spermidine *bis*-acridine used spermidine as the amine. Although this works quite well, we have found that the reaction is more easily completed using spermidine trihydrochloride.

References

1. Pardue, M. L. and Gall, J. G. (1969) Molecular hybridization of radioactive DNA to the DNA of cytological preparations. *Proc. Natl. Acad. Sci. USA* **64,** 600–604.
2. Gosden, J. R., Mitchell, A. R., Buckland, R. A., Clayton, R. P., and Evans, H. J. (1975) The location of four human satellite DNAs on human chromosomes. *Exp. Cell Res.* **92,** 148–158.
3. Gosden, J. R., Middleton, P. G., Rout, D., and de Angelis, C. (1986) Chromosomal localization of the human oncogene ERBA2. *Cytogenet. Cell Genet.* **43,** 150–153.
4. Bauman, J. G. J., Wiegant, J., Borst, P., and van Duijn, P. (1980) A new method fluorescence microscopical localization of specific DNA sequences by *in situ* hybridization of fluorochrome-labelled RNA. *Exp. Cell Res.* **128,** 485–490.
5. Brigati, D. J., Myerson, D., Leary, J. J., Spalholz, B., Travis, S. Z., Fong, C. K. Y., Hsiung, G. D., and Ward, D. C. (1983) Detection of viral genomes in cultured cells and paraffin-embedded tissue sections using biotin-labeled hybridization probes. *Virology* **16,** 32–50.
6. Landegent, J. E., Jansen in de Wal, N., Baan, R. A., Hoeijmakers, J. H. J., and Van der Ploeg, M. (1984) 2-Acetylaminofluorene-modified probes for the indirect hybridocytochemical detection of specific nucleic acid sequences. *Exp. Cell. Res.* **153,** 61–72.
7. Hopman, A. H. N., Wiegant, J., Tesser, G. I., and van Duijn P. (1986) A nonradioactive in situ hybridization method based on mercurated nucleic acid probes and sulfhydryl-hapten ligands. *Nucleic Acids Res.* **14,** 6471–6488.
8. De Frutos, R., Kimura, K., and Peterson K. R. (1989) In situ hybridization of Drosophila polytene chromosomes with digoxigenin-dUTP labeled probes. *Trends Genet.* **5,** 366.
9. Lichter, P., Chang Tang, C., Call, K., Hermanson, G., Evans, G. A., Housman, D., and Ward, D. C. (1990) High resolution mapping of human chromosome 11 by in situ hybridization with cosmid clones. *Science* **247,** 64–69.

10. Pinkel, D., Straume, T., and Gray, J. W. (1986) Cytogenetic analysis using quantitative, high sensitivity, fluorescence hybridization. *Proc. Natl. Acad. Sci. USA* **83,** 2934–2938.
11. Nederlof, P. M., Robinson, D., Abuknesha, R., Wiegant, J., Hopman, A. H. N., Tanke, H. J., and Raap, A. K. (1989) Three-color fluorescence in situ hybridization for the simultaneous detection or multiple nucleic acid sequences. *Cytometry* **10,** 20–27.
12. Heppel-Parton, A. C., Albertson, D. G., and Rabbitts, P. H. (1990) Ordering of polymorphic DNA markers critical for the delineation of the small cell lung carcinoma characteristic 3p deletion. *Proc. RMS* **25,** 266.
13. Koch, J. E., Kølvraa, S., Petersen, K. B., Gregersen, N., and Bolund, L. (1989) Oligonucleotidepriming methods for the chromosome-specific labelling of alpha satellite DNA in situ. *Chromosoma* **89,** 259–265.
14. Waye, J. S. and Willard, H. F. (1989) Human β satellite DNA: genomic organization and sequence definition of a class of highly repetitive tandem DNA. *Proc. Natl. Acad. Sci. USA* **86,** 6250–6254.
15. Rychlik, W. and Rhoads, R. E. (1989) A computer program for choosing optimal oligonucleotides for filter hybridization, sequencing and in vitro amplification of DNA. *Nucleic Acids Res.* **17,** 8543–8551.
16. Rychlik, W., Spencer, W. J., and Rhoads, R. E. (1990) Optimization of the annealing temperature for DNA amplification in vitro. *Nucleic Acids Res.* **18,** 6409–6412.
17. Hindkjaer, J., Koch, J., Mogensen, J., Pedersen, S., Fischer, H., Nygaard, M., Junker, S., Gregersen, N., Kølvraa, S., and Bolund, L. (1991) In situ labelling of nucleic acids for gene mapping, diagnostics and functional cytogenetics. *B. F. E.* **8,** 752–756.
18. Koch, J., Hindkjaer, J., Mogensen, T., Kølvraa, S., and Bolund, L. An improved method for chromosome-specific labelling of alpha satellite DNA in situ using denatured double stranded DNA probes as primers in a PRimed IN Situ labelling (PRINS) procedure. *Genetic Analysis: Techniques and Applications* **8,** 171–178.

CHAPTER 19

Electron Microscopic Localization of *in Situ* Hybrids

Sandya Narayanswami and Barbara A. Hamkalo

1. Introduction

In situ hybridization is used to map the position of DNA or RNA sequences relative to cytologically-identifiable landmarks. Although major progress has been made in sequence mapping at the light microscope (LM) level, there are inherent limits to resolution, notably when sequences are closely linked or when the target structure is very small. Mapping in such situations is facilitated by exploiting the resolution of the electron microscope (EM). The principles underlying *in situ* hybridization are the same regardless of the nature of the label (i.e., radioactive or nonisotopic) and the level of analysis (i.e., LM or EM). Cytological preparations fixed to a solid support are denatured for DNA detection followed by incubation in an appropriate buffer containing a labeled nucleic acid probe and salt at an appropriate temperature to affect hybridization between the target and probe. Hybridization to RNA does not require the denaturation step. After hybridization and removal of unhybridized probe, hybrid sites are located by either autoradiography for radioactive probes or via tagging with a visible detector. This chapter focuses on the use of probes labeled in vitro with a variety of nonisotopic tags that can be detected based on high-affinity interactions with specific ligands, such as antibodies, and then visualized in the EM by colloidal gold particles. Except for the smallest colloids (1–5 nm in diameter), particles are quite electron dense, ren-

From: *Methods in Molecular Biology, Vol. 29: Chromosome Analysis Protocols*
Edited by: J. R. Gosden Copyright ©1994 Humana Press Inc., Totowa, NJ

dering them readily identifiable even at low magnification (i.e., 2000×). This chapter describes a protocol for the preparation of metaphase chromosomes for EM *in situ* hybridization (EMISH) and details of the EMISH procedure itself.

2. Materials
2.1. Chromosome Preparation

1. 1% Nonidet P-40, pH 8–9, Millipore-filtered (0.22 μm pore size).
2. 1*M* Sucrose, pH 8–9, Millipore-filtered (0.22 μm pore size)
3. 0.4% Kodak Photoflo 200, pH 8.5, Millipore-filtered (0.22 μm pore size). Solutions 1 and 2 are stored in the refrigerator and are stable indefinitely provided they remain sterile. Solution 3 should be made fresh daily.

2.2. EMISH

1. 20X SSC: 3*M* NaCl, 0.3*M* Na citrate, pH 7.0. Stock solution is stored at room temperature; it is diluted to 2X SSC in dd H$_2$O followed by Millipore-filtering (0.22 μm pore size).
2. Glutaraldehyde: 8% stock (EM grade) is stored at 4°C. Stock is diluted to 0.1% in freshly prepared 2X SSC just prior to use. Opened ampules are tightly covered with parafilm, stored at 4°C, and used for no more than 1 wk.
3. Bovine serum albumin, 50 mg/mL (nuclease-free) stored at –20°C.
4. Carrier DNA, 2 mg/mL (*E. coli* or salmon sperm) stored at –20°C.
5. Formamide, 100%: Pass over a mixed bed ion-exchange resin, or recrystallize twice to remove decomposition products and then store at –20°C.
6. Hybridization buffer: Make 1.584-mL aliquots in disposable capped plastic tubes, and store at 4°C. The final concentrations given represent those in the final 2-mL hybridization mixture, which contains probe and tRNA.

Per 1.584-mL aliquot:	
200 mg dextran sulfate	(10%)
1 mL formamide	(50%)
4 μL 0.5*M* EDTA	(1 m*M*)
40 μL 0.5*M* Tris-HCl	(10 m*M*)
20 μL 2% Ficoll	(0.02%)
40 μL 50 mg/mL bovine serum albumin (BSA)	(1 mg/mL)
40 μL 2 mg/mL carrier DNA	(40 μg/mL)
240 μL 5*M* NaCl	(0.6*M*)

Mix the above components in a sterile tube. Dextran sulfate dissolves very slowly, but incubation at room temperature for 5–6 h is sufficient for solubilization. When dissolved, it increases the total volume by 200 µL.

7. Phosphate buffered saline (PBS): 0.2 g KCl, 0.2 g KH_2PO_4, 8.0 g NaCl, 1.14 g Na_2NPO_4 (anhydrous), made up to 1 L. Autoclave; pH should be 7–7.2; store at room temperature.

8. PBS/NaCl: Dilute $5M$ NaCl 1:10 in PBS, and filter through a 0.22 µm Millipore filter.

9. 1% BSA buffer: per liter   (final concentrations):
      21 mL $1M$ Tris-HCl, pH 8.0   (20 mM)
      10 g BSA (Fraction V powder)   (1%)
      9 g NaCl   (154 mM)
      5.24 mL 26% Na azide   (0.1%)

After dissolving BSA with stirring on a magnetic stirrer, filter through an 8-µm Millipore filter followed by a 0.22 µm filter. BSA can be replaced by cold-water fish gelatin (Sigma, St. Louis, MO), which is equivalently effective in reducing background.

3. Methods

3.1. Mitotic Chromosome Preparation

3.1.1. Established Cell Lines

Established cell lines represent an excellent source of large numbers of mitotic chromosomes.

1. Block logarithmic cells (50–75% confluent, depending on the line) in metaphase by treatment with colcemid (50–80 ng/mL) or nocodazole (100 ng/mL) for 6–18 h. The degree of confluence that gives maximum numbers of mitotic cells varies and must be determined empirically as described in Section 3.1.1., step 3.

2. Selectively detach and collect metaphase cells by gently shaking the culture flask. Pellet the cells in a 15-mL disposable conical centrifuge tube in a table-top centrifuge (740g), and resuspend in 0.1–0.2× the original vol of the same culture medium to a final concentration of about 1×10^5 cells/mL.

3. Lyse cells by the addition of 1% Nonidet P-40 (NP40). Place one drop of the cell suspension in one drop of 1% NP40 on a clean microscope slide and, after careful mixing, monitor cell lysis time and mitotic index by phase-contrast microscopy. At least 70% of the cells should be lysed, and chromosomes should be visible as individual structures. Lysis should

occur within 1–3 min, since longer exposure to detergent results in extensive chromation unfolding and chromosome clumping. Interphase nuclei are rapidly released from cells under the same conditions, but are not lysed.

3.1.2. Diploid Cells

Although established lines are ideal sources for large numbers of chromosomes, they are rarely diploid and, even if diploid, may have undergone chromosome rearrangements. A convenient source for diploid cells is a blood or spleen culture. In this case, cells grow in suspension, precluding separation of mitotic from interphase cells. As a result, there is a higher degree of contamination with nuclei, although it is possible to obtain a sufficient number of chromosomes for analysis. Cultures are generated and stimulated to proliferate by standard protocols, blocked with colcemid or nocodazole, and processed as described above.

3.2. Specimen Preparation

Deposit material by low-speed centrifugation *(1)* onto gold EM grids coated with a 1% parlodion-carbon support film. Gold grids are preferable to copper, since copper leaches into the hybridization solution and adversely affects the results. The chamber typically used for this step is diagrammed in Fig. 1. It is made out of Plexiglas™ to fit a 50-mL swinging bucket of any centrifuge; each chamber can be used to prepare up to four grids simultaneously.

1. Fill each well with $1M$ sucrose, pH 8.5, until a convex meniscus is formed. Dip grids, rendered hydrophilic by placing in 95% ethanol for 1 min, briefly in $1M$ sucrose, and drop into one of the four wells of the microcentrifugation chamber, carbon film side up; they should fall to the bottom and rest on the Plexiglas™ surface. Remove about half of the sucrose with a Pasteur pipet, forming a cushion in each well.
2. When the chambers are ready, lyse the cells in a siliconized test tube as described above. If necessary, mix the lysate carefully by pipeting with a siliconized Pasteur pipet to separate released chromosomes from each other. Layer a 30–50-μL aliquot of the chromosome suspension on top of the sucrose cushion in each well, and centrifuge chambers for 5 min at 2500g at 25°C in 50-mL swinging buckets in a table-top centrifuge. During centrifugation, chromosomes and nuclei adsorb to the grid film, whereas most other organelles and cytoplasm remain in suspension.

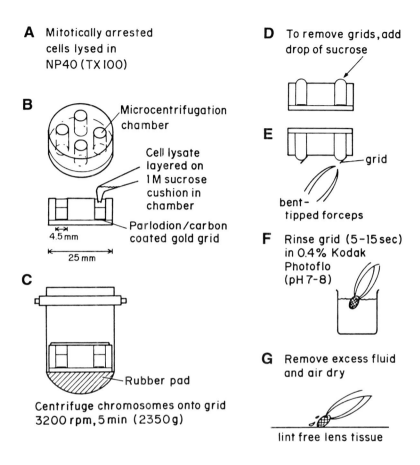

Fig. 1. Schematic representation of the procedure used for deposition of chromosomes and nuclei onto EM grids.

3. After centrifugation, add 1*M* sucrose to each well to form a convex meniscus. Invert the chamber. Grids should float away from the bottom of the well, to be held in the hanging droplet. Using forceps, pick individual grids from the droplets, and rinse in Photoflo solution (0.4% Kodak Photoflo 200, pH 8.5, Millipore-filtered) to reduce surface tension and remove residual sucrose. Air-dry the preparations.

4. Prior to carrying out EMISH, check each grid by phase contrast microscopy (40×) in order to evaluate chromosome morphology and density. Optimal preparations consist of well-spread groups of chromosomes, with few interphase nuclei. Approximately 1 metaphase/grid square is

an optimal density. Specimens, regardless of source, can be stored for at least 1 mo at 25°C without obvious loss of signal or morphology.

3.3. Prehybridization Treatments

Prehybridization treatments for EMISH are the same as those employed for LM *in situ* hybridization. Specimens are fixed and, if necessary, incubated with RNase A and/or proteinase K prior to DNA denaturation.

3.3.1. Fixation

1. Place grids in single grid holders (E. F. Fullam), and immerse in dilute glutaraldehyde in a beaker with stirring. Remove air bubbles on the grid surface by careful aspiration with a Pasteur pipet in order to ensure complete access of fixative to the specimen.
2. Fix grids for 20 min at 25°C with gentle stirring. Morphology is not improved with longer incubations or higher concentrations of glutaraldehyde. However, it is possible to fix for as little as 5 min, although chromosome morphology is less well preserved. Shorter fixation results in less crosslinking and, therefore, greater access of probe to targets.
3. After fixation, rinse each grid in the Photoflo solution and air-dry. Fixed specimens can be stored at 25°C for at least 3 mo without noticeable loss of signal or deterioration in chromosome morphology.

3.3.2. RNase A Digestion

When transcribed DNA sequences are to be localized, it may be necessary to remove nascent transcripts prior to hybridization. After fixation, incubate grids in 400 μg/mL of pancreatic RNase A (Sigma, dissolved in 2X SSC) for 30 min at 25°C. Place the grids in 50-μL droplets of enzyme on the surface of a clean Petri dish. Remove RNase by washing the grids in single-grid holders once in 2X SSC for 10 min at 25°C, followed by a Photoflo rinse and air-drying.

3.3.3. Proteinase K Digestion

A low hybridization signal may be owing to limited access of probe to target. Access can be increased by protease pretreatment.

Place grids in 50-μL droplets of 1 μg/mL autodigested proteinase K dissolved in 2X SSC for 30 min at 37°C in a Petri dish. Wash, rinse, and dry grids as in the previous step.

3.3.4. Denaturation

Denaturation is routinely achieved by incubation in alkaline 2X SSC. Although there are a variety of other denaturation solutions (Note 2), this method gives the largest *in situ* signal in our protocol despite the fact that there is some DNA loss. Denaturation times vary with the base composition of the target since (G + C)-rich DNAs (>60% G + C) require more extensive denaturation treatments (up to 30 min) to achieve a reproducible signal. Denaturation is carried out immediately prior to hybridization, since overnight storage of denatured preparations results in a reduced signal, presumably as a consequence of the reassociation of denatured DNA.

1. Perform denaturation at 25°C with the grids in single-grid holders. Prepare the denaturation solution just prior to use, by adding 24 drops of 10N NaOH to 100 mL of 2X SSC with a Pasteur pipet.
2. Immerse single-grid holders in this solution for 2–30 min. Remove air bubbles as described in Section 3.3.1., step 1.
3. Using forceps, remove each grid from the holder, rinse in Photoflo solution to remove alkali, and air-dry. The air-drying steps in the three preceding sections are not obligatory, but represent convenient stopping points.

3.4. Hybridization

3.4.1. Probes

A variety of probes and labeling regimens can be employed in EMISH. Details will be provided in this section for nick translation in the presence of biotin-dUTP and direct modification. Alternative labeling schemes will be referred to in Section 4. In all cases, labeled probes are stable for at least a year when stored frozen at –20°C.

3.4.1.1. NICK TRANSLATION WITH BIOTINYLATED NUCLEOTIDES

Several biotinylated nucleotides (dUTP, dATP, dCTP) containing linker arms of lengths ranging from C4 to C21 are available commercially. The shortest linker (C4) provides suboptimal labeling in some circumstances, but we have not seen major differences among the C11, C16, or C21 linker-containing nucleotides. However, in our experience, bio-dUTP is somewhat more efficiently incorporated than bio-dCTP in nick translation reactions (*see* Note 3). Commercially available nick translation kits are used routinely.

1. Monitor incorporation of biotinylated nucleotides by adding a small quantity of ^{3}HdATP to the reaction, and determine incorporation by measuring the counts in the TCA precipitable fraction of aliquots taken during the course of the reaction. A parallel reaction without Bio-dUTP is useful to assess the efficiency of nick translation with the modified nucleotide.

2. Lyophilize 20 µCi of ^{3}HdATP (Amersham Intl. [Bucks, UK] TRK 347, 17 Ci/mmol) per reaction in Eppendorf tubes, and place on ice.

3. Set up reactions on ice as per nick translation kit instructions. Each reaction should contain 2 µg of DNA in a reaction vol of 100 µL and 20–50 µM Bio-dUTP to ensure efficient incorporation of biotin.

4. Add 10 µL of the PolI-DNase I 10X stock solution to each tube. Mix well and incubate at 15°C for 90 min.

5. In order to determine the specific activity (cpm/µg DNA), place a 5-µL sample from each reaction on a GF/C filter (Whatman). Stop the reaction by adding 10 µL of STOP buffer and 2 µL of 5M NaCl. Dry the GF/C filter, and place it in cold 5% TCA for at least 1 h. Wash the filter with five changes of cold 5% TCA followed by two rinses in 95% ethanol. Air-dry. Calculate the specific activity of the reaction by liquid scintillation counting.

6. While the filters are drying, remove unincorporated nucleotides by Sephadex G-50 chromatography using the spin-column procedure of Maniatis et al. *(2)*. A 100-µL reaction can be loaded on a 1-mL Sephadex G-50 column. Measure the volume of the column eluate, and determine the amount of incorporated radioactivity by counting a 5-µL aliquot of the eluate. The amount of DNA recovered in the column eluate (µg) can be determined by dividing the total radioactivity in the eluate by the specific activity of the probe preparation as determined in Section 3.4.1.1., step 5. Dilute the probe to 4 µg/mL in either 100 mM NaCl, 10 mM Tris-HCl, pH 8.0, 1 mM EDTA, or distilled water. Omit this dilution step if the probe is to be used for multiple labeling.

3.4.1.2. Direct Probe Modification with AAF

Probes can be directly modified with the ligand *N*-acetoxy-2-acetylaminofluorene (AAF) as described in *(3)* and in detail below (*see* Note 4). AAF is carcinogenic and should be handled with appropriate precautions. However, once incorporated into a probe, it is innocuous. Although double-stranded DNA can be labeled, modification of single-stranded DNA provides a more reproducible *in situ* signal, possibly because the formation of intrastrand crosslinks during coupling *(4)* affects subsequent probe denaturation.

1. Digest DNA with DNase I to a mean length of about 3 kb. Denature the DNA by boiling at 100°C for 5 min. Fast cool the denatured DNA on ice.

2. Dilute the DNA to 0.2 mg/mL in 1.6 mM sodium citrate, pH 7, 20% (v/v) ethanol. Add AAF from a stock solution in DMSO (6 mg/mL) to a final concentration of 60 µg/mL (for approx 5% modification). The final con-

centration of AAF determines the amount of substitution of the DNA. However, the final concentration of DMSO should not exceed 0.8% (v/v). Levels of substitution above 5% result in significant reduction of the T_m of hybrids.

3. Run reactions for 1 h at 37°C in the dark. During this time, AAF covalently attaches to G-residues in DNA. Remove uncoupled AAF by extraction six times with water-saturated diethylether. Inactivate residues by adding bleach.
4. The ratio of A_{305}/A_{260} is used to calculate the percentage modification of the DNA based on a standard curve *(4)*.

3.4.2. Hybridization Reaction

The conditions described are for double-stranded (ds) DNA probes, regardless of the label.

1. Make up 100 µL of hybridization solution: Mix 79 µL of HB, 1 µL of yeast tRNA (phenol extracted, reprecipitated, and dissolved in dd H_2O at 7 mg/mL) and 20 µL of probe DNA (4 µg/mL) in a siliconized Eppendorf tube. Mix well. Use AAF probes at 5–10× greater concentration.
2. Denature the probe by boiling for 5 min, followed by rapid cooling on ice for 2 min. Spin tubes briefly in a microfuge (up to maximum speed and then down) in order to bring droplets of condensation to the bottom of the tube. Place probe on ice prior to use.
3. Pipet a 50-µL aliquot of the hybridization solution into a siliconized Reactivial (Kontes, Vineland, NJ).
4. Using watchmaker's forceps, place two grids, back to back (i.e., specimen side facing out) in each vial. Cap the vials, and incubate overnight in a water bath at the temperature selected for hybridization. The temperature normally used with the HB described is 30°C, but hybridizations to AAF-modified probes are done at 27°C because of the reduction in T_m that accompanies this modification.
5. After hybridization, place grids in individual grid holders and rinse in a beaker with stirring three times for 20 minutes each in 100 mL of 2X SSC at 25°C, to remove unhybridized probe. Keep grids moist between this and subsequent steps to retain antibody reactivity.

3.5. Hybrid Detection

Detection is effected by immunogold labeling. Although primary antibodies coupled to gold can be used, more intense labeling is obtained using the two-step procedure described here. Streptavidin or avidin can be used in place of antibodies to locate biotin-containing hybrids. Colloidal gold can be prepared in the laboratory with minimal equipment following the protocol described in *(5)*. Alternatively, colloidal gold and colloidal gold complexed with antibodies or streptavidin/avidin are commercially available in sizes from 1–80 nm.

3.5.1. Primary Antibody Reactions

1. Primary antibodies are diluted to an appropriate concentration in PBS supplemented with BSA and NaCl (*see* Note 5). The presence of BSA and high salt reduces nonspecific binding of antibodies to the grid film to virtually zero. Such nonspecific adsorption represented the major source of background observed during the development of this technique. Each antibody batch is titrated using a test system (in our case mouse satellite DNA and mouse metaphase chromosomes) in order to determine optimal antibody dilution and reaction time. The conditions given are suitable for multiple-step antibody sandwich reactions and multiple labeling.
2. Place grids, specimen side up, in 50-µL droplets of diluted affinity-purified primary antibody in Petri dishes, and incubate in a moist atmosphere for 4 h at 37°C. A plastic slide box lined with dampened paper towels makes a convenient moist chamber.
3. Remove unbound antibody by rinsing grids in single-grid holders at 25°C three times with 100 mL of PBS/NaCl for 10 min each in a beaker with stirring. Do not allow grids to dry between this step and the next.

3.5.2. Secondary Antibody / Gold Reactions

Details are provided for 15–20 nm gold particle labeling (*see* Note 5). These colloids are readily visible at low magnification. If smaller particles are used, centrifugation speeds are increased to ensure pelleting in step 1.

1. Pellet 0.5 mL of a 15–20 nm gold stock at 12,000*g* for 15 min at 4°C in a fixed-angle rotor. Pellet 5-nm gold stocks at 23,400*g* for 45 min to 1 h. This step is performed in order to remove unabsorbed protein, which will remain in the supernatant. In both cases, the pellet should be soft and loose in appearance.
2. Discard most of the supernatant except for a small quantity directly over the gold. Resuspend the remaining pellet in the original volume by adding an appropriate amount of either 1% BSA or 1% fish gelatin buffer *(6)*.
3. Dilute resuspended gold in 1% BSA to a concentration determined empirically for each batch. Follow by low-speed centrifugation of the diluted sample in a table-top centrifuge with a swinging bucket rotor (400–700*g* for 10 min at 25°C) in order to remove aggregates.

4. Using a micropipet, carefully remove 50-µL aliquots of the supernatant, and deposit as droplets in a clean Petri dish. Place one grid in each droplet, and incubate in a moist chamber at 25°C. Although overnight incubation is convenient, the time can be shortened based on that required to give a visible signal. Highly repeated sequences (e.g., mouse satellite) exhibit a good signal after as little as 2 h incubation in gold.

5. Rinse grids in single-grid holders at 25°C three times for 20 min each in 100 mL 1% BSA buffer in a beaker with stirring in order to remove unbound gold. Rinse in Photoflo and air-dry. Specimens can be viewed in the EM without further contrasting, since chromosomes and gold are sufficiently electron-dense. However, greater contrast can be obtained by staining or heavy metal shadowing. Figure 2 shows a representative *in situ* hybridization using the basic protocol described above. Metaphase chromosomes from a spleen lymphocyte culture of *Mus spretus* were hybridized on EM grids with the mouse minor centromeric satellite, which was biotin-labeled by nick translation. Signal detection was with 15 nm gold. The intensity of labeling is typical for a highly repeated sequence and is confined to the centromere, as expected.

3.6. Signal Amplification

It is possible to enhance a small signal easily by one of two amplification approaches.

3.6.1. Antibody Sandwich

This amplification scheme is applicable as described to any type of nonisotopic label provided that appropriate noncrossreacting antibodies are available.

1. After hybridization with bio-probes, incubate grids in antibiotin followed by incubation with biotin-coupled secondary antibody under the same conditions. Repeat these steps one or more times as necessary.

2. Amplified signals ultimately are detected with streptavidin gold. Although moderately repeated sequences (ca. 100 copies) are detectable without amplification, two cycles of amplification are sufficient to produce a signal that is visible in the light microscope *(7)*. One drawback of several rounds of signal amplification in EMISH is some loss of spatial resolution (Fig. 3).

3.6.2. Silver Intensification

The second approach to signal amplification is via silver intensification. This procedure involves increasing the size, and hence visibility, of individual particles *(8,9)*. Intensification is achieved by the

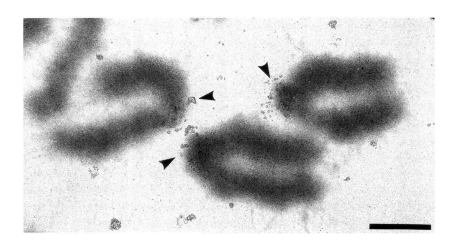

Fig. 2. Metaphase chromosomes from a *Mus spretus* lymphocyte culture after EMISH with biotin-substituted mouse minor centromeric satellite and labeling with 15 nm colloidal gold. Arrowheads denote labeling of centromere regions. Scale bar = 2 μm.

deposition of layers of metallic silver directly on colloidal gold particles. This amplification method is particularly useful when reduced accessibility dictates the use of very small particles, and it is imperative when 1 nm gold is used. The procedure is rapid and results in a severalfold increase in particle size within about 10 min. Intensification kits are commercially available (e.g., from Janssen Biochimica, Beerse, Belgium), which are used according to the supplier's instructions, without modification.

3.7. Multiple Labeling

Incorporation of minor modifications in the protocol described permits localization of multiple probes. If probes are cloned in the same vector, it is essential to purify the cloned insert from all but one probe so that vector sequences do not crosshybridize. In this case, inserts are prepared for probes that give the largest signals, because vector sequences allow network formation and hence signal enhancement. There are differences in the relative sensitivities of differently substituted DNA probes as assayed by EMISH. Although DNP- and Dig-labeled nucleotides are incorporated into DNA to similar levels to biotin (our observations), they give a severalfold lower hybridization signal com-

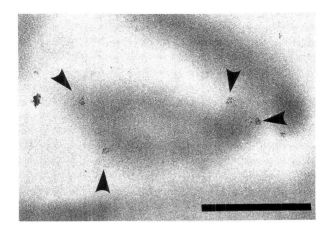

Fig. 3. Mouse chromosome after EMISH with a biotin-labeled telomere-specific oligonucleotide probe, signal amplification, and detection with 20 nm gold (arrowheads). The centromere proximal telomeres appear to contain more target than those at the long arm ends, which appear to be folded back into the chromosome arms. Scale bar = 2 μm.

pared to bio-labeled probes under equivalent conditions *(7)*. Thus, when targets are of different sizes, the probe for the sequence that is expected to give the smaller signal is biotin-labeled for maximal detectability. Nevertheless, these three labels can be used for the facile detection of highly and moderately repeated sequences by EMISH. AAF-labeled probes give substantially less signal under equivalent conditions but the lower signal can be compensated for by increasing probe concentration five- to 10-fold relative to biotinylated probes. There is some increase in background under these conditions, so that optimal reaction/detection conditions will vary with the probe, label, and target material. In addition, because direct labeling of probes is possible with AAF (as opposed to nick translation in the presence of DNase I and Pol I), AAF can be used to label relatively small pieces of DNA without degradation of the probe. Thus, AAF is useful when one of a pair or group of probes is smaller than the other(s).

Although all modifications reduce the thermal stability of hybrids, this effect is most pronounced with AAF, where each percent substitution is accompanied by a reduction in the T_m of 1°C *(3)*. Because of this, levels of substitution in the 5–10% range are routinely used. This is in contrast to bio-dUTP, where even totally substituted probes give specific and intense signals under normal hybridization conditions. A benefit of a reduction in T_m in all cases is the reduction in signal at crosshybridizing, nonidentical sites.

Probes are added to the hybridization mixture simultaneously and denatured together. As a result, probes used for multiple localizations should be at higher stock concentrations (ca. 20 µg/mL) than the 4 µg/mL recommended for a nick translated probe used alone. They can be stored without dilution after purification over Sephadex G50. Several probes can then be added to hybridization buffer without drastically changing the concentrations of buffer components. If even higher probe concentrations are necessary, they can be mixed and reprecipitated before adding to hybridization buffer. Primary antibodies are mixed and incubated with grids as described followed by mixed secondary antibody-gold incubation.

The choice of gold particle sizes for multiple-probe labeling depends on the expected signal size and the distance between sequences of interest. At the magnifications used to examine metaphase chromosomes, 5 nm gold is difficult to detect unless the signal is large. However, 10-, 15-, 20-, and 30-nm particles are all visible and distinguishable from each other in the EM. One-nanometer particles are most useful when accessibility is a problem. They are invisible at magnifications used routinely, but can be readily identified after silver intensification. Although we have carried out only double labeling to date, the availability of four modified probes and different sizes of gold should permit simultaneous detection of at least four loci. Figure 4 illustrates a typical double hybridization.

4. Notes

1. As in most laboratory protocols, essentially every step can be modified or varied to suit a particular system or problem. This section briefly describes variations on the theme described in detail above for EM *in situ* hybridization.
2. Denaturation at 70°C in 2X SSC/70% formamide results in better morphological preservation, but gives about a twofold lower signal. Denaturation with 70% ethanol/0.14M NaOH results in appreciably lower signals (about fourfold) than the standard alkali treatment.
3. As noted in Section 3.4.1.1., dATP, dCTP, and dUTP linked to biotin are available. Although DNA polymerase I incorporates bio-dUTP very

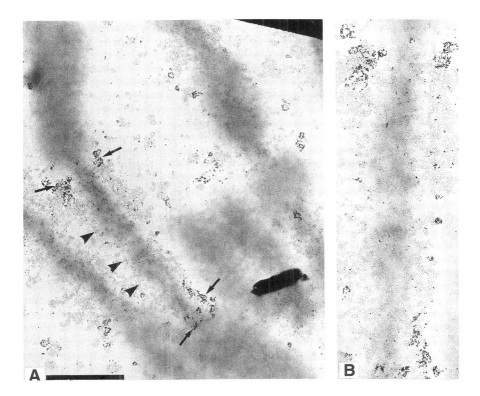

Fig. 4. **A.** Chromosome from a mouse L929 cell grown in the presence of Hoechst 33258, after double-label EMISH with a biotin-labeled ribosomal gene probe (detected with 20 nm gold) and DNP-labeled mouse major centromeric satellite DNA (detected with 5 nm gold). Arrowheads denote the extended centromere region and arrow sites of ribosomal gene clusters. Scale bar = 2 μm. **B.** Labeled region from A at higher magnification.

efficiently, this is not true for all enzymes used to label probes in vitro. When terminal deoxyribonucleotidyl transferase is used to end label probes, bio-dCTP should be used, since it is incorporated severalfold more efficiently than the other modified nucleotides *(10)*. In addition to nick translation and end labeling, it is possible to incorporate biotin into probes nonenzymatically via a photoactivable derivative of biotin, photobiotin, which is commercially available from several sources (e.g., Sigma) using a sunlamp for photocrosslinking. In addition, the powerful technique known as the polymerase chain reaction (PCR) is effective in generating a large amount of highly substituted probe. In this case, oligonucleotides typically are labeled with 30 cycles of standard

PCR, followed by 10 PCR cycles in the presence of bio dUTP. This protocol results in high levels of incorporation of the modified nucleotide. We have successfully used PCR-generated probes for EM localizations, but we found variability in signal strength from batch to batch. Figure 3 illustrates the pattern of hybridization in a metaphase chromosome from a mouse cultured cell line of an oligonucleotide probe for telomere repeats end labeled with biotin. These repeats are much less reiterated than the centromeric satellite illustrated in Fig. 2, resulting in a considerably lower signal. Nevertheless, hybridization is readily detectable at both ends of this chromosome. In this case, the signal was amplified by antibody sandwich and detected by streptavidin-gold as described in Section 3.6.1.

Based on the prototype biotin-coupled nucleotides, other ligands have been coupled to DNA bases for use as alternative labels. The two modified nucleotides we have experience with are dinitrophenol-dUTP *(11)* and digoxigenin-dUTP. Both of these can be incorporated enzymatically into probes in analogy to bio-dNTP. Biotin- and digoxigenin-coupled NTPs also are available commercially so that one can label RNA probes in vitro in situations where this is desirable, as, for example, to label selectively transcripts via antisense RNA.

4. As described in Section 3.4.1.2., it is possible to modify DNA directly with AAF. RNA can also be modified in an analogous reaction.

5. Beyond the issue of sensitivity, two problems have arisen that can be overcome. The first is background labeling of the grid film. It should be emphasized that this labeling does not compromise positive signal detection, because chromosomes are essentially free of this background. In extreme cases where films are covered with gold, chromosomes are surrounded by a halo devoid of gold, at least in part a consequence of repulsion between chromatin and gold. The source of this background is nonspecific adsorption of primary antibody to the film, and such nonspecific binding may not occur equivalently to chromosomes. Nevertheless, this source of background is reduced to nearly zero in standard two-step labeling when high salt and/or BSA are included during antibody incubations. However, it does occur to varying degrees when signals are amplified by antibody sandwiches. As a result, more extensive rinsing of such specimens may be necessary.

The other problem that arises occasionally appears to result from instability of gold colloids. In this case, one observes large aggregates of particles and/or gold particles coating the entire grid, including chromosomes. Although colloids usually are stable for up to a year when stored at 4°C, the instability noted is a function of the age of the colloid. The only solution to this problem is to discard the colloid.

Acknowledgments

We would like to thank the relevant individuals for probes, cell lines, chemicals, and antibodies, and Agnes Demetrescu for technical assistance. Research was supported by NIH GM23241 to BAH.

References

1. Rattner, J. B. and Hamkalo, B. A. (1978) Higher order structure in metaphase chromosomes. 1. The 250A fiber. *Chromosoma (Berl).* **69,** 363–372.
2. Maniatis, T., Fritsch, E. F., and Sambrook, J. (1982) *Molecular Cloning. A Laboratory Manual.* Cold Spring Harbor Laboratory, Cold Spring Harbor, NY, pp. 466,467.
3. Landegent, J. E., Jansen in de Wal, N., Baan, R. A., Hoeijmakers, J. H. J., and van der Ploeg, M. (1984) The use of 2-acetylaminofluorene modified probes for the indirect hybridocytochemical detection of specific nucleic acid sequences in microscopic preparations. *Exp. Cell. Res.* **153,** 61–72.
4. Fuchs, R. and Daune, M. (1972) Physical studies on deoxyribonucleic acid after covalent binding of a carcinogen. *Biochemistry* **11,** 2659–2666.
5. de Waele, M., de Mey, J., Moeremans, M., de Brabander, M., and Van Camp, B. (1983) Immunogold staining method for the light microscopic detection of leucocyte cell surface antigens with monoclonal antibodies. *J. Histochem. Cytochem.* **31(3),** 376–381.
6. Birrell, B. C., Hedberg, K. K., and Griffith, O. H. (1987) Pitfalls of immunogold labelling: Analysis by light microscopy, transmission electron microscopy, and photoelectron microscopy. *J. Histochem. Cytochem.* **35(8),** 843–853.
7. Narayanswami, S., Lundgren, K., and Hamkalo, B. A. (1989) Deoxyribonucleic acid sequence mapping on metaphase chromosomes by immunoelectron microscopy. *Scanning Microscopy Intl. Suppl.* **3,** 65–76.
8. Holgate, C. S., Jackson, P., Cowen, P. N., and Bird, C. C. (1983) Immunogold-silver staining: a new method of immunostaining with enhanced sensitivity. *J. Histochem. Cytochem.* **31,** 938–944.
9. Narayanswami, S. and Hamkalo, B. A. (1987) Hybridization to chromatin and whole chromosome mounts, in *Electron Microscopy in Molecular Biology. A Practical Approach* (Sommerville, J. and Scheer, U., eds.) IRL, Oxford, UK, pp. 215–232.
10. Moyzis, R. K., Buckingham, J. M., Cram, L. S., Dani, M., Deaven, L. L., Jones, M. D., Meyne, J., Ratliff, R. C., and Wu, J. R. (1988) A highly conserved repetitive DNA sequence, $(TTAGGG)_n$, present at the telomeres of human chromosomes. *Proc. Natl. Acad. Sci. USA* **85,** 6622–6626.
11. Narayanswami, S. and Hamkalo, B. A. (1991) DNA sequence mapping using electron microscopy. *GATA* **8(1),** 14–23.

CHAPTER 20

Protocols for Chromosome-Mediated Gene Transfer

Selection Strategies, Transgenome Analysis,
Enrichment Cloning, and Mapping

David J. Porteous

1. Introduction

Linkage studies in humans are strictly limited by such factors as family structure, the availability of material for study, and informative markers for linkage analysis. Parasexual approaches therefore have a particularly important role to play in human genetics *(1)*. A panoply of somatic cell genetic methods have been devised and exploited. These include (1) immortalizing experimental and clinical mutations and chromosome aberrations as lymphoblastoid cell lines (Chapters 5 and 17) and (2) segregating individual chromosome or subchromosome fragments one from another by cell fusion or gene transfer for (a) physical mapping of existing markers, and (b) as the starting material for enrichment cloning by one technique or another. I will focus here on the technique of chromosome-mediated gene transfer, a somatic cell genetic method that can bridge the gap between the functional and molecular analysis of single genes or whole chromosomes.

The ability to transfer genetic information by purified metaphase chromosomes to mammalian cells in culture was first described nearly two decades ago by McBride and Ozer *(2)*. I will refer to the technique throughout by the acronym CMGT, for chromosome-mediated gene transfer. Development of CMGT owes much to Ruddle and coworkers (reviewed in refs. *3* and *4*). The essential requirements are:

From: *Methods in Molecular Biology, Vol. 29: Chromosome Analysis Protocols*
Edited by: J. R. Gosden Copyright ©1994 Humana Press Inc., Totowa, NJ

1. Appropriate donor cells from which metaphase chromosomes can be prepared;
2. A recipient cell competent to take up metaphase chromosomes; and
3. A suitable selection assay, or effective screen, for successful transfer of genetic material from donor to recipient.

Early experiments relied extensively on the few biochemical selections, such as growth on HAT medium (hypoxanthine, aminopterin, and thymidine) to select for complementation by the donor chromosomes of recipient cells deficient in hypoxanthine phosphoribosyl transferase (HPRT) or thymidine kinase (TK) activity. These experiments demonstrated that chromosome fragments from subchromosomal-sized genes could be transferred apparently intact *(5)* and that markers known to be syntenic with the locus under selection were frequently cotransferred *(6,7)*. However, despite the obvious potential of this method *(1)*, lack of additional selection systems or molecular methods for structural analysis of the *trans*-genomes halted further exploitation. The method has been revived over the last few years by specifically addressing these two inherent limitations (reviewed in refs. *8–10*). The aim of this chapter is to outline the basic method, and to summarize and update the developments in selection strategies and analytical methods that have made this an effective enrichment cloning strategy and genome mapping tool.

2. Materials

2.1. Chromosome-Mediated Gene Transfer (CMGT)

2.1.1. Equipment

1. Sterile plastic 10-mL conical, 30-mL Universal, and 50-mL Falcon tubes.
2. A refrigerated bench centrifuge, e.g., Sorval RT6000, with buckets to accommodate each tube size, and an operating speed to generate 100–1600g.
3. Sterile disposable syringes (2–20 mL) and 21-gage needles.
4. Sterile disposable Pastets.
5. Access to a fluorescence microscope is preferable, but not absolutely essential.

2.1.2. Reagents

1. Colcemid (1000×): 1 mg/mL in sterile distilled water. Store in the dark at 4°C.
2. 0.075M KCl: Make up fresh in deionized water and filter sterilize.
3. Digitonin (Fluka AG, Buchs, Switzerland): Make up fresh as a 0.1%

suspension in 1X TCC and hold at 37°C (*see* Note 1).

4. 10X TCC: 150 mM Tris-HCl and 30 mM CaCl$_2$, pH 7.0. Store at –20°C.
5. 50% Sucrose: Sigma (St. Louis, MO) Tissue Culture quality dissolved in distilled water and sterilized by autoclaving. This is a 10X stock. Store at room temperature.
6. 2X HeBS: 50 mM HEPES, 280 mM NaCl, and 1.5 mM Na$_2$HPO$_4$, pH 7.15, at room temperature (*see* Note 2).
7. 2X CaCl$_2$: 250 mM CaCl$_2$ in distilled water, filter sterilized and stored at –20°C.
8. 100% Glycerol: Analar quality, sterilized by autoclaving. Store at room temperature.
9. Tissue culture medium is supplied by the manufacturer (e.g., Gibco-BRL, Paisley, Scotland) in liquid or powder form. Dulbecco's Minimal Essential Medium (DMEM) is suitable for most human, rat, and mouse fibroblast or epithelial cell lines, including EJ, MNNG-HOS, NIH3T3, C127, Cl 21, L, RAG, and Wg3H cells. Otherwise, use the medium recommended for the particular cell line (*see* Note 3).
10. Fetal calf serum is supplied sterile by the manufacturer (e.g., Gibco-BRL) and added to the medium as growth supplement at 2–10% v/v as required by the donor and recipient cell lines.
11. Seaplaque™ agarose (FMC Colloids Ltd.) is used to select for anchorage-independent growth in oncogenic transformation assays. Base agarose is 0.5% w/v, and top agarose is 0.25% w/v in tissue culture medium, autoclaved to sterilize. To prepare plates, melt the agarose/medium in a water bath at >70°C or in a microwave (low-power setting), and hold at 37°C to maintain liquid. Add 5 mL base agarose to a 35 mm diameter or 20 mL to a 100 mm diameter bacterial Petri dish, and set at 4°C. Resuspend cells in 2–3 mL of top agarose/35-mm dish or 10 mL per 100 mm dish at 37°C and overlay on base agarose. Allow to set at room temperature, and then incubate at 37°C.
12. Freezing medium is 10% fetal calf serum and 90% dimethyl sulfoxide (DMSO).
13. Optional reagents for determining chromosome yield and integrity by fluorescence microscopy: (a) Distamycin DAPI, 5 μg/mL, or (b) ethidium bromide, 10 μg/mL in TCC (*see* Note 4).

2.2. Selection Systems

2.2.1. Equipment

1. Fluorescent-activated cell sorter—*see* Chapter 13.
2. Antibody-coated magnetic beads (DYNABEADS M-450) and separator (DYNAL MPC) (Dynal [UK] Ltd.).

2.2.2. Reagents

1. HAT selection medium: 50X stock is 5 mM hypoxanthine, 20 µM aminopterin, and 500 µM thymidine, filter sterilized and stored at –20°C in convenient aliquots.
2. G418-Geneticin G418 (Gibco-BRL, Gaithersburg, MD) is made up as a 20 mg/mL stock in distilled water, filter sterilized, and stored at –20°C in convenient aliquots. Use at 200–1200 µg/mL tissue culture medium, depending on sensitivity of particular cell line.

2.3. Analytical Methods

2.3.1. In Situ *Hybridization*

See Chapters 25 and 26 for details.

2.3.2. Alu-*PCR*

2.3.2.1. Equipment

A PCR machine, e.g., Hybaid Thermal Reactor or Cetus Thermal Cycler, is the necessary equipment.

2.3.2.2. Reagents

1. Thermostable DNA polymerase: Cetus Ampli*Taq*I and Promega *Taq*I have proven reliable for generating strong multiband products suitable for "fingerprinting," "painting" (Chapter 26), and cloning. Hybaid Tth enzyme tends to produce more bands, each of lower intensity, and is therefore useful for "painting" and cloning, but less suitable for "fingerprinting." BCL and Amersham *Taq*I have also worked, but early batches tended to be rather variable. Best results (low background smear, multiple discrete bands) have been obtained using <2 U, and typically 1 U/assay.
2. PCR reaction buffer: The buffers recommended by the manufacturers work satisfactorily in most instances. However, the following buffer works well with all enzymes and all DNA samples tested to date: 50 mM KCl, 10 mM Tris-HCl, pH 8.4, 1.5 mM MgCl$_2$, 100 µg/mL gelatin, 0.01% Tween-20, 0.1% Triton X-100, and 0.1% Nonidet NP40, made up as a 10X stock, stored frozen, from titrated 1M stocks of KCl and MgCl$_2$, and from 10% stocks of detergent and 2% gelatin (autoclaved), all in ddH$_2$O.
3. Nucleotides: (from Pharmacia [Piscataway, NJ] 100 mM stock solutions) 200 µM GATC, stored separately and frozen as a 50X stock.
4. DNA: typically 100 ng, and not more than 1 µg of genomic DNA/50 µL vol reaction. Template DNA at 100 ng/µL is thoroughly heat denatured at 98°C for 5–10 min and then rapidly chilled on ice before adding to the PCR reaction mix.

5. Primers: Primers were synthesized on an ABI oligonucleotide synthesizer, ethanol precipitated direct from the column, stored in dH_2O or TE, and used at a final concentration of 0.5–1.0 μM in the PCR mix.
6. PCR reaction tubes: 0.5-mL microfuge tubes, Sigma cat. no. T5149.
7. Mineral oil: to overlay PCR samples, e.g., Sigma cat. no. 5OH-6125.

3. Methods
3.1. A Protocol for CMGT

1. Arrest donor cells in mitosis by the addition to the culture medium of colcemid at 0.1 µg/mL for 15–18 h (*see* Note 5).
2. For attached cells, shake off mitotic cells into suspension, and pellet from the medium by centrifugation at 200*g* for 7 min. If cells grow in suspension, then simply collect from the medium by centrifugation (*see* Note 6).
3. Resuspend to about 10^6/mL in fresh, filter-sterilized 0.75*M* KCl in deionized water (*see* Note 6). Leave to swell for 10–20 min at 37°C or 30–40 min at room temperature.
4. Chill on ice and spin down gently at 150*g* for 7 min at 4°C. Aspirate the supernatant, and resuspend to about 5×10^6/mL in freshly prepared 0.1% digitonin (Fluka AG) in 15 m*M* Tris-HCl and 3 m*M* $CaCl_2$, pH 7.0 (*see* Note 7). Maintain at 4°C through steps 5–7.
5. Gently draw the cell suspension three or four times through a 21-gage needle. Check for chromosome release and integrity by light microscopy or, preferably, by fluorescence microscopy of a sample stained with distamycin DAPI or ethidium bromide (*see* Note 4).
6. Centrifuge at 100*g* for 7 min to remove cell debris, whole cells, and nuclei. Dilute 10-fold in 15 m*M* Tris-HCl and 3 m*M* $CaCl_2$, pH 7.0, add sucrose to 5%, and pellet chromosomes by centrifugation at 1300*g* for 20 min.
7. Aspirate off all the supernatant, and gently resuspend in 10 vol 5% sucrose, 15 m*M* Tris-HCl, and 3 m*M* $CaCl_2$, pH 7.0, and repellet chromosomes by centrifugation at 1300*g* for 20 min.
8. Aspirate off all the supernatant, and resuspend the chromosomes gently and evenly in 50 m*M* HEPES, 280 m*M* NaCl, and 1.5 m*M* Na_2HPO_4, pH 7.15 (2X HeBS), at room temperature in a clear plastic tube (*see* Note 8). Resuspend at 5×10^6 mitotic cell equivalents/0.4 mL (*see* Note 9). Add an equal vol, dropwise, of 250 m*M* $CaCl_2$ while gently bubbling filtered air to mix through a disposable plastic pipet plugged with sterile cotton wool. A bluish and flocculent coprecipitate of chromosomes with $CaPO_4$ will form.
9. Aspirate the medium from the recipient cells. These should be seeded onto fresh 100 mm diameter Petri dishes about 18 h previously, i.e.,

about one cell generation) at a density to be approx one-third to one-half confluent at the time of chromosome transfection (*see* Note 10). Add 0.8 mL of the freshly formed precipitate/plate.

10. Leave the chromosome precipitate on the recipient cell monolayer at room temperature for 20 min with occasional agitation (*see* Note 11).

11. Add 10 vol of DMEM supplemented with fetal calf serum (2–10% as dictated by the recipient cell line), and incubate at 37°C for 6–8 h (*see* Note 12).

12. To shock cells into endocytosing membrane-bound chromosome precipitate, aspirate the medium plus chromosome precipitate and replace with 2–3 mL of 15% glycerol in HeBS for 2–3 min at 37°C. Aspirate off the glycerol, wash once with FCS-supplemented medium, and replace with same (*see* Note 13).

13. Leave the cells in nonselective medium for 24–48 h, thereafter, apply and maintain selection. Test cell populations or individual clones for successful CMGT by the assays and criteria set out below (*see* Note 14).

3.2. Selection Systems

3.2.1. Biochemical Markers

In the first CMGT experiments to be analyzed in any molecular detail, the basis for selection was the genetic complementation of biochemical deficiencies in DNA metabolism *(6,7)*. Transfer of normal metaphase chromosomes to recipient cells selected previously for (1) hypoxanthine phosphoribosyl transferase (HPRT) deficiency (resistance to 6-thioguanine) or (2) thymidine kinase (TK) deficiency (resistance to 5-Bromo-2-deoxyuridine), selects specifically for transfer of chromosome fragments encompassing (1) the HPRT locus at Xq26 or (2) the TK locus at 17q24 when subjected to HAT selection (100 μM hypoxanthine, 0.4 μM aminopterin, 10 μM thymidine).

A wide range of auxotrophs that lack enzymes involved in biosynthesis of aminoacids, purines, and pyrimidines, have been derived from Chinese hamster ovary (CHO) cells by Puck and Kao *(11)* and others, e.g., following mutagenesis with 5-bromodeoxyuridine plus visible light. These would serve as suitable recipients for genetic and biochemical complementation by CMGT with selection for growth on minimal medium.

3.2.2. Drug Resistance

Cell lines resistant to a variety of drugs important in cancer treatment and general medical care have been established or selected in culture. The genetic basis of drug resistance can take many forms, but is frequently associated with an increase or altered activity in a drug metabolizing enzyme, in turn associated with gene amplification. CMGT has an important advantage over DNA-mediated gene transfer (DMGT), in this context, where functional transfer of large amplicons may be necessary to transfer resistance. Examples include transfer of:

1. Elevated levels of dihydrofolate reductase from methotrexate-resistant Chinese hamster cells to sensitive mouse cells *(12);*
2. Elevated ribonucleotide reductase levels from hydroxyurea resistant to sensitive hamster cells *(13);*
3. Murine sodium, potassium ATPase α subunit conferring ouabain resistance to monkey CV-1 cells (14); and
4. Multidrug resistance from LZ Chinese hamster cells to drug-susceptible mouse LTA cells *(15).*

3.2.3. Oncogenes

The first molecular identification of the transforming principle in a human cancer was identified following tumor DMGT to immortalized, but nontransformed mouse NIH3T3 cells *(16,17).* Formation of transformed foci on a background of the contact-inhibited monolayer indicated individual clones derived from cells that had taken up, stably integrated, and expressed the tumor oncogene. The same principle can be applied to the closely related technique of CMGT. There is of course the absolute requirement that established lines or short-term tumor cultures are available as a source of metaphase chromosomes. NIH3T3 and Rat-1 cells are suitable recipients, but our preferred indicator is the C127 epithelial cell line derived from a RIII mouse mammary tumor. This line has a high plating efficiency and clones well. It normally grows as a flat monolayer, making it particularly easy to detect the formation of transformed foci (*see* Note 15). This is particularly valuable when selecting for weakly transforming oncogenes, such as SV40 *(18).* Plates seeded with 5×10^5 cells are split 1 in 4 at 24 h posttransfection. Foci will be first visible at about 10 d posttransfection, but may take up to 4 wk to establish. This is significantly longer than for DMGT foci and most likely reflects the process by which CMGT trans-genomes stabilize by establishing an autonomously replicating fragment or integrate into a recipient chromosome. Expect to see on average 1 focus/plate, i.e., per 10^5 cells transfected. C127 cells are also suitable for scoring oncogenic transformation by growth in soft agar; normal C127 cells are completely anchorage dependent for growth, but oncogenic transformants produce large colonies in Seaplaque™ agarose *(10,19)*. For initial screening, 10^4–10^5 cells should be plated in 10 mL of 0.25% top agarose/medium/100 mm diameter plate. For single-cell cloning, plate 10, 100, and 1000 cells on separate plates in 2–3 mL top agarose/medium/35 mm diameter dish to cover variation in plating efficiency. Individual well-separated colonies can be picked out of the soft agar with a sterile Pastet and transferred to liquid medium for mass culture.

Oncogenic transformants can also be selected directly or assayed secondarily by an immunosuppressed mouse tumor assay *(19)*. Primary transfection products (up to 10^7 cell/site) or selected transformants (as few as 10 cells, but typically 10^3–10^6/site) are inoculated subcutaneously, and the resultant tumors examined by molecular, biochemical, or histological methods *(19)* (*see* Notes 16 and 17).

Whereas a random selection of unrelated DNA sequences (summing to perhaps 1000 kbp in total) will be cotransferred along with the oncogene in each DMGT-derived clone, in CMGT, extensive contiguous lengths of chromatin are cotransferred *(20)*. The *trans*-genome may comprise as little as 200 kbp or as much as 100 Mbp of DNA *(20, 21)*. In particular, in CMGT, but not DMGT, extensive lengths of DNA sequence flanking the locus under selection can be cotransferred. Thus, the effect on oncogene expression of 5' and 3' controlling sequences can be studied *(10,19,22)*. Similarly, CMGT, but not whole-cell fusion or DMGT, can reveal syngeneic effects of syntenic sequences *(18)*. Oncogenes that have been analyzed and exploited in CMGT include HRAS1 from the EJ bladder carcinoma cell *(10,19,20)*, MET from the chemically mutagenized human osteosarcoma line MNNG-HOS *(23)*, and chromosomally integrated SV40 in the human chromosome 7-mouse somatic cell hybrid Cl 21 *(18)*.

3.2.4. Cell-Surface Markers

Species-specific monoclonal (or polyclonal) antibodies directed against cell-surface expressed antigens can be used to screen or select actively for the chromosomal locus in CMGT *(24)* in several ways.

3.2.4.1. LIVE CELL SORTING
ON A FLUORESCENT-ACTIVATED CELL SORTER

A single round of Fluorescent-Activated Cell Sorter (FACS) sorting will substantially enrich for a single clone expressing an immunoreactive cell-surface antigen out of a large population of negative cells. Positive cells are collected and propagated in culture. One or two further rounds of sorting on the FACS will be sufficient to give a pure population of expressing cells. A single-cell cloning step is advisable after the first round of sorting to show a significant peak of expressing cells. The FACS is a powerful and adaptable analytical and preparative tool that can be used to select for very uncommon events (Chapter 13), but in the context of CMGT suffers three intrinsic problems. First, there is an inherent bias toward selecting high-expression transfectants. These transfectants may be atypical, and carry amplified and grossly rearranged *trans*-genomes *(24)*. Second, independent transformants will tend to be lost through overgrowth by the dominant clone, unless the cells from the selected FACS window are single-cell cloned at an early stage. The third, but perhaps most significant, reason is that access to an FACS is the exception rather than the rule for most investigators. Fortunately, all these problems can be overcome by one or the other of three affordable and convenient alternatives.

3.2.4.2. ANTIBODY-COATED MAGNETIC BEADS

These offer a cheap alternative to the FACS for bulk cell sorting. Magnetic beads coated with antimouse Ig are commercially available (e.g., Dynal™ beads) and can be used to bind any monoclonal antibody directed to the desired cell-surface expressed antigen (Chapter 17). The transformants are mixed with the antibody-coated beads, placed in a tube next to a strong magnetic field, and the nonexpressing cells aspirated off. The bead-bound cells can then be removed from the magnetic field, resuspended, and washed in medium or PBS, and the process repeated once or twice. This simple and quick procedure efficiently and effectively removes all nonexpressing cells. Bead-bound cells are seeded into fresh wells and medium. The cells can be bulk cultured or single-cell cloned directly. To avoid selection of a dominant clone over other independent clones, primary transformants can be bead selected in small aliquots likely to contain only single CMGT events. Antibody-coated magnetic beads can be used to maintain actively expressing cultures by selecting for expressing cells at subsequent passages.

3.2.4.3. ROSETTING

If the transformants grow as individual attached cell clones, then expressing clones can be identified by "rosetting" with antibody conjugated to sheep red blood cells (SRBCs) or colored latex beads. In this way, individual transformants can be identified on the primary transfection dish and cloned directly. This procedure must be performed carefully and gently to avoid dislodging "rosettes" when washing off the vast excess of unattached antibody-conjugated SRBCs.

3.2.4.4. PANNING

This is a viable alternative to "rosetting" for isolating actively expressing clones and can be applied directly to suspension culture cells. Attached cells must first be suspended by gentle treatment with trypsin. In "panning," the transfected cells are allowed to bind to the surface of a tissue culture flask or Petri dish coated with antibody, and nonadherent cells gently washed off (Chapter 6). Individual transformants can thus be recovered directly.

3.2.5. Coselection
with Plasmid-Borne Biochemical Markers

Pritchard and Goodfellow *(25)* showed that coprecipitation of chromatin with plasmid DNA carrying a cloned selectable marker could be used to preselect for the small proportion of cells (1 in 1000 or less) taking up DNA and chromatin. This greatly aids the study of genetic factors not amenable to direct biochemical selection. Pritchard and Goodfellow *(25)* used this approach to enrich for clones expressing a cell-surface marker. Porteous et al. *(19)* used the same strategy to pre-select cells transfected with chromosomes from a bladder carcinoma cell line before selection for tumor growth in immunosuppressed mice. Alternatively, colony-based screening assays, including PCR-based DNA sequence assays, could be used to screen for cotransfer of chosen genetic factors.

3.2.6. Chromosomal Integration
of Dominant Selectable Markers

The laboratory of David Housman played a leading role in developing new selection strategies and molecular methods to exploit CMGT. Perhaps the most important was to use retroviruses carrying dominant selectable markers, e.g., neo or ecogpt, to infect mouse cells as a means for chromosomal insertion of a selectable tag *(26,27,* reviewed in ref. *8)*. Because the infection step is very efficient and, by superinfection, it is possible to obtain multiple independent integrations within one genome, it is practical to isolate many hundreds of viral transformants providing a resource in which at least one site will map close to any region in the mouse genome. It is then possible to screen in CMGT for cotransfer of an endogenous gene product, e.g., by expression of a cell-surface antigen *(27)*. The overriding limitation of this approach is of course the low frequency with which an integration site by chance will be closely linked to the unselectable locus of interest. In practice, cotransfer will occur only very infrequently. A solution would be to map the sites of retroviral integration first by rescue of DNA sequences flanking the integration sites or by *in situ* localization using retroviral vector as probe *(see* Section 3.2.7.), and select appropriate integrants for cotransfer studies. This is not a trivial exercise. A more elegant and direct approach that overcomes this limitation is outlined below.

3.2.7. Gene Targeting of Dominant Selectable Markers

DNA constructs incorporating a fragment of genomic DNA transfected into cultured cells tend to integrate randomly and recombine with the homologous site in the recipient genome perhaps only once in a thousand or more events. It is possible to design vectors that favor homologous recombination events by minimizing the possibility of random insertions. If the target gene is expressed, the most effective strategy is to build a construct devoid of promoter elements in which a portion of the target gene is placed upstream and in frame with just the coding segment of a selectable marker. Expression of the selectable marker relies on the endogenous promoter activity of the gene to be targeted. We have used this strategy to target with very high efficiency (>25% of G418-resistant clones correctly targeted) a neomycin cassette to two sites of SV40 on the chromosome 7 of a somatic cell hybrid, where this is the sole human component. CMGT with selection for G418 resistance gave rise to a set of reduced chromosome 7 hybrids nucleated around the targeted loci *(28–30)*.

The targeting strategy is not restricted to expressed genes. Positive negative selection (PNS) vectors have two selectable markers, a positive (P) selection marker (e.g., neo) between and a negative (N) selection marker (e.g., HSV-tk) flanking the cloned segments of the gene to be targeted *(31)*. Random insertion events tend to involve concatemers, and therefore, both P and N markers will be expressed. Cells expressing HSV-tk are specifically killed by addition of gancyclovir to the medium. Clones doubly resistant to G418 and gancyclovir will be enriched for homologous recombination events because the HSV-tk genes are clipped off and lost by the double-reciprocal recombination event, through which the neo is integrated. This general strategy for tagging chromosomes is only now being fully appreciated and exploited. The power and utility of this approach lie in the potential to target and thus manipulate by CMGT or other methods essentially any region of the genome for which a molecular clone of a few kilobase pairs in length is available *(32)*.

3.3. Analytical Methods

Development of CMGT as a useful genetic tool owes as much to the design and application of new analytical methods as to the exploitation of new selection strategies. The essential methods outlined below will provide a comprehensive picture of *trans*-genome complexity, organization, and origin. This is essential when assessing the potential of individual transfectants to serve as enrichment cloning resources and the interpretation for primary mapping purposes of cotransfer results obtained from a panel of CMGT hybrids.

3.3.1. In Situ Hybridization

In situ hybridization methods are described in detail elsewhere in this volume (Chapters 25 and 26). I will mention here only some of the key points of direct relevance to *trans*-genome analysis.

When we initiated our studies, it had been possible in a few exceptional cases to identify large donor chromosome fragments by cytogenetic staining against a background of the recipient karyotype *(5,6,20,21,32)*, but otherwise little was known about the organization of *trans*-genomes in CMGT hybrids. We started by using labeled total human DNA as probe to identify the human *trans*-genome in CMGT rodent hybrids. Initially *(33)*, we modified the guanine residues of our probe with *N*-acetyl-2-acetylaminofluorene (AAF). Hybridization was detected by indirect immunofluorescence after reaction first with a monoclonal antibody directed against AAF-modified guanine and then with an FITC-labeled antimouse IgG. This method gives a strong but discrete signal that allowed us to detect with ease *trans*-genomes estimated independently to have a molecular complexity of as little as 4 Mbp. It was apparent from these studies that stable hybrids fell into three general classes—those in which the *trans*-genome was maintained and segregated as an autonomously replicating fragment, hybrids in which the *trans*-genome was interstitially inserted as a single block in a rodent chromosome, and hybrids carrying two or more distinct fragments of human DNA at separate sites.

We wished to investigate further the structural organization of these various *trans*-genomes. We next developed a double-labeling procedure *(34)* that allowed us to visualize the location of the selectable marker superimposed on the total human component. We used biotinylation of total human DNA following nick translation to delineate the *trans*-genome (Chapter 26). Tritium-labeled pEJ plasmid was used to localize the HRAS1 gene within the *trans*-genome. Cohybridization and sequential visualization of human chromatin by FITC-labeled second antibody to anti-biotin IgG and HRAS1 by autoradiography established that all HRAS1-selected CMGT hybrids carried at least two copies of HRAS1, consistent with the idea that a single copy of activated oncogene is insufficient for full transformation *(10)*. Hybrids carrying multiple *trans*-genomes show HRAS1 hybridization to each independent fragment. Hybrids with single *trans*-genome fragments show two sites of HRAS1 hybridization consistent with a head-to-head or head-to-tail tandem duplication. These results are important for illuminating the process by which *trans*-genomes can rearrange, and are stabilized and maintained within the hybrid cell. Further studies on *trans*-genomes derived under different selection conditions are warranted. The preferred method now for dual (or multi) labeling would use two (or more) reporter molecules with distinguishable fluorescence spectra (Chapter 25).

Over and above the tandem reduplication of the whole *trans*-genome, molecular studies detailed below demonstrate that CMGT is often associated with intrachromosomal rearrangement *(8,20,25)*. Evaluation of the extent of rearrangement is limited by the depth of molecular analysis. It is therefore valuable to obtain a global picture of the chromosomal origin of *trans*-genomes. The method of choice is chromosome "painting" of normal human diploid metaphase spreads using a complex probe produced by *Alu*-PCR *(35)* amplification of the CMGT hybrids *(30* and Chapter 26). This provides a graphic of the *trans*-

genome origin that is in close agreement with that established by the more laborious process of extensive cotransfer analysis with previously mapped, or *trans*-genome-derived molecular probes or locus-specific PCR primers.

Finally, we have used vector specific probes to determine the chromosomal site of integration in gene-targeting experiments *(30)*. This is particularly important when the target site is a member of a gene or sequence family *(30,32)*, and is the method of choice for locating random sites of dominant selectable marker integration *(8)*.

3.3.2. Trans-Genome DNA "Fingerprinting"

3.3.2.1. INTERSPERSED REPEAT MAPPING

Housman and colleagues used probes that recognized a family of moderately repeated, interspersed DNA sequences to characterize the *trans*-genomes generated by transfer of retrovirally tagged mouse chromosomes to Chinese hamster or monkey cells. Independent hybrids derived from single integrant showed cotransfer of overlapping subsets of the repeat family *(8,26,27,36)*. We have developed a similar strategy for mapping human *trans*-genomes using L1 repeat probes.

3.3.2.2. L1 "FINGERPRINTING"

The L1 family of repeated sequence is dispersed throughout the human genome with one copy on average every 70–300 kbp. Although there are related sequences in all mammalian DNAs, probes are available that will specifically detect human DNA in a rodent background. The full-length repeat is 6.4 kbp long and is made up of four 5'–3' ordered *Kpn*I fragments of approx 1.8, 1.5, 1.2, and 1.8 kbp in length. Digestion of monochromosome or CMGT hybrid DNA with *Kpn*I and probing of Southern blots with any one *Kpn*I fragment produce a strong band of hybridization to the consensus band of either 1.8, 1.5, or 1.2 kbp (depending on the L1 subfragment used), plus a ladder of higher-mol-wt fragments. These act to provide a DNA "fingerprint" that is diagnostic for each CMGT hybrid. We coined the term restriction fragment length variants (RFLVs) *(20)* to denote these non-consensus fragments, which together comprise the "fingerprint." RFLVs occur because a proportion of L1 repeats have diverged from the consensus, are truncated (usually from the 5' end), or have lost one or more consensus restriction sites. Thus, the RFLVs are locus-specific markers mapping from a specific diverged L1 repeat to the nearest *Kpn*I site in the flanking DNA. The overall pattern and intensity of hybridization to L1 probes give a good estimate of the *trans*-genome complexity. Novel RFLVs in individual hybrids also provide direct evidence for molecular rearrangement accompanying the CMGT process. For maximum information, probes from the 5', central, and 3' ends of the L1 repeat should be used sequentially on several different digests. Preferred enzymes in addition to *Kpn*I are *Hind*III, *Bgl*II, and *Xba*I, all of which have consensus cutting sites in the repeat, but which generate informative "fingerprints." Five-microgram aliquots of DNA should be digested to completion, electrophoresed through 0.8% agarose, transferred to nitrocellulose or nylon membranes, and hybridized following standard procedures. Expect to obtain a good signal after 1–5 d, depending on the amount of DNA used and the complexity of the *trans*-genomes. In this way, hybrids with a human component ranging from about 1 Mbp to in excess of 100 Mbp can be analyzed.

3.3.2.3. *Alu*-PCR "Fingerprinting"

At an average reiteration frequency of 1 every 3–5 kbp, the *Alu* repeat characteristic of human DNA is too common to be of value for DNA hybridization "fingerprinting" other than for the very smallest *trans*-genomes. However, it has been possible to design oligonucleotide primers directed toward the consensus *Alu* repeat sequence, which will promote a polymerase chain reaction between closely spaced, inversely orientated *Alu* repeats. Since the original description of this idea *(35),* several primers and many applications have been described. I have designed a set of primers directed toward the *Alu* consensus sequence as compiled by Bains *(37),* which we find useful for "fingerprinting" CMGT hybrids and human YAC recombinants, for generating a complex probe for *in situ* localization of YAC recombinants, and "painting" of normal metaphase spreads with pooled *Alu*-PCR product from CMGT hybrids and enrichment cloning *(30* and Chapters 22 and 26) *(see* Notes 18 and 19). They have also been used in primed *in situ* hybridization (PRINS) (Chapter 18) *(see* Note 20). The following set is most suitable for *Alu*-PCR "fingerprinting" and cloning.

3.3.2.3.1. ALU-*PCR* PRIMERS

211 5' CCC.AAA.GTG.CTG.GCA.TTA.CAG.G, 3' Bottom strand, priming out to unique sequence from the 5' end of *Alu*.

239 5' CCC.AAA.GTG.CTG.GGT.CGA.CAG.G 3' Converts 211 to a *Sal*I site cloning primer.

152 5' GTG.AGC.CGA.GAT.CGC.GCC.ACT.GCA.CT 3' Top strand, priming out to unique sequence from the 3' end of *Alu*. Also known as 451 and 614. This primer overlaps partially at 5' end with TC-65, the original *Alu*-PCR primer described by Nelson et al. *(35)*.

476 5' GTG.AGC.CGA.GAG.CGC.GCC.ACT.GCA.CT 3' Converts 152 (451/614) to a *Bss*HII site cloning primer.

448 5' GAG.CCG.AGA.TCG.CGC.CAC.TGC.AC 3' Top strand, priming out to unique sequence from the 3' end of *Alu*. Truncation of 152 (451/614).

449 5' GTG.CAG.TGG.CGC.GAT.CTC.GGC.TC 3' Bottom strand, priming out to 5' unique sequence through *Alu,* from 3' end. Exact complement of 448.

3.3.2.3.2. ALU-*PCR* TEMPERATURE CYCLE PROGRAMS.

Buffer, nucleotides, primer, and enzyme are mixed and aliquoted prior to the addition of target DNA. Great care must be taken to avoid crosscontamination of reagents and samples. A set of pipetors should be set aside for aliquoting PCR templates and reagents. They should be regularly stripped down and steeped in $0.1M$ HCl and then glassware detergent, before washing extensively in fresh deionized water and finally alcohol to complete the decontamination procedure. All tubes and tips should be sterile virgin plastic and kept separate from all other laboratory procedures. Optimized programs for the Cetus Thermal Cycler and for the Hybaid Thermal Reactor are as follows (*see* Notes 18–22).

Cetus DNA Thermal Cycler
    1X 94°C, 3 min; 60–70°C, 1 min; 72°C, 1 min
    35X 94°C, 45 s;   60–70°C, 1 min; 72°C, 1 min, increasing
                                                        by 6 s/cycle
    1X 94°C, 45 s;   60–70°C, 1 min; 72°C, 10 min
Hybaid Thermal Reactor
    1X 94°C, 3 min; 60–70°C, 1 min; 72°C, 1 min
    5X 92°C, 20 s;   60–70°C, 1 min; 72°C, 1 min
    5X 92°C, 20 s;   60–70°C, 1 min; 72°C, 1.5 min
    5X 92°C, 20 s;   60–70°C, 1 min; 72°C, 2 min
    5X 92°C, 20 s;   60–70°C, 1 min; 72°C, 2.5 min

5X 92°C, 20 s; 60–70°C, 1 min; 72°C, 3 min
5X 92°C, 20 s; 60–70°C, 1 min; 72°C, 3.5 min
5X 92°C, 20 s; 60–70°C, 1 min; 72°C, 4 min
1X 92°C, 20 s; 60–70°C, 1 min; 72°C, 10 min

3.3.3. Enrichment Cloning and Mapping

Two important uses of CMGT are to produce reduced chromosome hybrids, which can serve as a source of new molecular markers for the immortalized region, and for fine-structure mapping by cotransfer analysis of these and preexisting markers using a panel of CMGT hybrids and conventional hybrids carrying clinical or experimental translocations or deletions *(38–40)*. All methods apply essentially standard molecular genetic procedures. The following comments aim to highlight aspects specific to CMGT analysis and exploitation.

3.3.3.1. GENOMIC LIBRARIES IN COSMID AND λ VECTORS

Standard procedures are used to construct and screen genomic libraries. Whole cosmid or λ recombinant clones can be used as a single-copy probe if it is radiolabeled by random priming or nick translation, and a large molar excess of unlabeled total human DNA or Cot1 fraction (Gibco-BRL) added to radiolabeled recombinants to suppress filter hybridization by repeated elements present in the probe. Recombinants can also be accurately localized by *in situ* hybridization (*3* and Chapter 25). It is noteworthy that of over 100 cosmid and λ clones isolated from a variety of CMGT hybrids, with one notable exception, all have mapped back to the chromosome under selection. The sole exception is a recombinant derived from an HRAS1-CMGT-derived breakpoint associated with elevated tumorigenicity (*22,* and Hirst and Porteous, unpublished). Thus, the rearrangements that characterize the CMGT process are almost entirely intrachromosomal.

3.3.3.2. *ALU*-PCR PROBES AND LIBRARIES

Alu-PCR reaction products can be conveniently cloned using primers 239 (*Sal*I compatible) or 471 (*Bss*HII compatible). These primers can be used directly on genomic template, but secondary amplification of 211 or 152 products, respectively, will maximize the set of products obtained. Direct cloning into TA cloning vectors (Invitrogen™) of *Alu*-PCR products by virtue of the propensity of the PCR to produce a 3' A tail is also effective. Since a portion of the *Alu* repeat is amplified in the course of the PCR, it is advisable to use suppression hybridization conditions for mapping. Individual bands can be cut from a preparative gel, and cloned or reamplified and labeled by *Alu*-PCR. *Alu*-PCR products from individual hybrids produced by one or more primer individually can be pooled and labeled by nick translation and used as a complex probe for *in situ* hybridization "painting" of normal metaphase chromosomes (Chapter 26), or to identify products shared between independent CMGT hybrids by Southern transfer hybridization (Leech and Porteous, unpublished).

3.3.3.3. CONTIG MAPPING

The contig mapping strategy—where recombinants from partial digest libraries are restriction mapped and compared for the presence of shared fragments indicating regions of partial overlap between independent recombinants and thus assembled into contiguous arrays— has been successfully applied to the relatively small genomes of *E. coli,* yeast, and *C. elegans.* However, the substantially greater complexity of the human genome means that a massive amount of data must be acquired and compared before any contigs will emerge, and it is questionable whether the method stringency is sufficient to avoid an unacceptable level of false contig assembly. However, CMGT *trans*-genomes are of a practical complexity for contig assembly with currently available procedures and analytical tools. Indeed, Weis et al. *(36)* showed that it was possible to link independent recombinants on the basis of shared restriction fragments by analyzing donor-specific recombinants isolated from a mouse *trans*-genome in which the MHC locus had been cotransferred with a retrovirally inserted dominant selectable marker. We have recently shown that it is possible without enormous effort to construct an extensive contig map for a subregion of human chromosome 11 immortalized in an HRAS1-CMGT hybrid *(41)*. Data acquisition can be largely automated and analysis computerized. The building of maps is accumulative rather than stepwise. Thus, the process is potentially much more efficient that other mapmaking procedures, such as library "walking." It has the enormous advantage of connectivity. For example, any number of previously unconnected defined markers can be incorporated into the "contig" and thus linked. Similarly, if markers are shown by physical or genetic linkage studies to flank a particular locus, placement on a "contig" map identifies directly a minimal set of cloned intervening DNA fragments that must encode the genetic marker for which we seek a molecular identity.

3.3.3.4. FINE STRUCTURE MAPPING BY COTRANSFER ANALYSIS

Although intrachromosomal rearrangement is commonly associated with CMGT, all of the evidence from several independent studies establishes quite clearly that closely linked markers tend to cosegregate *(5–7, 20,23,25, 38–40)*. Thus, having typed a set of defined markers to a panel of CMGT hybrids each carrying different chromosome fragment compositions, it is possible to assign new markers with great confidence to narrowly defined subchromosomal regions (Porteous, unpublished). Furthermore, since some CMGT hybrids contain DNA segments that have undergone local amplification and rearrangement, it is possible to incorporate evidence from hybridization analysis for (or against) close synteny into the confirmation or extension of "contig" maps (Porteous and Little, unpublished).

3.4. Summing Up

With the advent of new selection strategies for endogenous genes and the extraordinary potential of gene targeting for chromosome tagging, the CMGT strategy can be applied to the functional and molecular analysis of essentially any region of the mammalian genome.

Application of a range of new molecular and cytogenetic methods for analyzing *trans*-genome structure and organization has allowed CMGT to be exploited to great effect as an enrichment cloning *(36,38–42)* and fine structure mapping *(20,23,25,27,40)* method. These analyses have also highlighted the fact that frequent and complex rearrangements can accompany the CMGT process. It is not clear whether these are absolutely intrinsic to the process, or whether modifications to the methods for chromosome purification, transfection, and selection for stable transformants might materially affect the outcome.

Several commentators have compared CMGT unfavorably with radiation fusion as a method for establishing reduced chromosome hybrids. It is true that map order and length estimated on the basis of statistical analysis of marker cotransfer in large sets of radiation hybrids agree closely with independently deduced physical and genetic maps *(43)*. However, when individual radiation hybrids are analyzed in anything like the detail we have for CMGT, then a very similar picture emerges—radiation hybrids typically contain one or several blocks of chromosomes representing short stretches of preserved synteny, but with multiple and variable sized gaps (van Heyningen, Evans, Fletcher, and Porteous, unpublished). It is perhaps not surprising that the same commentators have viewed the propensity for rearrangements to accompany the CMGT process as a major limitation of the technique. Our view is that recognition and characterization of this feature is an attribute of CMGT (and radiation hybrids) that can be turned to great advantage *(39)*.

4. Notes
4.1. Reagents

1. Digitonin is a hazardous toxin. Handle with care. Dispense the required amount into a preweighed capped tube in a fume hood.
2. The pH of the 2X HeBS solution is critical and must be between pH 7.1 and 7.2. Mock coprecipitation with 2X $CaCl_2$ should give a fine precipitate with a bluish hue. 2X HeBS solution is made in bulk and stored frozen at $-20°C$ in convenient aliquots after testing.
3. A medium low in phosphate, such as DMEM, must be used during the primary transfection. An insoluble and cell lethal precipitate will form on addition of a $CaPO_4$ coprecipitate to media high in phosphate, such as RPMI 1640. The recipient cells must therefore be adapted to a suitable medium before transfection and maintained on the same for at least 24 h, with one medium change, posttransfection.
4. Ethidium bromide is a hazardous chemical carcinogen. The powder is absorbed by inhalation, and the liquid through the skin. Weigh, dispense, and dissolve in a fume cupboard. Handle with gloves at all times. Dispose of waste carefully by incineration of sealed samples.

4.2. CMGT Protocol

5. Donor chromosomes must be prepared from actively growing, mycoplasma-free cultures. The optimum period for colcemid arrest to maximize the yield of mitotic cells will be determined by the culture cell cycle time and should be determined empirically.
6. Steps 2–9 of the CMGT protocol (Section 3.1.) must be carried out under sterile conditions using sterile equipment and presterilized reagents. Some cells, e.g., the C127 line, require brief trypsin treatment prior to swelling with KCl for maximum chromosome recovery.
7. Chromosomes isolated in 15 mM Tris-HCl, 2 mM EDTA, 0.5 mM EGTA, 80 mM KCl, 20 mM NaCl, 14 mM β-mercaptoethanol, 0.5 mM

spermidine, and 0.2 m*M* spermine, pH 7.2, the buffer preferred for chromosome sorting on the FACS (Chapter 14), are biologically inactive, at least for HRAS1-mediated cellular transformation and transfection to G418 resistance by chromosomally integrated neo genes *(10)*. However, full activity can be restored by dialysis against 15 m*M* Tris-HCl and 3 m*M* CaCl$_2$, pH 7.0. Chromosomes stored in 0.1% digitonin, 15 m*M* Tris-HCl, and 3 m*M* CaCl$_2$, pH 7.0, on ice can retain their biological activity for at least 7 d.

8. **Do not use glass** test tubes or pipets, since DNA and chromatin will stick avidly to the glass.
9. The quantities given in the protocol correspond to between 2 and 10 mitotic cell equivalents of donor chromosomes/recipient cell. In a carefully conducted series of experiments *(12)*, Lewis et al. determined a linear relationship between chromosomes and transfectants up to at least 2 mitotic cell equivalents/recipient. Increasing the concentration of chromosomes to beyond $5 \times 10^6/0.8$ mL of precipitate in our hands leads to an excessively flocculent precipitate and a reduced transfection frequency.
10. Ensure that recipient cells are seeded evenly. The optimum number of cells per transfection dish will be determined by size and doubling time, e.g., 5×10^5 C127 cells or 2.5×10^6 mouse L-cells/100 mm diameter dish.
11. The precipitate, if swirled around the transfection dish, will be distributed unevenly and concentrate at the perimeter. Therefore, shake occasionally and firmly on a flat surface to ensure even spreading during the 20-min incubation period.
12. We have noted a marked cytotoxic effect if, as recommended in some DNA transfection protocols, the precipitate is left on overnight.
13. DMSO has been described as an alternative to glycerol for increasing the transfection frequency. In our experience, different recipient cells show marked variation in their tolerance of DMSO, and in some instances, this may reduce transfection frequencies dramatically. By contrast, most cells give a moderate, but positive (two- to fivefold increase) in transfection frequency following glycerol shock.
14. In general, the frequency of successful CMGT compares favorably with that for single-copy genomic DNA transfer *(12)*. The overall frequency is a compound of the transfectability of the recipient cell line (typically 1 in 10^3–10^4), the efficiency of the selection system (empiric), and the average fraction of the genome transferred to each transfectant (0.01–5%). Frequencies typically fall in the range of 1 in 10^5–10^7. By careful control of all parameters, Lewis et al. *(12)* reported transfection frequencies as high as 1 in 10^4 recipient cells.

4.3. Oncogene Selection

15. Although most established cell lines will grow happily on most fetal calf serums, special care must be taken in selecting a serum supplement for oncogenic transformation assays. Only certain batches of fetal calf serum will support and maintain a flat monolayer of contact inhibited indicator cells, e.g., NIH3T3 or C127 cells, thus allowing the outgrowth of foci of transformed cells induced by tumor gene transfer to be scored reliably. Samples of fetal calf serum must be tested regularly, and stocks of satisfactory batches purchased and held separately from those used for routine cell culture.

16. We use neonatally thymectomized, whole-body irradiated CBA mice, but genetically immunologically deprived mice, such as nu/nu or SCID mice, are also suitable, although they require more exacting animal husbandry for maintenance of stocks.

17. Experiments using protected species are governed by the Animals (Scientific Procedures) Act 1986, and application to and approval from the Home Office for a Personal and Project Licence to cover such work must be made before starting any experiments.

4.4. Alu-*PCR*

18. The annealing temperature largely determines the specificity of the reaction. There is a trade-off between specificity and yield, but it is essential for "fingerprinting" and cloning purposes that there is no amplification whatsoever from the rodent counterparts to the human *Alu* repeated sequence. Each of the above primers will give completely human specific amplification at elevated annealing temperatures. This is most critical for primers 211 and 239, for which the annealing temperature should be between 65 and 70°C. Human-specific amplification with the other primers should be possible at 60°C, but I usually use 65°C since the yield is still high.

19. Unlike locus-specific PCR, *Alu* primers are used individually. Simultaneous use of a 3' end and 5' end primer does not produce a "fingerprint" that is a compound and addition to that obtained with individual primers. This is most likely owing to competition within the PCR for amplification of inter-*Alu* fragments. However, each primer will give a distinct, but reproducible set of products for each template DNA and can be subsequently pooled to increase the complexity of "fingerprint" and probe.

20. The stringency requirements for "painting" purposes are less exacting, since a small fraction of nonspecific rodent DNA amplification will not interfere with the labeling of normal human metaphase spreads. This

has allowed us to design additional *Alu*-PCR primers notably for the 5'
end (Chapters 18 and 26). Primer 449 is suitable for "fingerprinting"
but not "painting" or cloning, because it results in the amplification of
most of the *Alu* repeat.

21. Analyze reactions by UV transilluminescence and photography after
electrophoresis through 1.5% agarose and staining with EtBr (*see* Note
4). Fragments ranging from 100 bp to 4 kbp are typically obtained, with
the majority falling in the 500 bp to 2 kbp range.

22. The Hybaid Thermal Reactor programs are on "Tube Control." The
lower denaturation temperature and times reflect the fact that the set
temperature on the Cetus Thermal Cycler is not reached in the tube.
The programs outlined above have been calibrated using a Hybaid
DataSentry thermocouple device.

References

1. Ruddle, F. H. (1981) A new era in mammalian gene mapping: somatic cell
genetics and recombinant DNA technologies. *Nature* **294,** 115–120.
2. McBride, O. W. and Ozer, H. L. (1973) Transfer of genetic information by
purified metaphase chromosomes. *Proc. Natl. Acad. Sci. USA* **70,** 1258–1262.
3. Klobutcher, L. A. and Ruddle, F. H. (1981) Chromosome mediated gene transfer. *Ann. Rev. Biochem.* **50,** 533–554.
4. McBride, O. W. and Peterson, J. L. (1980) Chromosome-mediated gene transfer in mammalian cells. *Ann. Rev. Genet.* **14,** 321–345.
5. Miller, C. L. and Ruddle, F. H. (1978) Co-transfer of human X-linked markers
into murine somatic cells via isolated metaphase chromosomes. *Proc. Natl.
Acad. Sci. USA* **75,** 3346–3350.
6. Willecke, K. and Ruddle, F. H. (1975) Transfer of human gene for hypoxan-
thine-guanine phosphoribosyltransferase via isolated human metaphase chromosomes into mouse L-cells. *Proc. Natl. Acad. Sci. USA* **72,** 1792–1796.
7. Klobutcher, L. A. and Ruddle, F. H. (1979) Phenotypic stabilization and integration of transferred material in chromosome-mediated gene transfer. *Nature*
280, 657–660.
8. Housman, D. E. and Nelson, D. L. (1986) Use of metaphase-chromosome transfer for mammalian gene mapping, in *Gene Transfer* (Kucherlapati, R., ed.),
Plenum, pp. 95–115.
9. Porteous, D. J. (1987) Chromosome mediated gene transfer: a functional assay
for complex loci and an aid to human genome mapping. *Trends Genet.* **3,**
177–182.
10. Morten, J. E. N., Hirst, M. C., and Porteous, D. J. (1987) The c-Harvey-*ras*-1
oncogene in chromosome mediated gene transfer. *Anticancer Res.* **7,** 573–588.
11. Puck, T. T. and Kao, F.-T. (1982) Somatic cell genetics and its application to
medicine. *Ann. Rev. Genet.* **16,** 225–271.

12. Lewis, W. H., Srinivasan, P. R., Stokoe, N., and Siminivitch, L. (1980) Parameters governing the transfer of the genes for thymidine kinase and dihydrofolate reductase into mouse L cells using metaphase chromosomes and DNA. *Somat. Cell Genet.* **6,** 333–347.
13. Lewis, W. H. and Srinivasan, P. R. (1983) Chromosome-mediated gene transfer of hydroxyurea resistance and amplification of ribonucleotide reductase activity. *Mol. Cell Biol.* **3,** 1053–1061.
14. Fallows, D., Kent, R. B., Nelson, D. L., Emanuel, J. R., Levenson, R., and Housman, D. E. (1987) Chromosome-mediated transfer of the murine Na,K-ATPase alpha subunit confers ouabain resistance. *Mol. Cell Biol.* **7,** 2985–2987.
15. Gros, P., Fallows, D. A., Croop, J. M., and Housman, D. E. (1986) Chromosome-mediated gene transfer of multidrug resistance. *Mol. Cell Biol.* **6,** 3785–3790.
16. Shih, C. and Weinberg, R. A. (1982) Isolation of a transforming sequence from a human bladder carcinoma cell line. *Cell* **29,** 161–169.
17. Goldfarb, M., Shimizu, K., Perucho, M., and Wigler, M. (1982) Isolation and preliminary characterisation of a human transforming gene from T24 bladder carcinoma cells. *Nature* **296,** 404–409.
18. Porteous, D. J., Dorin, J. D., Wilkinson, M. M., Fletcher, J. M., Emslie, E., and van Heyningen, V. (1990) SV40-mediated tumor selection and chromosome transfer to enrich for cystic fibrosis region. *Somat. Cell Molec. Genet.* **16,** 29–38.
19. Porteous, D. J., Morten, J. E. N., Foster, M. E., Cranston, G., Weir-Thompson, E., Bussutil, A., Bostock, C. J., and Steel, C. M. (1986) HRAS1-selected, chromosome-mediated transformants vary in phenotype in vitro and tumorigenic potential in vivo. *Int. J. Cancer* **38,** 603–612.
20. Porteous, D. J., Morten, J. E. N., Cranston, G., Fletcher, J. M., Mitchell, A., van Heyningen, V., Fantes, J. A., Boyd, P. A., and Hastie, N. D. (1986) Molecular and physical arrangements of human DNA in HRAS1-selected, chromosome-mediated transfectants. *Mol. Cell Biol.* **6,** 2223–2232.
21. Olsen, A. S., McBride, O. W., and Moore, D. E. (1981) Number and size of human X chromosome fragments transferred to mouse cells by chromosome-mediated gene transfer. *Mol. Cell Biol.* **1,** 439–448.
22. Hirst, M. C. and Porteous, D. J. (1991) Molecular cloning of a rearranged HRAS1 oncogene in chromosome mediated gene transfer associated with elevated tumorigenicity. *Oncogene* **6,** 153–157.
23. Scambler, P. J., Law, H-Y., Williamson, R., and Cooper, C. S. (1986) Chromosome mediated gene transfer of six DNA markers linked to the cystic fibrosis locus on human chromosome 7. *Nucleic Acids Res.* **14,** 7159–7174.
24. Pritchard, C. and Goodfellow, P. N. (1986) Development of new methods in human gene mapping: selection for fragments of the human Y chromosome after chromosome-mediated gene transfer. *EMBO J.* **5,** 979–985.
25. Pritchard, C. A. and Goodfellow, P. N. (1987) Investigation of chromosome-mediated gene transfer using the HPRT region of the human X chromosome as a model. *Genes Devel.* **1,** 172–178.

26. Nelson, D. L., Weis, J. H., Przyborski, M. J., Mulligan, R. C., Seideman, J. G., and Housman, D. E. (1984) Metaphase chromosome transfer of introduced selectable markers. *J. Molec. Appl. Genet.* **2,** 563–577.

27. Weis, J. H., Nelson, D. L., Przyborski, M. J., Chaplin, D. D., Mulligan, R. C., Housman, D. E., and Seidman, J. G. (1984) Eukaryotic chromosome transfer: linkage of the murine major histocompatibility complex to an inserted dominant selectable marker. *Proc. Natl. Acad. Sci. USA* **81,** 4879–4883.

28. Dorin, J. R., Inglis, J. D., and Porteous, D. J. (1989) Selection for precise chromosomal targeting of a dominant marker by homologous recombination. *Science* **243,** 1357–1360.

29. Dorin, J. R. and Porteous, D. J. (1991) Gene targeting for somatic cell manipulation, in *Methods in Molecular Biology, vol. #9, Protocols in Human Molecular Genetics* (Mathew, C., ed.) Humana, Clifton, NJ.

30. Dorin, J. D., Emslie, E., Hanratty, D., Farrall, M., Gosden, J., and Porteous, D. J. (1992) Gene targeting for somatic cell manipulation: rapid analysis of reduced chromosome hybrids by Alu-PCR fingerprinting and chromosome painting. *Human Molecular Genetics,* submitted.

31. Mansour, S., Thomas, K., and Capecchi, M. (1988) Disruption of the proto-oncogene int-2 in mouse embryo-derived stem cells: a general strategy for targeting mutations to non-selectable genes. *Nature* **336,** 348–352.

32. Porteous, D. J., Brookes, A., Arveiler, B., Gosden, J., Maule, J., Byrd, P., Dickinson, P., and Dorin, J. (1991) Gene targeting for somatic cell manipulation: an integrated approach to clinical and functional genome analysis. *Adv. Mol. Gen.* **4,** 9–17.

33. Mitchell, A. R., Ambros, P., Gosden, J. R., Morten, J. E. N., and Porteous, D. J. (1986) Gene mapping and physical arrangements of human chromatin in transformed, hybrid cells: fluorescent and autoradiographic in situ hybridization compared. *Somat. Cell Molec. Genet.* **12,** 313–324.

34. Gosden, J. R. and Porteous, D. J. (1987) HRAS1-selected, chromosome mediated gene transfer; in situ hybridization with combined biotin and tritium label localizes the oncogene and reveals duplications of the human transgenome. *Cytogenet. Cell Genet.* **45,** 44–51.

35. Nelson, D. L., Ledbetter, S. A., Corbo, L., Victoria, M. F., Ramirez-Solis, R., Webster, T. D., Ledbetter, D. H., and Caskey, C. T. (1989) Alu polymerse chain reaction: a method for rapid isolation of human-specific sequence from complex DNA sources. *Proc. Natl. Acad. Sci. USA* **86,** 6686–6690.

36. Weis, J. H., Seidman, J. G., Housman, D. E., and Nelson, D. L. (1986) Eucaryotic chromosome transfer: production of a murin-specific cosmid library from a neo^rlinked fragment of murine chromosome 17. *Mol. Cell Biol.* **6,** 441–451.

37. Bains, W. (1986) The multiple origins of human Alu sequences. *J. Mol. Evol.* **23,** 189–199.

38. Porteous, D. J., Bickmore, W., Christie, S., Boyd, P. A., Cranston, G., Fletcher, J. M., Gosden, J. R., Rout, D., Seawright, A., Simola, K. O. J., van Heyningen, V., and Hastie, N. D. (1987) Hras1-selected chromosome transfer generates

markers that colocalize aniridia- and genitourinary dysplasia-associated translocation breakpoints and the Wilms tumor gene within band 11p13. *Proc. Natl. Acad. Sci. USA* **84,** 5355–5359.

39. Bickmore, W., Christie, S., van Heyningen, V., Hastie, N. D., and Porteous, D. J. (1988) Hitch-hiking from HRAS1 to the WAGR locus with CMGT markers. *Nucleic Acids Res.* **16,** 51–60.

40. Xu, W., Gorman, P. A., Rider, S. H., Hedge, P. J., Moore, G., Pritchard, C., Sheer, D., and Solomon, E. (1988) Construction of a genetic map of human chromosome 17 by use of chromosome-mediated gene transfer. *Proc. Natl. Acad. Sci. USA* **85,** 8563–8567.

41. Harrison-Lavoie, K. J., John, R. M., Porteous, D. J., and Little, P. F. R. (1989) A cosmid clone map derived from a small region of human chromosome 11. *Genomics* **5,** 501–509.

42. Estivill, X., Farrall, M., Scambler, P. J., Bell, G. M., Hawley, K. M. F., Lench, N. J., Bates, G. P., Kruyer, H. C., Frederick, P. A., Stanier, P., Watson, E. K., Williamson, R., and Wainwright, B. J. (1987) A candidate for the cystic fibrosis locus isolated by selection for methylation-free islands. *Nature* **326,** 840–845.

43. Cox, D. R., Burmeister, M., Price, E. R., Kim, S., and Myers, R. M. (1990) Radiation hybrid mapping: a somatic cell genetic method for constructing high-resolution maps of mammalian chromosomes. *Science* **250,** 245–250.

CHAPTER 21

Construction of Chromosome-Specific Libraries of Yeast Artificial Chromosome Recombinants from Somatic Hybrid Cell Lines

Benoît Arveiler

1. Introduction

The Yeast Artificial Chromosome (YAC) *(1)* technology allows the cloning of large fragments of DNA (several hundreds of kilobase pairs, kbp) into the budding yeast *Saccharomyces cerevisiae,* and therefore bridges a gap between conventional cloning in bacteria (λ and cosmid cloning) and somatic cell hybridization techniques. This powerful cloning system has been used successfully for the construction of representative human *(2–5)*, mouse *(5–7), Drosophila (8),* and *Caenorrhabditis elegans (9)* genomic libraries.

The YAC cloning technology constitutes indeed a major breakthrough for the mapping of complex genomes: Markers several hundreds of kilobase pairs apart can be linked on a single clone, thus rendering the analysis of large genomic regions possible at once; chromosome walking and contig mapping *(10)* exercises are made faster and more efficient, since specific genomic regions can be covered with a limited number of clones (for instance, 500 YACs with an average size of 300 kbp would cover the 150 Megabase pairs [Mbp] of human chromosome 11, where 3500 cosmids would be necessary). The fact that YAC recombinants cover large regions of genomic DNA makes them an attractive reagent to screen cDNA libraries either by colony

From: *Methods in Molecular Biology, Vol. 29: Chromosome Analysis Protocols*
Edited by: J. R. Gosden Copyright ©1994 Humana Press Inc., Totowa, NJ

hybridization *(11,12)* or possibly by techniques based on coincident sequence cloning *(13)*.

In addition, the YAC cloning system benefits from the multiple possibilities offered by yeast genetics techniques: Taking advantage of the very high efficacy of homologous recombination in *Saccharomyces cerevisiae,* nested deletions have been introduced in YACs *(14,15)*, and partially overlapping YAC recombinants have been recombined so as to generate larger recombinants *(16,17)*. YACs can thus theoretically be tailored to contain the desired amount of genetic information and, subsequently, transformed into suitable mammalian cell lines for functional analysis both in vitro *(18–20)* and in vivo *(21,22)*. One can also anticipate that the analysis of YAC clones will help understanding the organization of complex eukaryotic genomes (distribution of genes and repetitive sequences, for instance *[23]*).

Most YAC libraries constructed so far cover whole genomes. A major problem encountered with such libraries, however, is the high frequency of chimeric clones resulting from the coligation of multiple noncontiguous fragments *(24)*. This phenomenon greatly complicates chromosome walking experiments *(16,25,26)* and constrains the potential for contig mapping technologies by fingerprint analysis. One way around this problem is to construct chromosome-specific libraries from somatic hybrid cell lines with a reduced human component *(27)*, reducing proportionally the probability of coligation of nonsyntenic human fragments. One can indeed calculate that if the human DNA content comprises approx 1% of the total, and assuming an overall coligation frequency of 40%, a figure that holds in widespread and now well-characterized libraries *(24)*, 99.6% of human recombinants will have single human inserts. A further advantage inherent to such libraries is that all the human clones map to the chromosome of interest. They are therefore of immediate mapping value by *in situ* hybridization to chromosome spreads *(28)* (*see* Chapter 26) and can directly be added to the contig maps of these chromosomes. Chromosome-specific libraries constructed from somatic hybrid cell lines with a reduced component thus constitute a cloning material of choice when the mapping of whole chromosomes or extended subchromosomal regions is to be undertaken.

The library of overlapping recombinants is organized for multiaccess, such that it can be screened through several routes and can be entered at various stages, depending on both the material available for screening (cDNA or genomic probes, PCR primers) and on the particular use(s) that is to be made of the library (screening for a specific locus; contig mapping; painting of the library with a collection of probes, such as *Alu*-PCR products or microdissection clones, covering a specific subchromosomal region in order to saturate that region with YACs; screening with motif-specific probes in order to identify YACs containing members of specific gene families; and so on).

2. Materials
2.1. Chemicals and Stock Solutions

1. Agarose, medium electroendosmosis.
2. β-Mercaptoethanol—Toxic; handle in a fume hood; wear gloves.
3. $CaCl_2$: $1M$ stock solution.
4. Dithioerythritol: $1M$ stock solution, filter sterilized, stored at –20°C.
5. Ethanol: absolute and 70%.
6. Ethidium bromide: 10 mg/mL stock solution. Toxic: Handle with gloves.
7. Ethylenediamine tetra-acetic acid, disodium salt, EDTA: $0.5M$ stock solution, pH 8.
8. Glycerol: 80% stock solution.
9. 2-Isopropyl alcohol.
10. Low-melting-point agarose (BRL Ultrapure).
11. $MgCl_2$: $1M$ stock solution.
12. NaCl: $5M$ stock solution.
13. NaOH: $5M$ stock solution.
14. Organic solvents: chloroform-isoamyl alcohol (24:1), phenol (saturated with 10 mM Tris-HCl, pH 7.5, 1mM EDTA).
15. Phenylmethylsulfonylfluoride, PMSF: Use fresh 100 mM solution made up in isopropanol. Extremely toxic: Wear gloves and face mask.
16. Potassium acetate: $5M$ stock solution.
17. Sodium dodecyl sulfate, SDS (BDH): 10% stock solution.
18. Sorbitol: $1M$ stock solution.
19. Spermidine trihydrochloride: 100 mM stock solution, filter sterilized, stored at –20°C.
20. Tris-HCl pH 7.5: $2M$ stock solution, stored at 4°C.

2.2. Solutions

1. 4% Sodium alginic acid, sodium salt (Sigma, St. Louis, MO), $1M$ sorbitol.
2. ES: $0.5M$ EDTA, 1% *N* sodium lauroyl sarcosinate.
3. PEGTC: 10 mM Tris-HCl, pH 7.5, 10 mM $CaCl_2$, 20% Polyethyleneglycol 6000 (BDH no. 29577 or 44271).

4. 1M Sorbitol, 100 mM EDTA.
5. SCE: 1M sorbitol, 0.1M trisodium citrate, 60 mM EDTA, pH 8.0.
6. STC:1M sorbitol, 10 mM Tris-HCl, pH 7.5, 10 mM CaCl$_2$.
7. 10 mM Tris-HCl, pH 7.5, 5 mM EDTA.
8. 10 mM Tris-HCl, pH 7.5, 2 mM EDTA.
9. 10 mM Tris-HCl, pH 7.5, 1 mM EDTA.
10. 10 mM Tris-HCl, pH 7.5, 0.5 mM EDTA.
11. 50 mM Tris-HCl, pH 7.5, 20 mM EDTA.
12. TEN: 10 mM Tris-HCl, pH 7.5, 0.5 mM EDTA, 25 mM NaCl.
13. TAENE: 1X TAE, 100 mM NaCl, 10 mM EDTA.

2.3. Biological Reagents

1. Agarase (Calbiochem).
2. Bacterial alkaline phosphatase (BAP).
3. Bovine serum albumin (20 mg/mL) (Boehringer Mannheim).
4. Carrier DNA for yeast transformation: sonicated human DNA (5 mg/mL) (size range: 200–500 bp).
5. Cot1 human DNA (Gibco BRL).
6. Lyticase (Sigma L5263).
7. Phage λ DNA concatemers *(29)*.
8. Proteinase K.
9. Random primed DNA labeling kit (Boehringer Mannheim).
10. Restriction enzymes: *Eco*RI (10 U/µL) and *Bam*HI (10 U/µL).
11. RNase A: 10 mg/mL stock solution, boiled 15 min to inactivate DNases, stored at −20°C.
12. Sonicated salmon sperm DNA (10 mg/mL).
13. Sonicated rodent DNA (10 mg/mL).
14. T4 DNA ligase (1 U/µL) (Boehringer Mannheim).
15. Total human DNA (high mol wt).
16. pYAC4 vector *(1)*.
17. Zymolyase 100T (ICN Immunochemicals).

2.4. Buffers

1. *Eco*RI restriction buffer without MgCl$_2$: 100 mM Tris-HCl, pH 7.5, 50 mM NaCl, 100 µg/mL bovine serum albumin, 10 mM β-mercaptoethanol.
2. Ligation buffer: 100 mM Tris-HCl, pH 7.5, 100 mM MgCl$_2$, 100 mM dithioerythritol, 6 mM ATP.
3. Prehybridization and hybridization buffer: 4X SSC, 4X Denhardt solution, 10% dextran sulfate, 0.5% SDS, 50 µg/mL sonicated salmon sperm DNA.
4. Phosphate-buffered saline, PBS.

5. 20X SSC: 3*M* NaCl, 0.3*M* trisodium citrate.
6. 20X TAE: 0.8*M* Tris-acetate, 20 m*M* EDTA.

2.5. Yeast Culture

1. α D(+) glucose: 40% stock solution, autoclaved.
2. Amino acids (*see* Appendix 2): Autoclaved stock solutions are kept at room temperature.
3. Bactopeptone.
4. Bacto-yeast nitrogen base without amino acids (Difco).
5. Select agar (Gibco BRL).
6. Yeast extract.

2.6. Strains

1. Propagation of the pYAC4 vector: *E. coli* DH5.
2. *Saccharomyces cerevisiae* strain AB1380.

2.7. Miscellaneous Materials

1. Hybond N 87 mm diameter disks (Amersham) or Pall Biodyne disks.
2. Kodak XAR films.
3. Ninety-six-well microtitration plates (flat bottom).
4. Petri dishes (243×243 mm^2) (Nunc).
5. Petri dishes (90 mm diameter).
6. UH 100/75 Ultra Thimbles (Schleicher and Schuell).
7. Whatman 3MM chromatography paper.
8. Whatman 17MM chromatography paper.

2.8. Equipment

1. Contour Clamped Homogeneous Electric Field (CHEF) apparatus *(30),* with cooling system.
2. Freezer (–70°C).
3. Fume hood.
4. Incubator-shaker at 30°C.
5. Incubator at 30°C.
6. Ninety-six prong replicator (Titertek).
7. Phase-contrast microscope.
8. Polymerase Chain Reaction (PCR) automat.
9. Safety cabinet (yeast culture).
10. Tap vacuum concentrator (Schleicher and Schuell).
11. Tissue culture facilities.
12. Vacuum oven at 80°C.

2.9. Appendicies

2.9.1. Appendix 1:
Manual High-Density Colony Replicator

The manual replicator is shown in Fig. 1. It comprises:

1. A lower part in which a sterile lid from a 96-well microtitration plate can be placed and locked. At each corner of this base part is a vertical rod with a spring.
2. An upper part: It has the same dimensions as the lower part and has four holes that fit the vertical poles at the corners of the base part; it sits on the springs and can therefore be actuated up and down manually.
3. A 96-prong device: This is a Titertek replicator, the pins of which have been machined to a diameter of 1 mm at their extremity. The replicator is mounted on a metal plate and can be suspended in the central frame of the upper part of the apparatus.
4. Two mobile spacers that allow placement of the 96-prong device in four distinct positions (1: upper left; 2: upper right; 3: lower left; and 4: lower right).

All parts are made from stainless steel.
The following details how to make replica filters:

1. Using sterile procedure, place an 8×11.3 cm^2 piece of sterile Hybond N membrane (Appendix 2) in a 96-well microtitration plate lid, and overlay. Lock the lid in the lower part of the replicator.
2. Ethanol flame the multiprong replicator, leave to cool down to room temperature, and dip it into microtitration plate no. 1.
3. Transfer the multiprong device into position 1 (*see above*) of the replicator, press down until the pins touch the surface of the Hybond N filter, and release the pressure.
4. Repeat 1–3 with another three microtitration plates, positioning the multiprong device in positions 2, 3, and 4, respectively.
5. Grow for 2–3 d on AHC agar at 37°C.

2.9.2. Appendix 2: Yeast Culture Media

1. YPD media: 1% yeast extract, 2% bactopeptone, 2% α D(+) glucose.
2. SD-U-T media: 0.67% bacto-yeast nitrogen base without amino acids, 2% glucose, adenine sulfate (20 mg/L), L-histidine-HCl (20 mg/L), L-arginine-HCl (20 mg/L), L-methionine (20 mg/L), L-tyrosine (30 mg/L), L-leucine (30 mg/L), L-isoleucine (30 mg/L), L-lysine-HCl (30 mg/L), L-phenylalanine (50 mg/L), L-aspartic acid (100 mg/L), L-glutamic acid (100 mg/L), L-valine (150 mg/L), L-threonine (200 mg/L), L-serine (400 mg/L). All amino acids are from 50–100X sterile stock solutions, stored at room

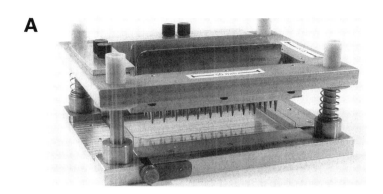

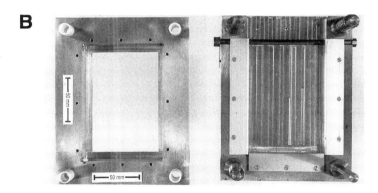

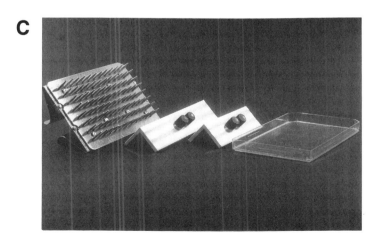

Fig. 1. Manual high density colony replicator: **A.** complete apparatus; **B.** upper (left) and bottom (right) parts: viewed from above; **C.** 96-prong device (left), spacers (middle), and tray (right).

temperature. The α D(+) glucose (40% stock solution), and the aspartic acid and threonine are added after autoclaving the media.

3. SD-U-T agar: same composition as SD-U-T, plus 2% bacto-agar.
4. Ca-SORB-U-T: same as SD-U-T agar, but containing 0.9*M* Sorbitol, 3% α D(+) glucose, and 10 m*M* $CaCl_2$.
5. AHC: 1.7g yeast nitrogen based without amino acids, 10 g casaminoacids, 50 mg adenine hemisulfate. Bring to 1 L and adjust to pH 5.8.
6. AHC agar: Same composition as AHC, but contains 1.8% agar.

3. Methods

3.1. Organization of the Library: General Scheme

There are two main levels in the library:

Level 1, the whole library, materializes as:

1. *n* Master plates (about 1000 colonies/plate), replica filters of which are stored frozen at –70°C;
2. A set of *n* replica filters corresponding to the *n* master plates of the library, for screening by hybridization; and
3. A set of *n* DNA samples prepared from the pooled colonies of each master plate, for screening by PCR (about 1000 recombinants/pool).

Level 2 is the collection of human chromosome-specific clones. The human clones are identified by screening the replica filters of the whole library with a total human DNA probe; they are picked individually, and ordered and propagated in 96-well microtitration plates. This collection of human-specific recombinants materializes as: (1) *m* 96-well plates stored at –70°C in triplicate; and (2) *m*:5 20 × 20 cm² replica filters corresponding to the *m* microtitration plates (replicas of five microtitration plates can be accommodated on a 20 × 20 cm²). High-density grids can also be generated using, for instance, the manufold device described in Appendix 1.

3.2. Preparation and Size Selection of the Target DNA, and Ligation to the Vector Arms

3.2.1. Preparation of High-Molecular-Weight Genomic DNA

1. Grow the somatic hybrid cells in culture, and collect them (*see* Chapter 5 for culture details).
2. Pellet the cells by centrifugation at 300*g* (1800 rpm in Sorvall RT6000), and wash them in 20 mL of PBS. All steps are done at room temperature.

3. Repeat step 2.
4. Pellet the cells as above, and resuspend them at a concentration of 4×10^7 cells/mL.
5. Add to the cell suspension an equal vol of 1% low-melting-point agarose (Ultrapure BRL) made up in PBS and cooled down to 50°C, and mix gently but thoroughly.
6. Aliquot the cells embedded in agarose per 100 μL in insert molds on ice; allow to set for 15 min, and transfer the agarose plugs to a $0.5M$ ES plus, 1 mg/mL proteinase K (ESP) solution (25 mL/50 agarose plugs); incubate at 50°C for 18 h.
7. Repeat the treatment with fresh ESP solution (*see* Note 1).
8. Wash the plugs three times for 20 min in 10 mM Tris-HCl, pH 7.5, 5 mM EDTA at 50°C.
9. Treat the plugs three times for 15 min in 10 mM Tris-HCl, pH 7.5, 0.5 mM EDTA, 0.5 mM PMSF at 50°C.

3.2.2. Partial Digestion with EcoRI

The digestion conditions hereafter provide a majority of digestion products in the size range between 200 and 500 kbp, as assessed by pulsed field gel analysis (*see* Fig. 2). (*See* Notes 2 and 3).

1. Twelve PMSF-treated plugs are equilibrated in 3 vol (3.6 or 4 mL) of *Eco*RI digestion buffer lacking MgCl$_2$ (100 mM Tris-HCl, pH 7.5, 50 mM NaCl, 100 μg/mL bovine serum albumin, 10 mM β-mercaptoethanol) at room temperature for 30 min. (*See* Note 4).
2. Incubate the plugs individually on ice in 130 μL of fresh digestion buffer lacking MgCl$_2$ in the presence of 2 or 5 U of *Eco*RI (Boehringer Mannheim) (six plugs each) for 1 h to allow the enzyme to penetrate uniformly into the plugs.
3. Finally, add MgCl$_2$ to a final concentration of either 1.5 mM (3 plugs) or 5 mM MgCl$_2$ (3 plugs), and incubate at 37°C for 1 h.
4. Stop the digestion by putting the samples on ice and adding 50 μL of $0.5M$ EDTA.

3.2.3. Preparation of the Vector Arms

1. Digest 100 μg of pYAC4 vector *(1)* to completion with both *Eco*RI and *Bam*HI in the restriction buffer: 100 mM Tris-HCl, pH 7.5, 50 mM NaCl, 5 mM MgCl$_2$, 100 μg/mL bovine serum albumin, 2 mM spermidin trihydrochloride, 10 mM β-mercaptoethanol (*see* Note 4).
2. Phosphatase the 5' termini with 2 U of bacterial alkaline phosphatase (Amersham, Arlington Heights, IL) at 65°C for 1 h in the restriction mixture.

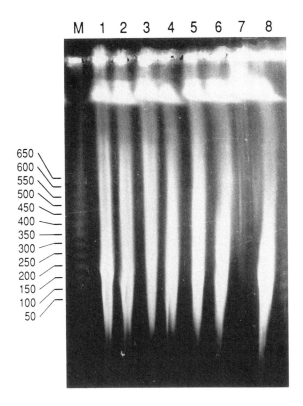

Fig. 2. *Eco*RI partial digestion of mammalian DNA embedded in agarose plugs. Digestion (*see* detailed protocol, Section 3.2.2.) was performed with varying amounts of *Eco*RI (expressed in units, U), in buffer containing varying concentrations of MgCl$_2$ (expressed in mM). Lane 1: 1.5 mM–5 U; lane 2: 1.5 mM–7 U; lane 3: 2.5 mM–1 U; lane 4: 2.5 mM–3 U; lane 5: 2.5 mM–5 U; lane 6: 2.5 mM–7 U; lane 7: 2.5 mM–0 U; lane 8: 2.5 mM–20 U. M: phage λ DNA concatemers; sizes are indicated in kbp on the left. Agarose plugs containing 1.5 × 10^6 cell of the somatic hybrid IWILA 4.9 *(27)* were used. Electrophoresis was performed through a 1% agarose gel in a CHEF apparatus *(30)* at 170 V, using 60-s pulse times for 20 h, followed by 100-s pulse times for 21 h, at 13°C.

3. Extract once with 2.5 vol of phenol-chloroform-isoamyl alcohol (25:24:1), once with 2.5 vol of chloroform-isoamyl alcohol (24:1), and once with 2 vol of diethyl ether.
4. Add NaCl (5M stock solution) to a final concentration of 0.25M, add 3 vol of cold absolute ethanol, mix well, and leave to precipitate at –20°C for at least 5 h.

5. Spin in a microfuge for 15 min at 4°C.
6. Remove the supernatant, and rinse the DNA pellet with 1 mL of 70% ethanol.
7. Spin in a microfuge for 10 min.
8. Remove the supernatant, and air-dry.
9. Resuspend in 50 μL of 10 m*M* Tris-HCl, pH 7.5, 1 m*M* EDTA.

3.2.4. Size Selection
of the EcoRI-Restricted Genomic DNA

1. Load 10 digested plugs next to each other in a large well. On each side, load one digested plug and one plug of concatenated phage λ DNA molecules.
2. Fractionate the *Eco*RI restricted DNA by pulsed field gel electrophoresis (PFGE) through a 1% low-gelling-temperature agarose gel (BRL Ultrapure) cast in a frame of 1% normal agarose (as suggested by Anand et al., 1989) *(31)* using a CHEF device *(30,32),* under electrophoretic conditions that allow the resolution of DNA fragments up to 300 kbp in size and that keep the compression zone close to the wells: typically, 25-s pulse time, 150 V, at 13°C for 12–18 h in 0.5X TAE with the apparatus described in *(30).*
3. Cut out the parts of the gel that contain the digest test sample and the λ ladder, and stain them with ethidium bromide (10 μg/mL), while the rest of the gel is kept in electrophoresis buffer at 4°C.
4. Check under UV that the electrophoretic separation is satisfactory, and note the position of the compression zone by indenting the agarose gel.
5. Slice out the region of the gel that contains the compression zone and the plugs (unstained with ethidium bromide) using ethanol-flamed scalpel and spatula, and transfer it to 30 mL of cold 10 m*M* Tris-HCl, pH 7.5, 0.5 m*M* EDTA, and 25 m*M* NaCl (TEN) solution, to equilibrate under gentle shaking for 15 min at 4°C. Repeat three times.

3.2.5. Ligation to the Vector Arms

1. Dilute the agarose slice with an equal volume of the same TEN solution, and melt thoroughly at 65°C.
2. Cool down to 37°C; add 100 μg of phosphatased vector arms (100-fold molar excess to the target DNA), a 1/10 vol of 10X ligation buffer (100 m*M* Tris-HCl, pH 7.5, 100 m*M* MgCl$_2$, 100 m*M* dithioerythritol, 6 m*M* ATP), and 60 μL of 1 U/μL DNA ligase, and mix gently with the pipet tip, keeping the mixture at a temperature of 30°C.
3. Aliquot by 100 μL with a cut 200 μL tip into plug molds, and leave to set at room temperature. Incubate for 18 h at room temperature (around 20°C).

3.2.6. Second Size Selection: Separation
of the Vector Arms (See Note 5)

1. Load the ligated DNA-containing plugs on a 1% low-gelling-temperature agarose gel made in 0.5X TAE, made and cast as described above
   (Section 3.2.4.). Load a λ DNA ladder-containing agarose plug on each
   side. The gel must fit into both a conventional electrophoresis and a
   CHEF apparatus.
2. Run under conventional electrophoretic conditions at low voltage: 25
   V for 6–8 h in 0.5X TAE.
3. Transfer the gel to a CHEF apparatus and run further under the same
   conditions as for the first size-selection step postrestriction.
4. Cut out and stain with ethidium bromide the parts of the gel that contain the λ ladders. Note the position of the compression zone. Slice the
   compression zone out that contains the ligated DNA, and estimate its
   volume (*see* Note 6).
5. In a 50-mL Falcon tube, equilibrate the gel slice in 40 mL of cold 1X TAE,
   100 mM NaCl, and 10 mM EDTA (TAENE) at 4°C under agitation for
   1 h. (*see* Note 7).
6. Replace by a fresh sample of TAENE equal to the volume of the gel slice.
7. Incubate at 68°C for 10 min in order to melt the agarose completely.
8. Cool the tube down to 37°C, and add 50 U of agarase (Calbiochem)
   (prediluted in 200 µL of TAENE at 37°C)/mL of molten gel, and mix
   gently with the pipet tip.
9. Incubate for 4 h at 37°C.
10. Add more agarase (25 U/mL), and continue the incubation for another
    12–16 h.
11. Add 1 vol of phenol (equilibrated in 10 mM Tris-HCl, 5 mM EDTA,
    and prewarmed to 37°C) slowly down the side of the tube, and deli-
    cately place the tube on its side for 20 min.
12. Spin at 400 rpm for 2 min.
13. Delicately remove the organic phase by pipeting with a sterile 10-mL
    pipet through the aqueous solution.
14. Gently add 1 vol of chloroform and isoamyl alcohol (24:1) (prewarmed
    at 37°C); leave the tube on its side for 20 min.
15. Spin at 400 rpm for 2 min.
16. Very slowly aspirate the aqueous phase using a sterile 10-mL pipet with
    an opening of at least 3 mm. The pipet is held on a retort stand, and the
    suction is applied using a 20 mL syringe connected to the upper end of
    the pipet with a piece of tubing.

17. Transfer to a UH 100/75 Ultra Thimble (Schleicher and Schuell) prewashed in water.
18. Concentrate to approx 500 μL using a Schleicher and Schuell tap vacuum concentrator against 10 m*M* Tris-HCl, pH 7.5, and 2 m*M* EDTA.
19. Transfer to a 1.5-mL microtube with a cut 1-mL pipet tip, and store at 4°C.

3.3. Transformation
into Saccharomyces cerevisiae

The protocol used is derived from Burgers and Percival *(33),* as modified by McCormick et al. *(34).*

1. Grow a 50-mL culture of the *S. cerevisiae* strain AB1380 in YPD *(see* Appendix 2) at 30°C in a shaker, to a density of 3×10^7 cells/mL.
2. Spin at 600*g* (3000 rpm in Sorvall RT6000) for 4 min to collect the cells. All the steps are carried out at room temperature.
3. Wash in 20 mL H_2O; spin as above.
4. Wash with 20 mL of 1*M* sorbitol; spin as above.
5. Resuspend in 30 mL of 1*M* sorbitol, 0.1*M* trisodium citrate, and 60 m*M* EDTA, pH 8.0 (SCE). The cell density must be around 7.5×10^7 cells/ mL; this is critical to ensure the next step of spheroplasting is efficient.
6. Add 30 μL of β-mercaptoethanol and 45 μL of 2 mg/mL 100T Zymolyase (ICN Immunobiologicals, High Wycombe, UK). Incubate for 20 min at 30°C under slow (50 rpm) agitation, the tube lying on its side. Check for spheroplasting under the microscope: Spread 10–20 μL of the suspension on a microscope slide covered with a cover slip, and add 30 μL of 10% sodium dodecyl sulfate (SDS). 80–90% of the cells should lyse. If the percentage of spheroplasts is lower, incubate for another 5–10 min and check again as above *(see* Note 8).
7. Collect the spheroplasts by centrifugation at low speed: 250*g* (1100 rpm in Sorvall RT6000) for 4 min. All centrifugations from now on are carried out at low speed because of the fragility of the spheroplasts.
8. Resuspend gently in 15 mL of 1*M* sorbitol, 10 m*M* Tris-HCl, pH 7.5, 10 m*M* $CaCl_2$ (STC), using an inoculation loop for instance, and centrifuge at low speed as above.
9. Repeat step 8.
10. Resuspend in 2 mL of STC. The spheroplasts are stable for 1 h at room temperature.
11. In a 4-mL polyethylene Falcon tube, dispense 5 μg of sonicated human DNA (carrier), 100 μL of spheroplasts in STC, and 1–10 μL of ligated DNA; mix gently and incubate for 10 min *(see* Notes 9 and 10).

12. Add 1 mL of PEGTC: 10 mM Tris-HCl, pH 7.5, 10 mM CaCl$_2$, 20% Polyethyleneglycol 6000 (*see* Note 11). Mix gently, but thoroughly. Incubate for 10 min.
13. Spin at 250g for 4 min. Decant carefully by pipeting the supernatant out.
14. Add 150 µL of SOS media: 1M sorbitol, 6.5 mM CaCl$_2$, 0.25% yeast extract, and 0.5% bactopeptone (*see* Note 11). Incubate at 30°C without shaking for 40 min.
15. Add 300 µL of 1M sorbitol, mix gently, and centrifuge at 250g for 4 min.
16. Remove the supernatant. Resuspend in 500 µL of 1M sorbitol.
17. Add 250 µL of 4% sodium alginate (Sigma, St. Louis, MO) made up in 1M sorbitol, and mix by pipeting back and forth (use a cut 1-mL tip).
18. Load onto a nylon membrane (Hybond N, Amersham, or Pall Biodyne) marked asymetrically (punch holes with a needle) and placed on a 90 mm diameter Ca-SORB-U-T agar plate (*see* Appendix 2), and spread evenly with a glass spreader. The alginate layer solidifies within 10 min. Wrap the plates with Parafilm™ in order to avoid dessication of the agar.
19. Incubate at 30°C for 3–4 d. (*see* Note 10).

3.4 Library Screening

3.4.1. Making Replica Filters of the Master Plates

After 3–4 d of growth at 30°C, the colonies stick out at the surface of the alginate layer.

1. Make three replica filters (RF 1, 2, and 3) (Hybond N, Amersham, or Pall Biodyne) of each master plate by pressing firmly and evenly between two sheets of Whatman 17MM paper (on RF1 and RF3, indicate the assymetric marks with a pen).
2. Place the replica filters on SD-U-T agar plates (*see* Appendix 2), and incubate for 1–2 d at 30°C in order to regenerate the colonies.

RF1s are then stored immediately at –70°C (*see* Section 3.5.1.). RF2s are used to pool the clones from each master plate for screening by polymerase chain reaction (PCR) *(35,36)* (Section 3.4.2.). RF3s are processed for screening the library by hybridization with radiolabeled probes (Section 3.4.3.).

3.4.2. PCR Screening (See Note 12)

1. Wash the colonies thoroughly from RF2i with a total of 7 mL of AHC liquid media, and collect the cells in a suitable tube.
2. Aliquot out 1 mL and store it away at –70°C in 20% (final concentration) of glycerol.

3. The rest of the cells are collected by centrifugation at 500*g* (3000 rpm in Sorvall RT6000), and processed to purify DNA from the pool of cells by the protocol of Sherman et al. *(37)*, as follows (*see* Note 13).

4. Resuspend in 0.5 mL of 1*M* sorbitol, 0.1*M* EDTA, pH 8.0, and transfer to a 1.5-mL microfuge tube.

5. Add 0.4 mg of Lyticase (i.e., 40-µL of a 10 mg/mL solution), mix well, and incubate at 37°C for 90 min. Mix the suspension now and again over that period.

6. Spin in microfuge for 1 min.

7. Resuspend the cells in 500 µL of 50 m*M* Tris-HCl, pH 7.5, 20 m*M* EDTA.

8. Add 50 µL of 10% SDS, and mix well by inverting the tube several times.

9. Incubate at 65°C for 30 min.

10. Add 200 µL of 5*M* potassium acetate, mix well by inverting the tube several times, and place on ice for 1 h.

11. Spin in microfuge for 5 min.

12. Transfer the supernatant to a fresh tube, and add 750 µL of isopropanol at room temperature. Mix well and leave at room temperature for 5 min.

13. Spin in microfuge for 1 min. Pour off the supernatant, and air-dry.

14. Resuspend (without vortexing) the pellet in 300 µL of 10 m*M* Tris-HCl, pH 7.5, 1 m*M* EDTA.

15. Add 1.5 µL of 10 mg/mL RNase A (Sigma) (boiled for 15 min) and incubate at 37°C for 30 min.

16. Add 15 µL of 5*M* NaCl, mix well, and add 900 µL of cold absolute ethanol; mix well. Let sit at room temperature for 5 min.

17. Spin in a microfuge for 5 min.

18. Pour off the supernatant, rinse with 1 mL of 70% ethanol, and spin for 1 min.

19. Pour off the supernatant, and air-dry. Resuspend in 500 µL of 10 m*M* Tris-HCl, pH 7.5, 1 m*M* EDTA.

20. Store at 4°C.

The DNA thus prepared is ready for PCR screening.

3.4.3. Screening by Hybridization (Adapted from Ref. 2)

1. In a 243 × 243 Petri dish (Nunc), place RF3*i* on a sheet of Whatman 3MM paper saturated with SCE containing 100 m*M* of β-mercaptoethanol and 160 U/mL of Lyticase. Make sure the replica filter itself is not soaked, so as not to wash the colonies away (this applies to steps 3–7 as well).

2. Seal the box in order to prevent evaporation, and incubate at 37°C for at least 6 h (and up to 18 h).

3. Transfer the replica filter to 3MM paper saturated with 10% SDS for 5 min. Steps 3–8 are carried out at room temperature.
4. Transfer briefly (3 s) to a dry 3MM paper sheet in order to remove any excess of 10% SDS, and then transfer to 3MM paper saturated with 0.5*M* NaOH for 5 min.
5. Remove any excess of NaOH by a rapid passage on dry 3MM paper, and transfer to 3MM paper saturated with 2X SSC for 5 min. Repeat this treatment twice (no need to remove the excess of liquid between the treatments).
6. Transfer to 3MM paper saturated with 0.2*M* Tris-HCl, pH 7.5, for 5 min. Repeat once.
7. Transfer to 3MM paper saturated with 0.2*M* Tris-HCl, pH 7.5, 100 µg/mL proteinase K for 30 min. (*see* Note 14).
8. Wash for 30 s in chloroform in a fume hood (*see* Note 15).
9. Air-dry thoroughly.
10. UV crosslink the DNA to the nylon matrix: 3.5 min on a 254–312-nm UV transilluminator, DNA side down.
11. Bake for 2 h at 80°C.

The filter is ready for hybridization with radiolabeled probes, using standard protocols.

3.4.4. Screening for Human Clones

1. Label 30 ng of either total human DNA or human Cot1 DNA (Gibco BRL, Gaithersburg, MD) by random priming *(38)* (Boehringer Mannheim [Mannheim, Germany] Random Prime Labeling Kit).
2. Prehybridize replica filter RF3*i* for 1 h at 68°C in 4X SSC, 4X Denhardt solution, 10% dextran sulfate, 0.5% SDS, and 50 µg/mL sonicated salmon sperm DNA.
3. Hybridize the denatured probe to the RF3*i* filters at 68°C for a minimum of 16 h in the same solution as for the prehybridization, complemented with 40 µg/mL of sonicated rodent DNA as a competitor.
4. Wash in 0.2X SSC, 0.1% SDS, twice at room temperature, and twice at 65°C.
5. Expose with an autoradiographic Kodak XAR film and an intensifying screen at –70°C.
6. Report the assymetric marks on the autoradiograph.

3.5. Propagation and Storage of the Library

3.5.1. Storage of the Replica Filters of the Library

Each Replica Filter 1 (*see* Section 3.4.1.) is treated separately.

1. Place RF1*i* on a Whatman 3MM paper saturated with YPD media (Appendix 2) containing 20% glycerol. Make sure no free liquid washes the colonies away. Leave to impregnate for 15 s.

2. In the same way, prewet a Hybond N or Pall Biodyne disk of the same size as RF1*i*.
3. Place RF1*i* on a piece of Whatman 17MM paper, colonies side up. Carefully overlay with the prewet disk (freed of any excess liquid).
4. Place a piece of Whatman 17MM paper on the top, and press firmly and evenly. Punch holes with a needle at the position of the marks.
5. Store between two sheets of 3MM paper at −70°C in a nylon bag.

3.5.2. Storage of the Collection of Human Recombinants

1. Align the marks present on both the autoradiograph and either the master plate (if it is recent enough), or the RF1*i* filter stored at −70°C.
2. Either the positive colonies are picked from the master plate, or the corresponding areas are cut from the stored RF1*i* filter and transfered to a 96-well microtitration plate containing 200 μL per well of AHC media (*see* Appendix 2).
3. Grow the plate at 30°C for 2 d (*see* Note 15).
4. Inoculate three fresh microtitration plates (containing 150 μL of SD-U-T media/well) with 50 μL of each well, using a multichannel pipet. Grow to high density (2–3 d) at 30°C.
5. To these three plates, add 65 μL of 80% glycerol, and mix well (20% final).
6. Immediately store at −70°C.

3.6. Screening the Collection of Human Recombinants

1. At step 3 of Section 3.5.2., make replicas of the microtitration plates on 8 × 12 cm² pieces of Hybond N (Amersham) or Pall Biodyne membrane using a 96-prong replicator (Titertek). Fourfold density grids can be produced using the manual device presented in Appendix 1: Four microtitration plates are replicated on an 8 × 11.3 cm² piece of Hybond N or Pall Biodyne membrane, and five such filters are grown on agar in a 22 × 22 cm² Petri dish. 20 × 20 cm² replica filters are then produced in turn, which bear 1920 clones each (96 × 4 × 5 = 1920) (*see* Note 16).
2. Grow on AHC agar (*see* Appendix 2) for 2 d at 30°C.
3. Process the filters as described in Section 3.4.3. for screening by hybridization.
4. Replica filters can also be stored as described in Section 3.5.1. (optional).

4. Notes

1. The plugs can then be stored at 4°C virtually indefinitely after replacing the E.S.P. solution with 0.5*M* EDTA. Prior to digestion with *Eco*RI

(Section 3.2.2.), the agarose plugs will have to undergo steps 8 and 9 of Section 3.2.1.

2. The purified DNA (about 15–20 µg/100 µL) is partially digested in the agarose plugs with *Eco*RI, using limiting amounts of restriction enzyme and of MgCl$_2$, as suggested by Albertsen et al. *(39)*. Optimal conditions (concentration of MgCl$_2$, amount of *Eco*RI, incubation time) must be established for each batch of agarose plugs used, mainly because of DNA concentration differences, and depending on the size range of restriction products desired.

3. Some batches of low-melting point agarose need to be purified before they are used for embedding cells *(40)*. It also seems that using β-mercaptoethanol instead of dithioerythritol as a reducing agent in restriction buffers improves the restriction of DNA in agarose, thus rendering the purification of the agarose unnecessary (personal observations).

4. It is important to perform *Eco*RI digestions in a well-buffered solution (100 m*M* Tris-HCl, pH 7.5) in order to avoid the star activity sometimes observed with *Eco*RI. This buffer is also used for the double restriction of the vector with *Eco*RI and *Bam*HI (Section 3.2.3.).

5. Apply a second size selection, in order both to elute the unligated vector arms and possibly contaminating circular vector molecules, and to perfect the sizing of the DNA before transformation into the yeast host. This is ideally achieved by fractionation first through an agarose gel under conventional electrophoretic conditions and then under PFGE conditions *(34)*. This results in a far better separation of the vector arms than if the first step of conventional electrophoresis was omitted (*see* Fig. 3A,B).

6. At this stage, it is advised to run an aliquot of the size-selected ligated DNA on a pulsed field gel under conditions allowing the separation of DNA molecules up to 1 mbp in size (typically 90-s pulse times, for 40 h) in order to check that the sizing of the ligated material is satisfactory. Blot and hybridize with a pBR322 probe; after washes at medium stringency (0.5X SSC, 0.1% SDS at 65°C), an autoradiographic smear will indicate that the ligation has been effective.

7. Steps 5–19 of Section 3.2.6. are adapted from Anand et al. *(31)*.

8. The zymolyase must be titrated. Perform tests with 100 ng of circular YAC vector DNA, using various amounts of Zymolyase 100T for various incubation times (the expected efficiency is about 1000 colonies/100 ng of pYAC4). I found, for instance, that the Zymolyase 100T produced by ICN Immunobiologicals works best using half as much as would be required with the Zymolyase 100T produced by Miles (Rexdale, Ontario, Canada), but slightly longer incubations at 30°C are

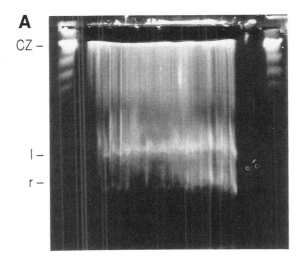

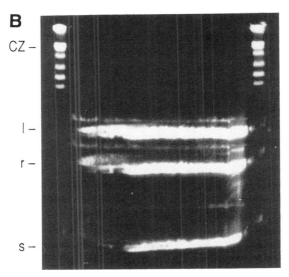

Fig. 3. Separation of the vector arms from the ligated material. **A.** *Eco*RI digested DNA (not size fractionated) was ligated to the pYAC4 vector *(1)* arms and fractionated through a 1% LMP agarose gel, using a CHEF design *(30)*, using pulse times of 15 s for 18 h at 150 V. Phage λ concatemers were loaded on both sides. CZ: compression zone (excised); l and r: vector's left and right arms. **B.** *Eco*RI-digested, size-fractionated, DNA was ligated to the pYAC4 arms and fractionated through a 1% LMP agarose gel for 8 h at 25 V under conventional electrophoresis conditions, and for 16 h in a CHEF device *(26)*: pulse time: 18 s, 150 V. Phage λ concatemers were loaded on both sides. CZ, l and r are as in A.

necessary (25–30 min instead of 20 min). Batch dependent variations are also observed.

9. Various protocols have been described where ligated DNA is kept in low-melting-point agarose and is either just melted *(34)* or agarased *(4,5)* before the transformation. The addition of polyamines to the transformation mixtures has been reported to improve the transformation efficiency when agarose-embedded ligation samples are used *(5,34)*. Also, some data suggest that the transformation efficiency can be improved by the addition of Lipofectin™ (Gibco BRL) *(41);* these data, however, are the result of tests performed with plasmids, and it remains to be proven that the same effect is observed with large linear molecules, such as YACs, as is the case in *Schizosaccharomyces pombe (41)*.

10. It is advised to titrate the ligation product, so as to obtain about 1000 colonies/filter.

11. The choice (mol wt, grade, and manufacturer) of the PEG is crucial, since some PEGs cause the lysis of the spheroplasts. The PEGTC solution is sterilized through a 0.2- or 0.4-µm DynaGard™ syringe filter (Microgon, Inc.). The SOS solution is sterilized by autoclaving without the $CaCl_2$; sterile $CaCl_2$ is added before use.

12. Principle of the PCR screening: The whole library is composed of n master plates, to which correspond n RF2 filters. The colonies of each RF2i filter are collected to constitute pool i. DNA is purified from the n pools separately; locus-specific PCR is then carried out on the n DNA samples; when a positive pool p is identified, the corresponding RF3p filter is screened by hybridization in order to identify the positive clone.

13. Alternatively, the cells can be embedded in low-melting-point agarose (Ultrapure BRL), and high-mol-wt DNA prepared by the protocol described in Chapter 14. The agarose plugs must then be treated with PMSF as described above (Section 3.2.1., steps 8 and 9), and equilibrated in 10 mM Tris-HCl, pH 7.5, 1 mM EDTA (TE) (several washes in 5 vol of TE). They are finally diluted fivefold with TE, and melted at 65°C for 10 min. The DNA is then ready for screening by PCR.

14. This step is dispensable and can be replaced by a third 5-min treatment with 0.2M Tris-HCl, pH 7.5. In that case, the wash in chloroform (step 8) is not performed.

15. At this stage, one can also make replica filters of the collection of human clones for screening by hybridization (Section 3.6.). The replica filters can alternatively be made at a later stage from one of the microtitration plates stored at –70°C: The plate is thawed and replica filters prepared as described in Section 3.6. The 96-well microtitration plate is frozen again at –70°C.

16. Note that if the YAC inserts average 300 kbp in size, this figure represents four equivalents of a medium-size human chromosome, such as chromosome 11.

Acknowledgments

I wish to thank D. J. Porteous for fruitful discussions and for his continuous support and encouragement, Douglas Finlayson for constructing the manual high-density replicator, and S. Bruce, N. Davidson, and D. Stuart for preparing the figures. This work was supported by the Wellcome Trust and by the Medical Research Council of the UK. I dedicate this chapter to the memory of my former colleague Isabelle Oberlé.

References

1. Burke, D. T., Carle, G. F., and Olson, M. V. (1987) Cloning of large segments of exogenous DNA into yeast by means of artificial chromosome vectors. *Science* **236,** 806–812.
2. Brownstein, B. H., Silverman, G. A., Little, R. D., Burke, D. T., Korsmeyer, S. J., Schlessinger, D., and Olson, M. V. (1989) Isolation of single-copy human genes from a library of yeast artificial chromosome clones. *Science* **244,** 1348–1351.
3. Anand, R., Riley, J. H., Butler, R., Smith, J. C., and Markham, A. F. (1990) A 3.5 genome equivalent multi access YAC library: construction, characterisation, screening and storage. *Nucleic Acids Res.* **18,** 1951–1955.
4. Albertsen, H. M., Abderrahim, H., Cann, H. M., Dausset, J., Le Paslier, D., and Cohen, D. (1990) Construction and characterization of a yeast artificial chromosome library containing seven haploid human genome equivalents. *Proc. Natl. Acad. Sci. USA* **87,** 4256–4260.
5. Larin, Z., Monaco, A. P., and Lehrach, H. (1991) Yeast artificial chromosome libraries containing large inserts from mouse and human DNA. *Proc. Natl. Acad. Sci. USA* **88,** 4123–4127.
6. Burke, D. T., Rossi, J. M., Leung, J., Koos, D. S., and Tilghman, S. M. (1991) A mouse library of yeast artificial chromosome clones. *Mammalian Genome* **1,** 65.
7. MacMurray, A. J., Weaver, A., Shin, H.-S., and Lander, E. S. (1991) An automated method for DNA preparation from thousands of YAC clones. *Nucleic Acids Res.* **19,** 385–390.
8. Garza, D., Ajioka, J. W., Burke, D. T., and Hartl, D. L. (1989) Mapping the *Drosophila* genome with yeast artificial chromosomes. *Science* **246,** 641–646.
9. Coulson, A., Waterson, R., Kiff, J., Sulston, J., and Kohara, Y. (1988) Genome linking with yeast artificial chromosomes. *Nature* **335,** 184–186.
10. Coulson, A., Sulston, J., Brenner, S., and Karn, J. (1986) Toward a physical map of the genome of the nematode *Caenorhabditis elegans. Proc. Natl. Acad. Sci. USA* **83,** 7821–7825.

11. Elvin, P., Slynn, G., Black, D., Graham, A., Butler, R., Riley, J., Anand, R., and Markham, A. F. (1991) Isolation of cDNA clones using yeast artificial chromosome probes. *Nucleic Acids Res.* **18,** 3913–3917.
12. Kinzler, K. W., Nilbert, M. C., Su, L.-K., Vogelstein, B., Bryan, T. M., Levy, D. B., Smith, K. J., Preisinger, A. C., Hedge, P., McKechnie, D., Finniear, R., Markham, A., Groffen, J., Boguski, M. S., Altschul, S. F., Horii, A., Ando, H., Myioshi, Y., Miki, Y., Nishisho, I., and Nakamura, Y. (1991) Identification of FAP locus genes from chromosome 5q21. *Science* **253,** 661–665.
13. Brookes, A. J. and Porteous, D. J. (1991) Coincidence sequence cloning. *Nucleic Acids Res.* **19,** 2609–2613.
14. Pavan, W. J., Hieter, P., and Reeves, R. J. (1990) Generation of deletion derivatives by targeted transformation of human-derived yeast artificial chromosomes. *Proc. Natl. Acad. Sci. USA* **87,** 1300–1304.
15. Campbell, C., Gulati, R., Nandi, A. K., Floy, K., Hieter, P., and Kucherlapati, R. S. (1991) Generation of a nested series of interstitial deletions in yeast artificial chromosomes carrying human DNA. *Proc. Natl. Acad. Sci. USA* **88,** 5744–5748.
16. Green, E. D. and Olson M. V. (1990) Chromosomal region of the Cystic Fibrosis gene in yeast artificial chromosomes: a model for human genome mapping. *Science* **250,** 94–98.
17. Silverman, G. A., Green, E. D., Young, R. L., Jockel, J. I., Domer, P. H., and Korsmeyer, S. J. (1990) Meiotic recombination between yeast artificial chromosomes yields a single clone containing the entire BCL2 gene. *Proc. Natl. Acad. Sci. USA* **87,** 9913–9917.
18. Pachnis, V., Pevny, L., Rothstein, R., and Costantini, F. (1990) Transfer of a yeast artificial chromosome carrying human DNA from *Saccharomyces cerevisiae* into mammalian cells. *Proc. Natl. Acad. Sci. USA* **87,** 5109–5113.
19. Pavan, W. J., Hieter, P., and Reeves, R. H. (1990) Modification and transfer into an embryonal carcinoma cell line of a 360-kilobase human-derived yeast artificial chromosome. *Mol. Cell. Biol.* **10,** 4163–4169.
20. Fernandez-Luna, J. L., Matthews, R. J., Brownstein, B. H., Schreiber, R. D., and Thomas, M. L. (1991) Characterization and expression of the human leukocyte-common antigen (CD45) gene contained in yeast artificial chromosomes. *Genomics* **10,** 756–764.
21. Jacobovits, A., Moore, A. L., Green, L. L., Vergara, G. J., Maynard–Currie, C. E., Austin, H. A., and Klapholtz, S. (1993) Germ-line transmission and expression of a human-derived yeast artificial chromosome. *Nature* **362,** 255–258.
22. Schedl, A., Montoliu, L., Kelsey, G., and Schütz, G. (1993) A yeast artificial chromosome covering the tyrosinase gene confers number-dependent expression in transgenic mice. *Nature* **362,** 258–261.
23. Arveiler, B. and Porteous, D. J. (1992) Distribution of Alu and L1 repeats in human YAC recombinants. *Mammalian Genome* **3,** 661–668.
24. Green, E. D., Riethman, H. C., Dutchik, J. E., and Olson, M. V. (1991) Detection and characterization of chimeric yeast artificial chromosome clones. *Genomics* **11,** 658–669.

25. Bonetta, L., Kuehn, S. E., Huang, A., Law, D. J., Kalikin, L. M., Koi, M., Reeve, A. E., Brownstein, B. H., Yeger, H., Williams, B. R. G., and Feinberg, A. P. (1990) Wilms Tumor Locus on 11p13 defined by multiple CpG island-associated transcripts. *Science* **250,** 994–997.
26. Silverman, G. A., Jockel, J. I., Domer, P. H., Mohr, R. M., Taillon-Miller, P., and Korsmeyer, S. J. (1991) Yeast artificial chromosome cloning of a two-megabase-size contig within chromosomal band 18q21 establishes physical linkage between BCL2 and Plasminogen Activator Inhibitor Type-2. *Genomics* **9,** 219–228.
27. Arveiler, B., Murray, I., Stevenson, B., and Porteous, D. J. (1991) Construction of a library enriched for human chromosome 11 and Xp YAC recombinants. *Mammalian Genome* **1,** 265–266.
28. Breen, M., Arveiler, B., Murray, I., Gosden, J. R., and Porteous, D. J. (1992) YAC mapping by FISH using Alu-PCR generated probes. *Genomics* **13,** 726–730.
29. van Ommen, G. J. B. and Verkerk, J. M. H. (1986) Restriction analysis of chromosomal DNA in a size range up to two million base pairs by pulsed field gradient electrophoresis, in *Analysis of Human Genetic Diseases* (Davies, K., ed.) IRL, Oxford, pp. 113–133.
30. Maule, J. C. and Green, D. K. (1990) Semi-conductor controlled contour-clamped homogeneous electric field apparatus. *Anal. Biochem.* **191,** 390–395.
31. Anand, R., Villasante, A., and Tyler-Smith, C. (1989) Construction of yeast artificial chromosome libraries with large inserts using fractionation by pulsed-field gel electrophoresis. *Nucleic Acids Res.* **17,** 3425–3433.
32. Chu, G., Vollrath, D., and Davis, R. W. (1986) Separation of large DNA molecules by contour-clamped homogeneous electric fields. *Science* **234,** 1582–1585.
33. Burgers, P. M. and Percival, K. J. (1986) Transformation of yeast spheroplasts without cell fusion. *Anal. Biochem.* **163,** 390–395.
34. McCormick, M. K., Shero, J. H., Connelly, C. J., Antonorakis, S. E., and Hieter, P. (1990) Methods for cloning large DNA segments as artificial chromosomes in *S. cerevisiae. Technique* **2,** 65–71.
35. Saiki, R. K., Gelfand, D. H., Stoffel, S., Scharf, S. J., Higuchi, R., Horn, G. T., Mullis, K. B., and Ehrlich, H. A. (1988) Primer-directed enzymatic amplification of DNA with thermostable DNA polymerase. *Science* **239,** 487–491.
36. Green, E. D. and Olson, M. V. (1990) Systematic screening of yeast artificial chromosome libraries by use of polymerase chain reaction. *Proc. Natl. Acad. Sci. USA* **87,** 1213–1217.
37. Scherman, F., Fink, G. R., and Hicks, J. B. (1983) *Methods in Yeast Genetics Laboratory Manual,* Cold Spring Harbor Laboratory, Cold Spring Harbor, NY.
38. Feinberg, A. P. and Vogelstein, B. (1984) A technique for radiolabeling DNA restriction endonuclease fragments to high specific activity. *Anal. Biochem.* **137,** 266–267.
39. Albertsen, H. M., Le Paslier, D., Abderrahim, H., Dausset, J., Cann, H., and Cohen, D. (1989) Improved control of partial DNA restriction enzyme digest in agarose using limiting concentrations of Mg^{++}. *Nucleic Acids Res.* **17,** 808.

40. Arveiler, B., Vincent, A., and Mandel, J.-L. (1989) Toward a physical map of the Xq28 region in man: linking color vision, G6PD, and coagulation Factor VIII genes to an X-Y homology region. *Genomics* **4,** 460–471.

41. Allshire, R. C. (1990) Introduction of large linear minichromosomes into *Schizosaccharomyces pombe* by an improved transformation procedure. *Proc. Natl. Acad. Sci. USA* **87,** 4043–4047.

CHAPTER 22

Yeast Artificial Chromosome Recombinants in a Global Strategy for Chromosome Mapping

Amplification of Internal and Terminal Fragments by PCR, and Generation of Fingerprints

Benoît Arveiler

1. Introduction

The large cloning capacity of Yeast Artificial Chromosomes (YACs) *(1)* makes them a powerful reagent for long-range mapping and cloning toward contiguous chromosomal maps. Full value is to be attained through an integrated, global strategy (Fig. 1), including both

1. Genetic mapping techniques *(2,3):* The characterization of VNTRs *(4,5)* or microsatellites *(6,7)* (found approx every 30 kbp in the human genome) in a limited number of randomly selected chromosome-specific YACs (90 and 20 in the case of human chromosomes 1 and 22, respectively) will allow the construction of 2-cM (centimorgans) chromosomal maps; and
2. Physical mapping technologies, such as long-range restriction mapping by pulsed field gel electrophoresis *(8,9),* elaboration of contigs *(10),* nonisotopic high-resolution *in situ* hybridization to chromosome spreads *(11,12)* (subchromosomal localization, detection of chromosome breakpoints of translocations, inversions, and so on), somatic cell hybridization, analysis of panels of somatic hybrids with reduced genetic components, and crosslibrary screening (painting of YAC libraries with complex probes derived from somatic hybrids with a reduced genetic component, cDNA library screening, and so forth) *(13,14).*

From: *Methods in Molecular Biology, Vol. 29: Chromosome Analysis Protocols*
Edited by: J. R. Gosden Copyright ©1994 Humana Press Inc., Totowa, NJ

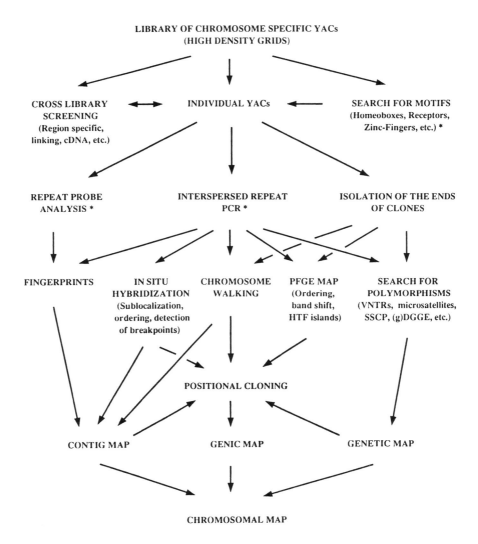

Fig. 1. YACs in a global strategy toward genome mapping. VNTR: variable number of tandem repeats; SSCP: single-strand conformation polymorphism; DGGE: denaturing gradient gel electrophoresis; gDGGE: genomic DGGE. An asterisk indicates insight into the organization of the genome.

Whereas most YAC libraries available to date are derived from total genomes *(15–19),* it becomes widely accepted that the cost-effective success of genome mapping projects relies on the use of chromosome-specific ordered libraries constructed from somatic hybrid cell lines with a reduced foreign component (*see* Chapter 21). There are several reasons for this:

1. YAC recombinants constitute complex probes, and aspecific crossreactions (owing mainly to the presence of repeat elements) render their use by *in situ* hybridization to chromosome spreads sometimes difficult; clones issued from chromosome-specific libraries, by essence, map to the chromosome of interest, and are therefore more readily sublocalized by hybridization to chromosome spreads from normal individuals or from monochromosome somatic hybrids;
2. The clones can be added immediately to the contig map of the chromosome of interest;
3. YACs from total genome libraries suffer from the presence (at high frequency in some libraries) of chimeric clones resulting from the coligation of multiple nonsyntenic fragments *(20–23)*. This phenomenon greatly complicates chromosome walking experiments and constrains the potential for contig mapping technologies by fingerprint analysis. These problems are largely circumvented with chromosome-specific recombinants, since, in the case of a human chromosome-specific library, virtually all human DNA-containing clones contain a single human fragment, the coligated segment originating from the rodent background in more than 99% of the cases; also, the presence and extent of the chimerism are very simply estimated by hybridization with a total rodent DNA probe, whereas in the case of YACs from whole genome libraries, this necessitates lengthy processes, such as *in situ* hybridization, analysis of both ends of the clone, and extensive restriction mapping; and
4. Chromosome-specific libraries can be made available on a restricted number of replica filters, thus making their propagation, screening, and management both highly practical and efficient.

Putting the YAC technology in the prospect of genome mapping projects implies the ability to:

1. Derive single copy internal probes for DNA transfer analysis, *in situ* hybridization to chromosome spreads, and crosslibrary screening;
2. Create highly polymorphic markers for genetic mapping;
3. Isolate the ends of the clones for bidirectional chromosome walking; and
4. Generate fingerprints diagnostic of each clone, and detect overlaps between clones for contig mapping.

In this chapter, I present the use of the *Alu*-PCR technique *(24)* to amplify essentially unique sequences that are specific to human YACs, and I describe a method for isolating specifically either end of YACs by inverse PCR (I-PCR) *(25).* Both types of products can be sequenced to create Sequence Tagged Sites (STSs) *(26),* or landmarks along the chromosomal map, and can be screened for the presence of sequence or conformational polymorphisms *(4–6,27–31).* I finally propose to generate fingerprints of human YACs either by *Alu*-PCR or by repeat sequence analysis.

Although the emphasis is put here on recombinants of human origin, all the techniques presented are either directly applicable (amplification of end fragments, fingerprinting by repeat probe analysis) or at least adaptable to clones derived from other organisms (the interspersed repeat PCR technique, for instance, applies to all organisms with highly reiterated sequence families, and has indeed been shown recently to be effective in the mouse) *(32).*

2. Materials
2.1. Chemicals and Stock Solutions

1. Agarose, medium electroendosmosis.
2. Ammonium persulfate: 10% stock solution, stored at 4°C.
3. β-mercaptoethanol: Toxic; handle in a fume hood, and wear gloves.
4. Deoxyadenosine, deoxycytosine, deoxyguanosine, and deoxythymidine triphosphate: 100 mM stock solutions stored at –20°C.
5. Dithioerythritol: 1M stock solution, filter sterilized, stored at –20°C.
6. Ethanol: absolute and 70%.
7. Ethidium bromide: 10 mg/mL stock solution. Toxic; handle with gloves.
8. Ethylenediamine tetra-acetic acid, disodium salt, EDTA: 0.5M stock solution, pH 8.
9. HCl, concentrated: Wear gloves, and handle in a fume hood.
10. 2-Isopropyl alcohol.
11. MgCl$_2$: 1M stock solution.
12. NaCl: 5M stock solution.
13. NaOH: 5M stock solution.
14. Organic solvents: chloroform, isoamylalcohol (24:1), phenol (saturated with 10 mM Tris-HCl, pH 7.5, 1 mM EDTA).
15. Sodium dodecyl sulfate, SDS (BDH): 10% stock solution.
16. Sorbitol: 1M stock solution.
17. Spermidine trihydrochloride: 100 mM stock solution, filter sterilized, and stored at –20°C.
18. *N,N,N',N'* tetramethylethylenediamine (TEMED).
19. Tris-HCl, pH 7.5, 8, and 8.3: 2M stock solutions; stored at 4°C.

2.2. Solutions

1. Acrylamide—*N,N'* methylene*bis*-acrylamide (29:1) solution: 29 g acrylamide, 1 g *bis*-acrylamide, 100 mL H_2O. Both acrylamide and *N,N'* methylene*bis*-acrylamide are neurotoxic: Wear gloves and face mask.
2. ES: 0.5*M* EDTA, 1% *N* sodium lauroyl sarcosinate.
3. 1*M* Sorbitol, 100 m*M* EDTA.
4. 1*M* Sorbitol, 100 m*M* trisodium citrate, 60 m*M* EDTA.
5. 10 m*M* Tris-HCl, pH 8, 0.45*M* EDTA, 7.5% β-mercaptoethanol (add the β-mercaptoethanol just before use).
6. 10 m*M* Tris-HCl, pH 7.5, 5 m*M* EDTA.
7. 10 m*M* Tris-HCl, pH 7.5, 1 m*M* EDTA.
8. 50 m*M* Tris-HCl, pH 7.5, 20 m*M* EDTA.

2.3. Biological Reagents

1. Bovine serum albumin (20 mg/mL) (Boehringer Mannheim, Mannheim, Germany).
2. Cot1 human DNA (Gibco BRL, Paisley, Scotland).
3. Lyticase (Sigma [Dorset, UK] L5263).
4. Phage λ DNA concatemers (ref. *33,* and Chapter 14).
5. Proteinase K.
6. Random primed DNA labeling kit (Boehringer Mannheim).
7. Restriction enzymes: *Eco*RI, *Eco*RV, *Hae*III, *Hind*III, *Nhe*I, *Pst*I, *Rsa*I, and *Taq*I.
8. RNase A: 10 mg/mL stock solution, boiled for 15 min to inactivate DNases, and stored at –20°C.
9. Sonicated salmon sperm DNA (10 mg/mL).
10. Total human DNA: both high-mol-wt (30 ng/μL) and sonicated (10 mg/mL) (size range: 200–500 bp).
11. Total rodent DNA: both high-mol-wt (30 ng/μL) and sonicated (10 mg/mL) (size range: 200–500 bp).
12. T4 DNA ligase (1 and 8 U/μL).
13. Zymolyase 100T (ICN Immunochemicals, Bucks, UK).
14. *Taq* DNA polymerase.

2.4. Buffers

1. Ligation buffer: 100 m*M* Tris-HCl, pH 7.5, 100 m*M* $MgCl_2$, 100 m*M* dithioerythritol, 6 m*M* ATP.
2. PCR buffer: 10 m*M* Tris-HCl, pH 8.3, 50 m*M* KCl, 0.01% gelatin, 1.5 m*M* $MgCl_2$, 0.01% Tween 20, 0.1% Triton X-100, 0.1% Nonidet NP40, 200 μ*M* of each dATP, dCTP, dGTP, dTTP.

3. Prehybridization and hybridization buffer: 4X SSC, 4X Denhardt solution, 10% dextran sulfate, 0.5% SDS, and 50 µg/mL sonicated salmon sperm DNA.
4. 20X SSC: 3M NaCl, 0.3M trisodium citrate.
5. 20X TAE: 0.8M Tris-acetate, 20 mM EDTA.
6. 5X TBE: 0.45M Tris-borate, 10 mM EDTA.

2.5. Yeast Culture

1. α D(+) glucose: 40% stock solution, autoclaved.
2. Casaminoacids.
3. Bacto-yeast nitrogen base without amino acids (Difco).
4. AHC: 17 g yeast nitrogen based without amino acids, 10 g casaminoacids, 50 mg adenine hemisulfate. Bring to 1 L and adjust to pH 5.8.

2.6. Miscellaneous Materials

1. Hybond N (Amersham).
2. Kodak XAR films.

2.7. Equipment

1. Contour Clamped Homogeneous Electric Field (CHEF) apparatus *(34),* with cooling system.
2. Freezer (–70°C).
3. Fume hood.
4. SE600 Hoefer vertical gel electrophoresis apparatus.
5. Incubator-shaker at 30°C.
6. Polymerase Chain Reaction (PCR) automat.
7. Safety cabinet (yeast culture).
8. Vacuum oven at 80°C.

3. Methods

3.1. Estimation of the Size of YAC Recombinants

3.1.1. Preparation of Yeast Chromosomes for Electrophoretic Karyotyping

3.1.1.1. PREPARATION OF 50 AGAROSE PLUGS

1. Grow the YAC in 50 mL of AHC media to late logarithmic phase (about 5×10^8 cells/mL) at 30°C.
2. Purify chromosome-size DNA in agarose plugs by the method described in *(35),* as detailed in Chapter 14.

3.1.1.2. PREPARATION OF SMALL NUMBERS OF AGAROSE PLUGS

As a general rule, one can prepare 1 agarose plug/mL of culture grown to high density (about 5×10^8 cells/mL). The technique described in Chapter 15 is scaled down proportionately.

To make three agarose plugs:

1. Grow the YAC in 3 mL of AHC to late logarithmic phase (about 5×10^8 cells/mL) at 30°C.
2. Collect the cells by centrifugation at 300*g* (1500 rpm in Sorvall RT6000) for 4 min.
3. Resuspend the cells in 1 mL of cold 50 m*M* EDTA on ice, and spin as above.
4. Repeat step 3.
5. Resuspend in 120 μL of 50 m*M* EDTA at room temperature.
6. Add 30 μL of solution 1 (1 mL of 1*M* sorbitol, 0.1*M* trisodium citrate, 60 m*M* EDTA, 50 μL β-mercaptoethanol, 1 mg of Zymolyase 100T), and mix gently but thoroughly.
7. Immediately add 150 μL of 1% low-melting-point agarose (Ultrapure BRL) made up in 0.125*M* EDTA and cooled down to 50°C. Mix well, and aliquot by 100 μL into plug molds placed on ice.
8. Allow to set for 10–15 min, and transfer to 3 mL of solution 2: 0.45*M* EDTA, 10 m*M* Tris-HCl, pH 8, 7.5% β-mercaptoethanol. Incubate for 16 h at 37°C.
9. Transfer to 3 mL of solution 3: 0.5*M* EDTA, 1% *N* sodium lauroyl sarcosinate, 1 mg/mL proteinase K. Incubate at 50°C for 20 h.
10. Repeat step 9 with fresh solution 3.
11. Store in 3 mL of 0.5*M* EDTA.

3.1.2. Fractionation of the Yeast Chromosomes by Pulsed Field Gel Electrophoresis

1. Equilibrate one plug in 1 mL of 0.5X TAE electrophoresis buffer for 1 h at room temperature under agitation.
2. Load on a 1% agarose gel made in 0.5X TAE. Run under electrophoretic conditions resolving all 17 chromosomes of *Saccharomyces cerevisiae* (*see* Note 1). Use concatemers of phage λ DNA (*33,* and Chapter 15) and *S. cerevisiae* chromosomes prepared from the strain used to construct the library as standard size markers.
3. Stain the gel with ethidium bromide (10 μg/mL) for 20 min. Destain in water for 20 min.

3.1.3. Detection of the YAC

1. Examination of the gel under UV illumination will show an extra band when compared to the parent yeast strain karyotype. The YAC's size can then be directly estimated. Sometimes, however, the YAC is not visible, either because it is hidden by an endogenous chromosome or because it has been lost in a proportion of the cells. In any case, it is necessary to blot the gel in order to check that the clone contains a single YAC and to detect any chimerism.
2. Depurinate the DNA in-gel by two treatments of 10 min each in 0.25*M* HCl.
3. Wash three times briefly in demineralized water.
4. Denature, neutralize, and transfer onto a nylon membrane (Hybond N, Amersham, for instance) according to the manufacturer's instructions.
5. Prehybridize the blot for 1 h at 68°C in 4X SSC, 4X Denhardt solution, 10% dextran sulfate, 0.5% SDS, 50 μg/mL sonicated salmon sperm DNA.
6. Hybridize simultaneously with radiolabeled total or Cot1 human DNA and phage λ DNA probes for 16 h at 68°C in the same solution as for the prehybridization, complemented with 40 μg/mL of sonicated rodent DNA as a competitor.
7. Wash in 0.2X SSC, 0.1% SDS, twice at room temperature, and twice at 65°C, and expose with an autoradiographic Kodak XAR film at –70°C. (*see* Note 2).

3.1.4. Detection of Chimerism (Case of a Library Constructed from a Somatic Hybrid Cell Line with a Reduced Human Component)

1. Strip the signal from the blot.
2. Prehybridize as described above, and hybridize with a total rodent DNA probe in the presence of 40 μg/mL of sonicated total human DNA as a competitor.
3. Wash as in Section 3.1.3., and put down with an autoradiographic film.
4. A positive signal at the position of the YAC band indicates a coligation event.

3.1.5. Estimation of the Extent of Chimerism (Case of a Library Constructed from a Somatic Hybrid Cell Line with a Reduced Human Component)

1. Purify total DNA from the YAC clone, grown to high density in 15 mL AHC, by the method detailed in Chapter 21 (Section 3.4.2.). The cells are collected by centrifugation, resuspended in 1 mL of 1*M* sorbitol and

0.1*M* EDTA, and incubated with 0.4 mg of Lyticase at 37°C for 90 min. Then follow the protocol exactly until the end, where the DNA is resuspended in 300 μL of 10 m*M* Tris-HCl, pH 7.5, 1 m*M* EDTA. The DNA concentration should be about 100 ng/mL.

2. Digest 500 ng of YAC DNA to completion with a 6-bp cutting restriction enzyme (*Eco*RI, *Pst*I, *Hind*III, and so on).
3. Fractionate through a 0.9% agarose gel, transfer onto a nylon membrane, hybridize with a total rodent DNA probe, using total human DNA as a competitor, wash at high stringency (*see* Section 3.1.3.), and expose with an autoradiographic film.
4. The number of rodent bands detected allows the estimation of the extent of the chimerism; for instance, 1 band is detected per 25–30 kbp of mouse DNA digested with *Pst*I.

3.2. Amplification
of Internal Single-Copy Sequences by Alu-PCR

1. Use 50–100 ng of total YAC DNA (purified as described in Section 3.1.5.)/PCR reaction, in the following buffer: 10 m*M* Tris-HCl, pH 8.3, 50 m*M* KCl, 0.01% gelatin, 1.5 m*M* MgCl$_2$, 0.01% Tween 20, 0.1% Triton X-100, 0.1% Nonidet NP40, and 200 μ*M* of each dATP, dCTP, dGTP, and dTTP. Two hundred and fifty nanograms of either or both 5' and 3' consensus *Alu*-repeat primers are added to the reaction (*see* Note 3 for the sequence and position of the primers in the *Alu* repeat). Carry out the reactions in a final vol of 50 μL with 1 U of Cetus Ampli*Taq*. (The PCR buffer and the *Taq* polymerase supplied by Promega can be used instead.)
2. The optimized program used with a Perkin Elmer Cetus DNA Thermal Cycler is subdivided into three segments as follows: segment 1: 94°C, 3 min; 60°C, 1 min; 72°C, 1 min (1 cycle); segment 2: 92°C, 45 s; 60°C, 1 min; 72°C, 1 min, with an increment of 6 s/cycle (35 cycles); segment 3: 92°C, 45 s; 60°C, 1 min; 72°C, 10 min (1 cycle) (*see* Note 4).
3. Load 10 μL of each sample on a vertical composite 3% polyacrylamide and 0.25–1% agarose (PA-Ag) gel, and run at 200 V in 1X TBE electrophoresis buffer in a SE600 Hoefer apparatus *(36)* (*see* Note 5). Prepare 50 mL of 3% PA:1% Ag gel as follows: Mix 5 mL of acrylamide-*bis*-acrylamide (29:1), 14.65 mL of distilled water, and 5 mL of 5X TBE, and prewarm to about 50°C; add this solution to 25 mL of 2% agarose made up in 1X TBE (cooled down to 50°C), while mixing with a magnetic stirrer; immediately add 350 μL of 10% ammonium persulfate and 25 μL of TEMED, and pour the gel between prewarmed glass plates using a 25-mL or 50-mL syringe.

4. Stain the gel for 30 min with ethidium bromide (10 µg/mL), and destain for 30 min. Figure 2 shows *Alu*-PCR products from three YAC recombinants (*see* Note 6).

3.3. Amplification of End Fragments by Inverse-PCR (37)

3.3.1. Preparation of the Template for Inverse-PCR (I-PCR) (See Note 7)

1. Digest 500 ng of DNA to completion with 5–10 U of the appropriate enzyme (*see* Notes 8 and 9) in 20 µL of restriction buffer (1X KGB buffer is suitable; ref. *38*) containing 2 mM spermidine. Do not incubate the DNA for too long (3 h proved to be sufficient), since overdigestion will result in the degradation of the cohesive ends and thus reduce the efficiency of circularization at a later stage.
2. Extract with organic solvents twice: first with 50 µL of phenol, chloroform, isoamylalcohol (25:24:1), and then with 50 µL of chloroform and isoamylalcohol (24:1).
3. Add 1 µL of 5M NaCl (0.2M final), mix, add 3 vol (about 60 µL) of cold absolute ethanol, and vortex; leave to precipitate at –20°C for at least 5 h.
4. Spin in microfuge for 15 min at 4°C; discard the supernatant, and rinse the DNA pellet with 500 µL of cold 70% ethanol.
5. Spin for 5 min at 4°C; air-dry the DNA pellet thoroughly, and resuspend it in 10 µL of distilled H$_2$O.
6. Heat up at 65°C for 10 min, and put on ice; immediately aliquot out 1 µL into 9 µL of 1X ligation buffer (10 mM Tris-HCl, pH 7.5, 10 mM MgCl$_2$, 10 mM dithioerythritol, 0.6 mM ATP); add 1 U of T4 DNA ligase (Boehringer Mannheim), and incubate at 14°C for 16 h. The remaining 9 µL of purified restriction digest are stored at –20°C. (*see* Notes 10 and 11).
7. Purify with organic solvents, ethanol-precipitate, and rinse with 70% ethanol as described above postrestriction; air-dry thoroughly and resuspend in 20 µL of distilled H$_2$O; store at –20°C.

3.3.2. Inverse Polymerase Chain Reaction (I-PCR)

1. Aliquot out 1 µL of purified ligation product (corresponding to approx 500 pg of template DNA) into a microfuge tube suitable for PCR.
2. Add 49 µL of the following PCR buffer containing 1 U of Cetus Ampli*Taq* DNA polymerase and 250 ng of each primer of the appropriate pair (*see* Note 8).
3. PCR program: same as in Section 3.2., using a Perkin Elmer Cetus DNA Thermal Cycler. This program is effective for the amplification of fragments up to 4 kb (*see* Note 12).

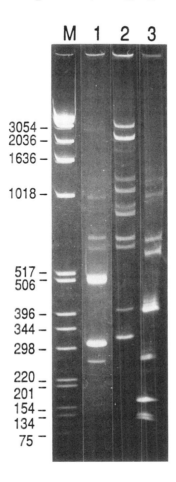

Fig. 2. Analysis of human YAC recombinants by *Alu*-PCR. Two YACs were analyzed as described in Section 3.2., and the *Alu*-PCR products fractionated through a composite 3% polyacrylamide, 0.25% agarose gel in 1X TBE at 200 V for 1.5 h in a SE600 Hoefer apparatus. Lane 1: YAC 257G1, primer 450; lane 2: YAC VI1, primer 451; lane 3: YAC VI1, both primers 450 and 451. M: size marker (1 kbp ladder, Gibco BRL). Sizes are indicated in bp.

3.3.3. Analysis of the Amplified End Fragments

1. Run 10 µL of the I-PCR on a 1.3% agarose gel.
2. Stain with ethidium bromide (10 µg/mL), and examine under UV illumination. A unique band should be visible in each sample. Multiple bands are sometimes observed, mainly because of partial digestion before the ligation (*see also* Note 13).

3. Transfer onto a nylon membrane.
4. Hybridize with YAC arm-specific kinase-labeled oligonucleotides that are internal to the primers used for the amplification (*see* Note 14).
5. Wash in 4X SSC and 0.1% SDS, once at room temperature, and three times at 50°C, for 5 min each, and put down with an X-ray film.
6. Only genuine end products will show positive signals (*see* Notes 15 and 16).

3.4. Fingerprinting of YAC Recombinants

3.4.1. Fingerprinting by Interspersed Repeat PCR

The pattern of fragments generated by *Alu*-PCR is clone-specific, and thus constitutes fingerprints of human YACs. The PCR products amplified with various consensus *Alu* primers either alone or in combination can be fractionated either separately or pooled in order to produce the most complex fingerprint of each YAC on a high-resolution gel (Fig. 3). This may, however, result in the loss of some information owing to comigration of unresolved fragments.

Up to 30 major bands could be amplified from YACs derived from a library with an average insert size of 150 Kbp *(39)*. This corresponds to 1 band/10–15 kbp of cloned DNA and should provide sufficient interclone overlap information for contig mapping procedures. In the case of *Alu*-poor YACs, a combination of interspersed repeat primers can be used (L1-L1 or *Alu*-L1 PCR) *(40)* to amplify supplementary sequences and improve the fingerprint (the *Alu* richness of YACs and the complexity of *Alu*-PCR fingerprints are indeed strongly correlated; ref. *41*).

Additional fingerprint information can be gained by DNA transfer analysis of the interspersed repeat products with various types of oligonucleotides, such as di-, tri-, or tetranucleotide repeats. All the information is then stored in a data base and treated for pattern comparison.

3.4.2. Fingerprinting by Repeat Probe Analysis

1. Digest 500 ng of YAC DNA to completion with a 6-bp cutter (*Hind*III for instance) and fractionate through a 0.9% agarose gel. Alternatively, the 4-bp cutter *Rsa*I can be used, and the digested DNA fractionated through a 2% agarose gel (*see* Note 17).
2. Transfer onto a nylon membrane.
3. Hybridize sequentially with radiolabeled total human DNA or its Cot1 fraction (Gibco BRL), with an *Alu* repeat-specific probe (for instance BLUR8) *(42)* and L1 probes that cover the full length of L1 repeats *(43)*.

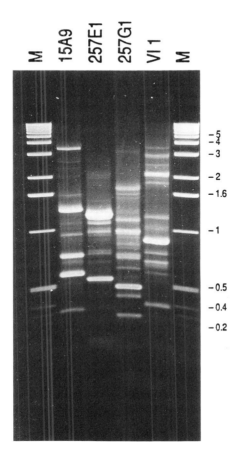

Fig. 3. Fingerprinting human YACs by *Alu*-PCR. Four YACs *(39)* were *Alu*-PCRed using primers 450 and 451 either alone or in combination (Section 3.2.). The three amplification products were then pooled and fractionated through a 1.5% agarose gel at 100 V in 1X TBE. Lane 1: YAC 15A9; lane 2: YAC 257E1; lane 3: YAC 257G1; lane 4: YAC VI1. M, the size marker is as in Fig. 2; sizes are indicated in kbp.

4. Wash in 1X SSC and 0.1% SDS, twice at room temperature and twice at 65°C.
5. Expose with an X-ray film for autoradiography.

The analysis of *Hind*III digests of six YACs isolated from the library described in *(39)* is shown in Fig. 4. Total or Cot1 human DNA detects on average 1 band/10–15 kbp in 4-bp cutter digests, and 1 band/15–20 kbp in 6-bp cutter digests. This again should allow the detection of mod-

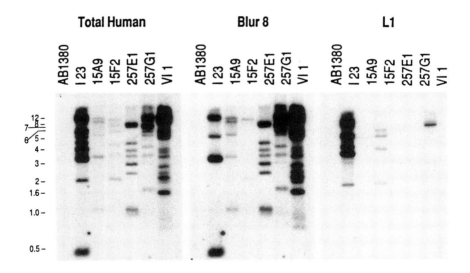

Fig. 4. Fingerprints of human YACs by repeat probe analysis. The YAC DNAs were digested with HindIII and fractionated through a 1% agarose gel. Probes are indicated above each panel. Probe BLUR8 is from *(41);* the L1 probe used was BK(1.2)11 from *(42).* Sizes are indicated in kbp on the left.

erate (10–20%) overlaps between clones. Very specific fingerprints can be generated by integrating the data obtained with the various probes. A combination of multiple digests and additional repeat- or motif-specific probes, together with records of the densitometric analysis of the autoradiograms, will further increase the information content of the fingerprints (important intensity differences are indeed observed between bands, reflecting the number of repeat copies accommodated in individual restriction fragments).

3.4.3. Comparison
of the Two Fingerprinting Techniques

There is merit to both strategies for fingerprinting YAC recombinants: The repeat probe analysis maximizes the potential information, but requires relatively large amounts of purified DNA and lengthy processing; by contrast, interspersed repeat PCR is quick and requires minimal amounts of DNA, but the information may be limited in the case of repeat-poor clones. Importantly, both techniques are amenable to standardization and automation for handling large numbers.

The interspersed repeat PCR technique also has the important advantage of generating molecularly pure fragments of insert DNA that can be:

1. Screened for polymorphisms *(4–6,27–31);*
2. Used directly as probes; or
3. Sequenced to create Sequence Tagged Sites *(26).*

4. Notes

1. An accurate estimation of the YAC's size is best achieved by a second fractionation under optimal conditions resolving the desired size-range.
2. The blot may have to be hybridized with a total yeast DNA probe in order to estimate the size of large YACs more accurately. All the endogenous chromosomes of the YAC clone will then light up as well.
3. The sequences of the four primers are as follows:
   153: 5'GGGATTACAGGCGTGAGCCAC 3'
   154: 5'TGCACTCCAGCCTGGGCAAC 3'
   450: 5'AAAGTGCTGGCATTACAGG 3'
   451: 5'GTGAGCCGAGATCGCGCCACTGCACT 3'

   They correspond, respectively, to bases 27–47 (bottom strand), 248–267 (top strand), 37–55 (bottom strand), and 228–253 (top strand) of the *Alu* consensus sequence as compiled and analyzed by Bains *(44)*. These primers are derived from the 5' (153 and 450) and 3' (154 and 451) sequences, the most conserved throughout the family of *Alu*-repeat elements. Using one primer at a time leads to the amplification of sequences between inversely oriented *Alu* repeats. Using a pair of primers derived from both ends of the repeat allows the amplification of sequences between *Alu* repeats in the same orientation. Although primers 153 and 450, on one hand, and primers 154 and 451, on the other hand, overlap partially, they give rise to the amplification of different sets of products, thus reflecting the sequence divergence between *Alu* repeats. This shows that using multiple primers, separately or in combination, leads to the amplification of additional sequences by hitting a higher number of *Alu* elements, thereby providing a probe of greater total length that covers the YAC insert more thoroughly.

   Most products generated are repeat-free, as assessed by Southern blot analysis with the *Alu* specific probe BLUR8 *(42)* and with probes covering the full length of L1 repeats *(43)*. The pooled *Alu*-PCR products can thus be used as probes under suppression hybridization conditions for both DNA *in situ* hybridization (Chapter 26, and ref. *45)* and DNA transfer analysis.
4. No amplification is observed under these conditions with total genomic mouse, hamster, or yeast DNA.

5. Polyacrylamide (3%), 0.25–1% agarose composite gels provide excellent resolution of fragments in the 100–3000-bp size range *(36),* as typically required for the analysis of *Alu*-PCR fragments. In addition, all bands are very sharp regardless of their size (Fig. 2). No diffusion is observed even after storage at 4°C overnight. This gel matrix is very robust and can be processed for DNA transfer analysis without deformation of the gel.

Agarose gels (1.5%) can be used instead, but the resolution and sharpness of the bands are far poorer, especially in the lower mol-wt domain. Agarose gels must be run fast, and the electrophoresis buffer cooled, if possible, so as to minimize diffusion.

6. The number of bands amplified in individual YACs is very variable and reflects the uneven distribution of *Alu* repeats in the human genome *(41,46,47).* YACs derived from *Alu*-poor regions give rise to very few products. If the amount of internal sequences thus amplified is not satisfactory, L1-PCR or L1-*Alu*-PCR amplification can be performed *(40).*

7. The first generation of YAC vectors *(1,48,49)* are not designed for easy subcloning of end fragments (although the vector arm that carries the ampicillin resistance gene and the *E. coli* origin of replication could be used for isolating the corresponding end). The protocol described here allows the selective amplification of either end of any first-generation YAC recombinant by Inverse-PCR (I-PCR) *(25)* with a set of primers derived from the arms of the pYAC4 vector *(1). See* ref. *37* for representative examples.

8. The clone's end that carries the TRP1 complementation gene is referred to as the left end, and that which carries the URA3 gene as the right end. For the left arm (*Taq*I), the primers are 372 (5'GAATTGATCCA CAGGACGGG 3') (located 25 bp away from the *Taq*I site at position 5407 in pYAC4, and derived from the bottom strand) and 373 (5'GCCAAGTTGGTTTAAGGCGC 3') (25 bp from the cloning site in pYAC4, top strand). For the right arm, enzymes *Pst*I or *Hind*III can be used; if the YAC DNA is restricted with *Pst*I, use primers 374 (5'GGAAGAACGAAGGAAGGAGC 3') (90 bp from the *Pst*I site at position 6980 in pYAC4, top strand) and 556 (5'GCCCGATCTCAA GATTACG 3') (immediately adjacent to the *Eco*RI cloning site at position 5615 in pYAC4, bottom strand); if the DNA is cut with *Hind*III, the primers are 375 (5'AAACTCAACGAGCTGGACGC 3') (71 bp away from the *Hind*III site at position 8599 in pYAC4, top strand) and 556.

9. Other restriction enzymes can be used to produce end fragments with the primers described in Note 8, although resulting in the coamplification of larger adjacent vector sequences. These are, in increasing order of

distance from the primers: *Hae*III, *Nhe*I, *Eco*RV, and *Rsa*I (at positions 5363, 5296, 5252, and 5231 in pYAC4, respectively) for the left end (using primers 372 and 373), and *Rsa*I and *Eco*RV (at positions 7118 and 7189, respectively) for the right end (using primers 374 and 556).

10. At this concentration (1–2.5 ng/μL, assuming an overall loss of 50–80% of the material through the purification procedure of the digestion product), intramolecular ligation events resulting in the circularization of the DNA fragments are favored over intermolecular ligation events.

11. Since blunt ends ligate far less efficiently than cohesive ends, more T4 DNA ligase has to be added if the enzymes *Eco*RV, *Hae*III, or *Rsa*I were used to restrict the YAC DNA. The ligation is then performed in a total of 20 μL with 1 μL of 8 U/μL T4 DNA ligase (Boehringer Mannheim) for 24 h at 14°C. The reaction is continued for another 2 d by adding the same amount of ligase every 24 h.

12. An equivalent program for Hybaid Thermal Reactors is as follows:
    Segment 1: 94°C, 2 min 30 s; 60°C, 1 min; 72°C, 1 min (1 cycle)
    Segment 2: 90°C, 20 s; 60°C, 1 min; 72°C, 1 min, with an increment of 30 s every five cycles (35 cycles)
    Segment 3: 90°C, 20 s; 60°C, 1 min; 72°C, 10 min (1 cycle).

13. A fragment of about 550 bp in size is amplified up in the *Hind*III I-PCR sample of every YAC; this fragment hybridizes to the internal oligonucleotide 769. The origin of this fragment is unknown.

14. Oligonucleotide 768 (5'ACTACGCGATCATGGCGACC 3') is used for assessing the left-end fragments, 769 (5'GGTAAAGCTCATCA GCGTGG 3') for the *Hind*III-generated right-end fragments, and 770 (5'GTTGGGTTAAGAATACTGGGC 3') for the *Pst*I-, *Rsa*I-, and *Eco*RV-generated right-end fragments.

15. It should be noted that, considering the relative positions of the various primers to the cloning site (*Eco*RI in the case of pYAC4) and to the recognition sites for the enzymes used to restrict the YAC DNA prior to I-PCR, vector DNA sequences are coamplified with the insert's end fragments; left arm: 90 bp (*Taq*I), 200 bp (*Nhe*I), 244 bp (*Eco*RV), 256 bp (*Hae*III), and 265 bp (*Rsa*I); right arm: 129 bp (*Pst*I), 266 bp (*Rsa*I), 337 bp (*Eco*RV), and 110 bp (*Hind*III). The vector sequences can readily be removed by double restriction both at the cloning site (*Eco*RI in the case of pYAC4) and at the site used for I-PCR; the end-fragment can then be purified, cloned, and sequenced to produce an STS *(26),* and screened for polymorphisms *(4–6,27–31).*

It is worth noting that about 5.5% of *Eco*RI sites in the human genome are found in L1 repeats. Therefore, 11% of YAC recombinants isolated from *Eco*RI partial libraries will have L1 repetitive sequences at one end. This is corroborated by the analysis of human chromosome 11-specific YAC recombinants *(41)*. About the same proportion (10%) would be observed in partial *Bam*HI libraries, and an even higher proportion (about 14.5%) in partial *Bgl*II libraries. This has important implications for chromosome walking exercises, in which single copy probes must be derived from sequences close to the ends of the clones for further library screening.

16. The I-PCR technique has a success rate very similar to the "vectorette" system proposed by Riley et al. *(50),* which is also constrained by the maximum length of DNA that can be amplified with current PCR protocols (4–4.5 kb). Both approaches are universally applicable to YACs inserted in first-generation vectors. Note that the yield of large PCR products can be improved by adding gene 32 protein to the reaction *(51)*.

17. *Rsa*I cuts less frequently than other 4-bp cutters (*Hin*fI, *Sau*3A), and thus provides larger, less diffusible, fragments. Furthermore, this enzyme does not cut in the consensus *Alu*-repeat sequence. It seems, therefore, preferable for fingerprint analysis to other very frequent cutters. In addition, since this enzyme provides more complex fingerprints than 6-bp cutters do, it may prove very useful, especially when the YAC analyzed are small.

Acknowledgments

I wish to thank D. J. Porteous for fruitful discussions and for his continuous support and encouragement, and S. Bruce, N. Davidson, and D. Stuart for preparing the figures. This work was supported by the Wellcome Trust and by the Medical Research Council of the UK. I dedicate this chapter to the memory of my former colleague Isabelle Oberlé.

References

1. Burke, D. T., Carle, G. F., and Olson, M. V. (1987) Cloning of large segments of exogenous DNA into yeast by means of artificial chromosome vectors. *Science* **236**, 806–812.

2. Morton, N. E. (1955) Sequential tests for the detection of linkage. *Amer. J. Hum. Genet.* **7**, 277–318.

3. Lathrop, G. M., Lalouel, J. M., Julier, C., and Ott, J. (1985) Multilocus linkage analysis in humans: detection of linkage and estimation of recombination. *Amer. J. Hum. Genet.* **37**, 482–498.

4. Jeffreys, A. J., Wilson, V., and Thein, S. L. (1985) Hypervariable "mini-satellite" regions in human DNA. *Nature* **314**, 67–73.

5. Nakamura, Y., Leppert, M., O'Connell, P., Wolff, R., Holm, T., Culver, M., Martin, C., Fujimoto, E., Hoff, M., Kumlin, E., and White, R. (1987) Variable number of tandem repeat (VNTR) markers for human gene mapping. *Science* **235**, 1616–1622.

6. Weber, J. L. and May, P. E. (1989) Abundant class of human DNA polymorphisms which can be typed using the polymerase chain reaction. *Amer. J. Hum. Genet.* **44,** 388–396.

7. Weber, J. L. (1990) Informativeness of human (dC-dA)n·(dGdT)n polymorphisms. *Genomics* **7,** 524–530.

8. Schwartz, D. A. and Cantor, C. R. (1984) Separation of yeast chromosome-sized DNAs by pulsed field gradient gel electrophoresis. *Cell* **37,** 67–75.

9. Carle, G. F. and Olson, M. V. (1984) Separation of chromosomal DNA molecules from yeast by orthogonal-field alternation gel electrophoresis. *Nucleic Acids Res.* **12,** 5647–5664.

10. Coulson, A., Sulston, J., Brenner, S., and Karn, J. (1986) Toward a physical map of the genome of the nematode *Caenorhabditis elegans. Proc. Natl. Acad. Sci. USA* **83,** 7821–7825.

11. Pinkel, D., Straume, T., and Gray, J. W. (1986) Cytogenetic analysis using quantitative, high sensitivity, fluorescence hybridization. *Proc. Natl. Acad. Sci. USA* **83,** 2934–2938.

12. Trask, B., Pinkel, D., and van den Engh, G. (1989) The proximity of DNA sequences in interphase cell nuclei is correlated to genomic distance and permits ordering of cosmids spanning 250 kilobase pairs. *Genomics* **5,** 710–717.

13. Monaco, A. P., Lam, V. M. S., Zehetner, G., Lennon, G. G., Douglas, C., Nizetic, D., Goodfellow, P. N., and Lehrach, H. (1991) Mapping irradiation hybrids to cosmid and yeast artificial chromosome libraries by direct hybridization of Alu-PCR products. *Nucleic Acids Res.* **19,** 3315–3318.

14. Elvin, P., Slynn, G., Black, D., Graham, A., Butler, R., Riley, J., Anand, R., and Markham, A. F. (1991) Isolation of cDNA clones using yeast artificial chromosome probes. *Nucleic Acids Res.* **18,** 3913–3917.

15. Brownstein, B. H., Silverman, G. A., Little, R. D., Burke, D. T., Korsmeyer, S. J., Schlessinger, D., and Olson, M. V. (1989) Isolation of single-copy human genes from a library of yeast artificial chromosome clones. *Science* **244,** 1348–1351.

16. Anand, R., Riley, J. H., Butler, R., Smith, J. C., and Markham, A. F. (1990) A 3.5 genome equivalent multi access YAC library: construction, characterisation, screening and storage. *Nucleic Acids Res.* **18,** 1951–1955.

17. Albertsen, H. M., Abderrahim, H., Cann, H. M., Dausset, J., Le Paslier, D., and Cohen, D. (1990) Construction and characterization of a yeast artificial chromosome library containing seven haploid human genome equivalents. *Proc. Natl. Acad. Sci. USA* **87,** 4256–4260.

18. Larin, Z., Monaco, A. P., and Lehrach, H. (1991) Yeast artificial chromosome libraries containing large inserts from mouse and human DNA. *Proc. Natl. Acad. Sci. USA* **88,** 4123–4127.

19. Burke, D. T., Rossi, J. M., Leung, J., Koos, D. S., and Tilghman, S. M. (1991) A mouse library of yeast artificial chromosome clones. *Mammalian Genome* **1,** 65.

20. Green, E. D., Riethman, H. C., Dutchik, J. E., and Olson, M. V. (1991) Detection and characterization of chimeric yeast artificial chromosome clones. *Genomics* **11,** 658–669.

21. Green, E. D. and Olson, M. V. (1990) Chromosomal region of the Cystic Fibrosis gene in yeast artificial chromosomes: a model for human genome mapping. *Science* **250,** 94–98.
22. Bonetta, L., Kuehn, S. E., Huang, A., Law, D. J., Kalikin, L. M., Koi, M., Reeve, A. E., Brownstein, B. H., Yeger, H., Williams, B. R. G., and Feinberg, A. P. (1990) Wilms Tumor Locus on 11p13 defined by multiple CpG island-associated transcripts. *Science* **250,** 994–997.
23. Silverman, G. A., Jockel, J. I., Domer, P. H., Mohr, R. M., Taillon-Miller, P., and Korsmeyer, S. J. (1991) Yeast artificial chromosome cloning of a two-megabase-size contig within chromosomal band 18q21 establishes physical linkage between BCL2 and Plasminogen Activator Inhibitor Type-2. *Genomics* **9,** 219–228.
24. Nelson, D. L., Ledbetter, S. A., Corbo, L., Victoria, M. F., Ramirez-Solis, R., Webster, T. D., Ledbetter, D. H., and Caskey, C. T. (1989) Alu polymerase chain reaction: a method for rapid isolation of human-specific sequences from complex DNA sources. *Proc. Natl. Acad. Sci. USA* **86,** 6686–6690.
25. Ochman, H., Gerber, A. S., and Hartl, D. L. (1988) Genetic applications of an Inverse Polymerase Chain Reaction. *Genetics* **120,** 621–623.
26. Olson, M., Hood, L., Cantor, C., and Botstein, D. (1989) A common language for physical mapping of the human genome. *Science* **245,** 1434,1435.
27. Botstein, D., White, R. L., Skolnick, M., and Davis, R. W. (1980) Construction of a linkage map in man using restriction fragment length polymorphisms. *Amer. J. Hum. Genet.* **69,** 201–205.
28. Myers, R. M., Fischer, S. G., Maniatis, T., and Lerman, L. S. (1985) Modification of the melting properties of duplex DNA by denaturing gradient gel electrophoresis. *Nucleic Acids Res.* **13,** 3111–3129.
29. Abrams, E. S., Murdaugh, S. E., and Lerman, L. S. (1990) Comprehensive detection of single base changes in human genomic DNA using denaturing gradient gel electrophoresis and a GC clamp. *Genomics* **7,** 463–475.
30. Orita, M., Iwahana, H., Kanazawa, H., Hayashi, K., and Sekiya, T. (1989) Detection of polymorphisms of human DNA by gel electrophoresis as single-strand conformation polymorphisms. *Proc. Natl. Acad. Sci. USA* **86,** 2766–2770.
31. Burmeister, M., di Sibio, G., Cox, D. R., and Myers, R. M. (1991) Identification of polymorphisms by genomic denaturing gradient gel electrophoresis: application to the proximal region of human chromosome 21. *Nucleic Acids Res.* **19,** 1475–1481.
32. Simmler, M.-C., Cox, R. D., and Avner, P. (1991) Adaptation of the interspersed repetitive sequence polymerase chain reaction to the isolation of mouse DNA probes from somatic cell hybrids on a hamster background. *Genomics* **10,** 770–778.
33. van Ommen, G. J. B. and Verkerk, J. M. H. (1986) Restriction analysis of chromosomal DNA in a size range up to two million base pairs by pulsed field gradient electrophoresis, in *Analysis of Human Genetic Diseases* (Davies, K., ed.) IRL, Oxford, UK pp. 113–133.
34. Maule, J. C. and Green, D. K. (1990) Semi-conductor controlled contour-clamped homogeneous electric field apparatus. *Anal. Biochem.* **191,** 390–395.

35. Carle, G. F. and Olson, M. V. (1985) An electrophoretic karyotype for yeast. *Proc. Natl. Acad. Sci. USA* **82,** 3756–3760.
36. Arveiler, B. and Porteous, D. J. (1992) Polyacrylamide-agarose composite gels for high resolution of fingerprints. *Trends Genet.* **8,** 82.
37. Arveiler, B. and Porteous, D. J. (1991) Amplification of end fragments of YAC recombinants by inverse-polymerase chain reaction. *Technique* **3,** 24–28.
38. McClelland, M., Hanish, J., Nelson, M., and Patel, Y. (1988) KGB: a single buffer for all restriction enzymes. *Nucleic Acids Res.* **16,** 364.
39. Arveiler, B., Murray, I., Stevenson, B., and Porteous, D. J. (1991) Construction of a library enriched for human chromosome 11 and Xp YAC recombinants. *Mammalian Genome* **1,** 265–266.
40. Ledbetter, S. A., Nelson, D. L., Warren, S. T., and Ledbetter, D. H. (1990) Rapid isolation of DNA probes within specific chromosome regions by interspersed repetitive sequence polymerase chain reaction. *Genomics* **6,** 475–481.
41. Arveiler, B. and Porteous, D. J. (1992) Distribution of Alu and L1 repeats in human YAC recombinants. *Mammalian Genome* **3,** 661–668.
42. Deininger, P. L., Jolly, D. J., Rubin, C. M., Friedmann, T., and Schmid, C. W. (1981) Base sequence study of 300 nucleotide renatured repeated human DNA clones. *J. Mol. Biol.* **151,** 17–33.
43. Shafit-Zagardo, B., Brown, F. L., Maio, J. J., and Adams, J. W. (1982) KpnI families of long, interspersed repetitive DNAs associated with the human beta-globin gene cluster. *Gene* **20,** 397–407.
44. Bains, W. (1986) The multiple origin of human Alu sequences. *J. Mol. Evol.* **23,** 189–199.
45. Breen, M., Arveiler, B., Murray, I., Gosden, J. R., and Porteous, D. J. (1992) YAC mapping by FISH using Alu-PCR generated probes. *Genomics* **13,** 726–730.
46. Korenberg, J. R. and Rykowski, M. C. (1988) Human genome organization: Alu, Lines, and the molecular structure of metaphase chromosome bands. *Cell* **53,** 391–400.
47. Moyzis, R. K., Torney, D. C., Meyne, J., Buckingham, J. M., Wu, J. R., Burks, C., Sirotkin, K. M., and Goad, W. B. (1989) The distribution of interspersed repetitive sequences in the human genome. *Genomics* **4,** 273–289.
48. Cooke, H. and Cross, S. (1988) pYAC4Neo, a yeast artificial chromosome vector which codes for G418 resistance in mammalian cells. *Nucleic Acids Res.* **16,** 11,817.
49. Marchuk, D. and Collins, F. S. (1988) pYAC-RC, a yeast artificial chromosome vector for cloning DNA cut with infrequently cutting restriction endonucleases. *Nucleic Acids Res.* **16,** 7743.
50. Riley, J., Butler, R., Ogilvie, D., Finniear, R., Jenner, D., Powell, S., Anand, R., Smith, J. C., and Markham, A. F. (1990) A novel, rapid method for the isolation of terminal sequences from yeast artificial chromosome (YAC) clones. *Nucleic Acids Res.* **18,** 2887–2890.
51. Schwartz, K., Hansen-Hagge, T., and Bartram, C. (1990) Improved yields of long PCR products using gene 32 protein. *Nucleic Acids Res.* **18,** 1079.

CHAPTER 23

Chromosome Dissection and Cloning

Steven D. M. Brown and Alyson H. Carey

1. Introduction

Microdissection and microcloning involve the physical removal of chromosome fragments and the cloning of the collected DNA using specialized microprocedures. Microdissection represents the most direct method for recovery of cloned DNA from an individual chromosome region providing banks of microclones for the genome analysis of the targeted region. A number of chromosome regions have been microdissected and successfully microcloned from a wide range of species, including human *(1–5)*, mouse *(6–8)*, *Drosophila (9)*, and, most recently, plants *(10)*.

The classical techniques of microdissection and microcloning involved the direct cloning of the DNA recovered from dissected chromosomes. Because of the small amounts of DNA recovered (picogram quantities), the microcloning took advantage of λ based vectors, principally λgt10, and the high rate of clone recovery obtainable through the use of λ in vitro packaging systems to recover recombinant DNA molecules *(11)*. For *Drosophila*, the availability of polytene chromosomes enhanced the ability to recover relatively large quantities of chromosomal DNA with the minimum of dissection, and thus, *Drosophila* pioneered the way in the application of eukaryotic chromosome dissection *(11)*. With the dissection of a greater number of chromosomes, the technique also proved successful in recovering sufficient DNA from individual regions of mouse or human chromosomes to produce several hundred

From: *Methods in Molecular Biology, Vol. 29: Chromosome Analysis Protocols*
Edited by: J. R. Gosden Copyright ©1994 Humana Press Inc., Totowa, NJ

clones originating from the dissected regions *(1,6–8).* Nevertheless, the production of microclones from these experiments was close to the limit of the recovering power of the cloning systems. In addition, all the early experiments on mammalian chromosomes used unstained metaphase spreads observed with phase-contrast microscopy, and the dissections were performed under oil, limiting optical conditions and therefore the accuracy of the dissection.

Most recently, the techniques of microdissection and microcloning have been extended to the dissection of stained chromosomes coupled with the use of the polymerase chain reaction (PCR) to enhance the recovery of DNA from the dissected region *(2).* We describe here the various experimental steps for the dissection and collection of stained chromosome fragments, and the steps required for microligation of the recovered DNA into a vector suitable for PCR. We briefly summarize the steps required to PCR the ligated DNA, prior to cloning, although these molecular techniques, which are in common use, are not described in detail. It should be noted that the described procedures are equally suitable for the microdissection of stained chromosome fragments and their microligation into a λ vector prior to in vitro packaging for the recovery of microclones as in the classical techniques. Equally, the described procedures are suitable for the microdissection and microligation of DNA from *Drosophila* polytene fragments, although, of course, in this case, the chromosomes are not stained.

2. Materials

2.1. Glass Materials
for the Preparation of Microneedles

Microneedles can be prepared from standard soda glass rods, 2 mm in diameter.

2.2. Glass Materials
for the Preparation of Micropipets

Micropipets can be prepared from Pasteur pipets or standard glass 1-mm microcapillaries.

2.3. Siliconization Solutions
for Microinstruments

2% Dimethyl dichlorosilane in 1,1,1 trichloroethane 1 mM Na$_2$EDTA.

2.4. Collection Drop

Tris-HCl (10 mM, pH 7.5), 10 mM NaCl, 0.1% SDS, 1% glycerol, and 500 µg/mL proteinase K.

2.5. Micromanipulation Oil

Spectroscopic-grade paraffin oil (Merck [Rahway, NJ] no. 7161) equilibrated with *Rsa*I buffer (*see* Section 2.7.).

2.6. Phenol for Extraction of Collection Drop

Phenol equilibrated with *Rsa*I buffer (*see* Section 2.7.).

2.7. Enzyme Buffer
for Digestion of Collection Drop

10X *Rsa*I buffer: 50 mM NaCl, 25 mM Tris-HCl (pH 8), 10 mM MgCl$_2$, 1 mM DTT, and 100 µg/mL bovine serum albumin.

2.8. Ligation Reaction

Polyethylene glycol (relative molecular mass, 8000). T4 DNA ligase buffer: 50 mM Tris-HCl, pH 7.8, 10 mM MgCl$_2$, 1 mM ATP, and 50 µg/mL bovine serum albumin.

3. Methods

3.1. Preparation
of Chromosome Metaphase Spreads
for Microdissection

Although it is not within the scope of this chapter to discuss in detail the methods for the preparation and staining of metaphase chromosome spreads, it is worth considering two major points relating to the preparation of chromosome spreads that affect their use for chromosome dissection and microcloning.

3.1.1. Depurination
of DNA During Acid Fixation of Chromosomes

The standard methanol–acetic acid fixative used in the preparation of metaphase chromosomes probably causes significant hydrolysis of the incumbent DNA that presumably results from acid depurination of DNA and subsequent base hydrolysis when chromosome material is restored to neutral pH *(12)*. It has been estimated that using standard fixation conditions of methanol–acetic acid 3:1 (pH 1.8) and fixation times of around 1 h, hydrolytic events may be as frequent as 1 every 100 nucleotides *(12)*. Such a high level of hydrolysis may account in part for, first, the relatively low yields of microclones produced in traditional microcloning experiments and, second, the relatively small size of clones (<400 bp) recovered; those restriction fragments carrying hydrolytic events are unclonable. It is to be noted that in one experiment where fixation times were reduced to 5–20 min, the yield of microclones was raised along with their average size *(13)*. In addition, hydrolyzed and depurinated microdissected DNA is likely to be a poor substrate for successful and faithful PCR. For this reason, microdissection and microcloning experiments involving PCR have made use of the single-cell pipet method for the production of metaphase spreads *(14)*, where individual cells in division are fixed for a minimum period of time (10–20 s). In addition, it is important to use freshly prepared metaphase spreads for dissection, since this minimizes the effects of any residual fix that is not removed from the chromosome preparations.

3.1.2. Giemsa Banding
of Metaphase Spreads Prior to Microdissection

The use of Giemsa banding has dramatically improved the accuracy of microdissection of chromosome material for microcloning *(2,3)* and does not appear to interfere with subsequent microligation steps. The method most widely used involves the use of trypsin. It is pertinent to make a number of comments here relating to the suitability of banded chromosome preparations for microdissection. First, too extended a trypsinization can lead to rather hard chromosome material, which is difficult to dissect. At the other extreme, too short a trypsinization can lead to rather sticky chromosome material. In this case, it is difficult to make a clean cut with the dissection needle, and fragments of surrounding chromosome material may be drawn along with the material from the dissected region. There are no hard and fast rules for the preparation of adequate G-banded material for microdissection; rather, each set of chromosome preparations must be examined critically for its suitability for dissection by trial experiment.

3.2. Preparation of Microinstruments

In classical dissection and microcloning methods, all manipulations were carried out on the underside of cover slips inverted over an oil chamber. This involved the fashioning of complex microinstruments on a microforge *(11)*. However, it appears there is no impediment to dissecting banded metaphase spreads in air followed by their immediate transfer to a collection drop held in an adjacent moist chamber (*see* Section 3.3.2.). This has simplified the production of microneedles. Although micromanipulation of the collected DNA must occur in an oil chamber, again, relatively simple micropipets are required.

3.2.1. Needles (See Note 1)

1. Needles can be drawn on a simple pipet puller from lengths of 2 mm soda glass.
2. Each needle is siliconized by briefly immersing in 2% dimethyl dichlorosilane, followed by air-drying. Each needle is then briefly washed in 1 mM Na$_2$EDTA.

3.2.2. Micropipets (See Notes 2–4)

Traditionally, micropipets were forged from capillaries on a microforge that included the fashioning of a bulb for measurement of volume carried and extruded. This was a complex and time-consuming procedure. However, given that microdrops that are manipulated on a siliconized surface take on a hemispherical shape, drop volume can be readily estimated from drop size observed in the microscope and adjusted accordingly.

1. Micropipets can be drawn from Pasteur pipets on a pipet puller, the diameter of the pipet opening being in the range 10–70 μm.
2. Alternatively, micropipets can be produced by heating 1 mm capillary tubing on a microforge. Use an alcohol flame to introduce a hook to one end of the capillary. Attach a weight to the hook. Apply gentle heat from the microforge filament to the capillary. The weight begins to pull the capillary into a fine neck. Continue to apply gentle heat until the capillary breaks, leaving a flush end. The amount of weight attached to the capillary determines the width of the pipet opening and is best judged empirically.
3. Attach some tubing and a syringe to the micropipets, and draw in some 2% dimethyl dichlorosilane. Leave for a few moments before expelling and allowing to air-dry. Subsequently, draw in some 1-mM Na$_2$EDTA and expel.

3.3. Microdissection and Microcloning

3.3.1. Microdissection Equipment

An inverted microscope (for example, IM Zeiss), magnification 1250X, with the aid of a micromanipulator, is used for the microdissection and microcloning procedures. The inverted microscope should have a rotating platform. Suitable micromanipulators include the pneumatic De Fonbrunne micromanipulator or the MR MOT Zeiss electronic micromanipulator. Micropipets are connected to a 1-mL Hamilton syringe via a three-way adaptor.

3.3.2. Setting Up the Dissection Area

1. The stage of the microscope is set up in the following way: Two cover slips are placed in a glass Petri dish that has a rectangle cut out of the bottom, and this is placed on the rotating platform of the microscope (*see* Fig. 1). One cover slip holds the metaphase spreads, whereas the other holds the collection drop.
2. Using a micropipet, dispense a 1-nL collection drop to the cover slip (*see* Notes 5–7).
3. The collection drop is surrounded by a small moist chamber consisting of an Eppendorf screw-cap lid with wet tissue inside. The size of the drop can be increased by increasing the humidity inside the chamber, which is achieved by turning up the intensity of the microscope light beam. If this is done after every dissection, the drop will never evaporate.

3.3.3. Chromosome Dissection

1. A microneedle is inserted into the clamp attached to the micromanipulator and positioned next to the chromosome band of interest. The chromosome should be lying in a position such that its telomeres are pointing north/south.
2. The microneedle is moved through the chromosome in an east/west direction until the chromosomal material becomes attached to the tip (*see* Fig. 2 for illustration of a dissected chromosome).
3. The chromatin is then deposited into the collection drop on the other cover slip. This process is repeated with 10–20 chromosomes.
4. When all the dissections have been completed, the collection drop is taken up into a micropipet and transferred to a small, siliconized watch dish (1.5 cm diameter) that lies within a Petri dish filled with oil equilibrated with *Rsa*I reaction buffer, and the drop covered. All subsequent micromanipulations are performed under oil.

3.3.4. Proteinase K and SDS Treatment

An equal vol (1 nL) of collection solution is added, and the drop incubated for 90 min at 37°C in a large humidity chamber to prevent evaporation. The chamber consists of three Petri dishes of increasing size inside one another with tissue and water on the base of each.

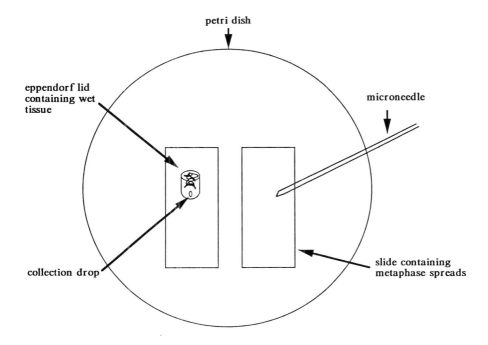

Fig. 1. Layout of stage for microdissection on an inverted microscope.

3.3.5. Phenol Extractions (See Note 8)

Four phenol extractions are performed in the following way.

1. An equal vol (2 nL) of phenol equilibrated in *Rsa*I buffer is added to the collection drop. The phenol surrounds the collection drop and is left for 5 min before being removed by micropipeting.
2. The residual phenol is removed by diffusion by changing the oil in the Petri dish and incubating overnight at 4°C in a humidity chamber. The oil is changed again, this time incubating for 1 $^{1}/_{2}$ h.

3.3.6. Digestion with Rsa*I*

1. The dissected DNA is digested with *Rsa*I by fusion with a drop of equal vol (2 nL) of *Rsa*I in a 2X reaction buffer and incubation in a humidity chamber for 2 $^{1}/_{2}$ h at 37°C.
2. This is repeated with a second aliquot (4 nL) of *Rsa*I in 1X reaction buffer.
3. The digested DNA is phenol extracted four times as previously described, to inactivate the enzyme.

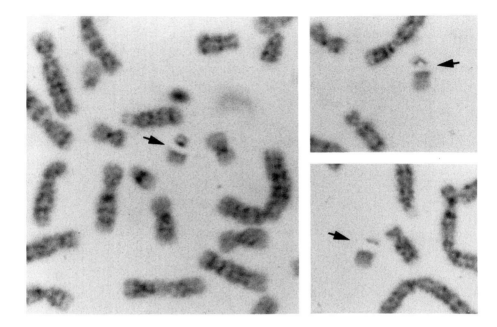

Fig. 2. Microdissection of Giemsa-stained human chromosomes. The dissection of human chromosome 22 band q11 is shown.

3.3.7. DNA Ligation

1. The drop containing the DNA is now 8 nL in vol.
2. To this is added 8 nL (8.5 ng) of *Sma*I-cut pUC vector. (The pUC vector used has been modified to incorporate a single *Sma*I site [*see* Fig. 3] flanked by two *Eco*RI sites, and its construction is described in ref. 2). The drop is left for 5 min.
3. Polyethylene glycol (40%) (relative molecular mass 8000) is added twice (16 and 32 nL) to give a final concentration of 15% in the ligation mixture (*see* Note 9).

Fig. 3. *(opposite page)* A modified pUC vector used for microligation of microdissected *Rsa*I fragments as constructed by Lüdecke et al. *(2).* A synthetic *Eco*RI–*Sma*I linker was cloned into *Eco*RI-cut M13mp7 to yield a simple *Eco*RI–*Sma*I–*Eco*RI polylinker. The encompassing 320-bp *Pvu*II fragment from this M13 derivative was used to replace the corresponding fragment from pUC19. The *Sma*I-cut pUC vector is used for blunt-ended microligation of *Rsa*I fragments from microdissected DNA. In the process, the *Sma*I site is destroyed. The pUC sequencing and reverse-sequencing primer sites are used for PCR amplification of ligated inserts, which are subsequently released from the adjacent priming sites by *Eco*RI digestion. PCR products can then be cloned in standard *Eco*RI-cut pUC vectors.

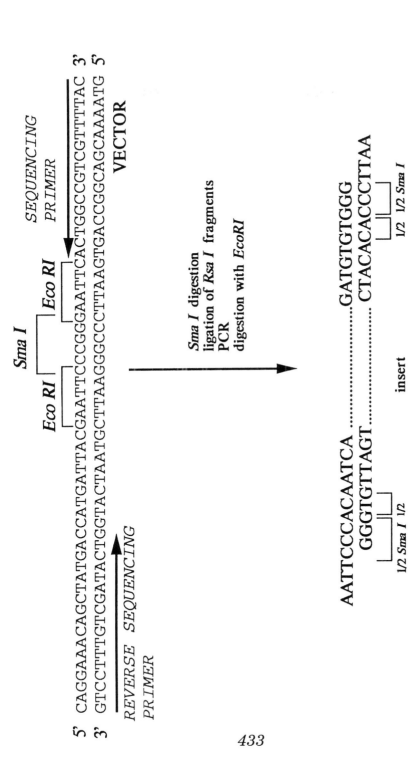

4. An equal vol (64 nL) T4 DNA ligase in ligation buffer (at 6 U/µL) is added, and the mixture incubated overnight at 12°C in a humidity chamber.
5. The microdrop is then taken up in 2 µL water and transferred to an Eppendorf tube for the amplification steps. The DNA ligase is inactivated by heating for 5 min at 65°C.

3.3.8. PCR and Construction of Clone Bank

We do not describe in detail here subsequent steps for the PCR and cloning of the ligated microdissected DNA. We summarize the basic steps, which are all standard molecular biological methods.

1. The high vector:insert ratio used in the ligation of the dissected DNA fragments encourages the formation of nonrecombinant polylinker sequences, which PCR amplifies better than the sequences containing inserts. The nonrecombinant sequences are therefore removed prior to PCR amplification by *Sma*I digestion, which does not cut the recombinant molecules because they have lost the recognition site after the *Rsa*I ligation (*see* Fig. 3).
2. A PCR is performed on this sample using standard methods, the M13/pUC sequencing, and reverse-sequencing primers (*see* Fig. 3).
3. The amplified DNA inserts are released by *Eco*RI digestion, and the primers removed. The mixture is spun through two successive Sepharcyl S-200 columns, equilibrated with ligation buffer, at 500*g* for 2 min to separate the inserts from the primers and unincorporated nucleotides, and the eluate collected.
4. Seventeen microliters of a total of 150 µL column eluate are used in a standard ligation reaction with *Eco*RI-cut pUC 13 DNA. An aliquot of the ligation mixture is used to transform commercial competent cells (DH5α) using standard methods.

4. Notes

1. Each needle fashioned must be tested empirically for its size and suitability for dissection of the appropriate chromosome area.
2. Each pipet should be used for only one solution.
3. Too fine a pipet opening and liquid is difficult to draw up or expel; too coarse a pipet opening and the flow of liquid can be difficult to control. It is best to test each pipet before use.
4. If it is required to introduce a bend into a microneedle or micropipet to aid ease of manipulation, this can be achieved by gentle heating on a microforge.
5. When handling *small* volumes in the micropipet, it is helpful to introduce some paraffin oil into the micropipet before and after taking up a microdrop to prevent evaporation.

6. A 1-nL drop is estimated by size diameter when viewed in the microscope.
7. Each subsequent addition to the collection drop involves the supplementation of the drop with an equal volume; a drop of similar size is dispensed along side the current working drop, and the two drops merged by pushing together with the micropipet.
8. All subsequent phenol extractions are carried out in this way.
9. The use of polyethylene glycol encourages the formation of long concatemers of insert and vector.

References

1. Bates, G. P., Wainwright, B. J., Williamson, R., and Brown, S. D. M. (1986) Microdissection and microcloning from the short arm of human chromosome 2. *Mol. Cell Biol.* **6,** 3826–3830.
2. Lüdecke, H.-J., Senger, G., Claussen, U., and Horsthemke, B. (1989) Cloning defined regions of the human genome by microdissection of banded chromosomes and enzymatic amplification. *Nature* **338,** 348–350.
3. Lüdecke, H.-J., Senger, G., Claussen, U., and Horsthemke, B. (1990) Construction and characterisation of band-specific DNA libraries. *Hum. Genet.* **84,** 512–516.
4. Buiting, K., Neumann, M., Lüdecke, H.-J., Senger, G., Claussen, U., Antich, J., Passarge, E., and Horsthemke, B. (1990) Microdissection of the Prader-Willi syndrome chromosome region and identification of potential gene sequences. *Genomics* **6,** 521–527.
5. Fielder, W., Clausse, U., Lüdecke, H.-J., Senger, G., Horsthemke, B., Van Kessel, A. G., Goertzen, W., and Fahsold, R. (1991) New markers for the Neurofibromatosis-2 region generated by microdissection of chromosome 22. *Genomics* **10,** 786–791.
6. Rohme, D., Fox, H., Herrmann, B., Frischauf, A.-M., Edstrom, J.-E., Mains, P., Silver, L. M., and Lehrach, H. (1984) Molecular clones of the mouse t complex derived from microdissected metaphase chromosomes. *Cell* **36,** 783–788.
7. Fisher, E. M. C., Cavanna, J. S., and Brown, S. D. M. (1985) Microdissection and microcloning of the mouse X chromosome. *Proc. Natl. Acad. Sci. USA* **82,** 5846–5849.
8. Greenfield, A. J. and Brown, S. D. M. (1987) Microdissection and microcloning from the proximal region of mouse chromosome 7: isolation of clones genetically linked to the Pudgy locus. *Genomics* **1,** 153–158.
9. Scalenghe, F., Turco, E., Edstrom, J.-E., Pirotta, V., and Melli, M. L. (1981) Microdissection and cloning of DNA from a specific region of *Drosophila melanogaster* polytene chromosomes. *Chromosoma* **82,** 205–216.
10. Sandery, M., Forster, J. W., Macadam, S. R., Blunden, R., Neil Jones, R., and Brown, S. D. M. (1991) Isolation of sequences common to A- and B-chromosomes of Rye (*Secale cereale*) by microcloning. *Plant Mol. Biol. Reporter* **9,** 21–30.

11. Edstrom, J.-E., Kaiser, R., and Rohme, D. (1987) Microcloning of mammalian metaphase chromosomes, in *Methods in Enzymology* vol. 151 (Gottesman, M. M., ed.) Academic, London, UK, pp. 503–516.
12. Brown, S. D. M. and Greenfield, A. J. (1987) A model to describe the size distribution of mammalian genomic fragments recovered by microcloning. *Gene* **55,** 327–332.
13. Weith, A., Winking, H., Brachmann, B., Boldyreff, B., and Traut, W. (1987) Microclones from a mouse germ line HSR detect amplification and complex rearrangements of DNA sequences. *EMBO J.* **6,** 1295–1300.
14. Claussen, U., Klein, R., and Schmidt, M. (1986) A pipette method for rapid karyotyping in prenatal diagnosis. *Prenatal Diagn.* **6,** 401–408.

CHAPTER 24

Molecular Analysis of Chromosome Aberrations in Hematological Malignancies

Southern Hybridization

David L. Saltman, Stephen P. Hunger, and Gillian E. Turner

1. Introduction

Since the first reports of the Philadephia chromosome in chronic myelogenous leukemia (CML), nonrandomly occurring chromosome abnormalities have been described in a number of leukemias and lymphomas *(1,2)*. The identification of the DNA sequences that span the translocation breakpoints in several hematological malignancies, and the cloning and sequencing of the immunoglobulin and T-cell receptor genes, have created the ability to reliably diagnose and monitor these diseases with molecular-based techniques that complement the analysis of banded metaphase chromosomes *(3)*.

One of the pivotal steps in many of the molecular approaches that are used to analyze chromosome aberrations is Southern hybridization *(4)*. This technique involves the transfer and immobilization of DNA fragments separated by agarose gel electrophoresis to a membrane that can be hybridized with a labeled probe complementary to the DNA. This chapter will outline methods to detect DNA rearrangements in hematological malignancies using high-mol-wt genomic DNA cleaved with restriction endonucleases. All of these procedures

From: *Methods in Molecular Biology, Vol. 29: Chromosome Analysis Protocols*
Edited by: J. R. Gosden Copyright ©1994 Humana Press Inc., Totowa, NJ

can easily be performed in a laboratory equipped with standard molecular biology reagents and instruments. Southern hybridization can be divided into the following steps:

1. Isolation of DNA: Procedures are described for the extraction of high-mol-wt DNA from peripheral blood and bone marrow cells. The extraction of DNA from lymph nodes and other soft tissues will be discussed in the Notes.
2. Restriction enzyme digestion: High-mol-wt DNA can be cleaved into fragments by restriction endonucleases. The enzymes most commonly used to analyze chromosome aberrations recognize a specific sequence of 4–6 nucleotides and produce a double-stranded cleavage within this sequence.
3. Gel electrophoresis: DNA fragments resulting from endonuclease digestion can be size-fractionated by agarose gel electrophoresis. The concentration of the agarose, the length of time the gel is run, and the voltage gradient will all determine the resolution of the DNA fragments.
4. DNA transfer: DNA fragments that have been separated in an agarose gel are transferred to a nitrocellulose or nylon membrane. Double-stranded DNA will not be retained by the membrane unless it is first denatured with sodium hydroxide. The DNA is then fixed to the membrane by either baking at 80°C or ultraviolet (UV) irradiation, depending on the type of membrane. The capillary transfer method will be described. Alternative transfer techniques will be mentioned in the Notes.
5. Labeling of probes: DNA fragments that have been separated by electrophoresis, transferred, and trapped on a membrane can be identified using radiolabeled probes. The random hexanucleotide primer technique will be described. Alternative labeling techniques will be discussed in the Notes.
6. Hybridization and autoradiography: Membranes are incubated with a solution that prevents the nonspecific binding of single-stranded DNA, but does not interfere with the specific annealing of labeled complementary sequences. Membranes are then hybridized with the labeled probe, washed in a low-salt solution, dried, and exposed to X-ray film.

2. Materials
2.1. Isolation of High-Molecular-Weight DNA
1. Ficoll-Hypaque (Pharmacia, Piscataway, NJ).
2. Phosphate-buffered saline (PBS): 137 mM NaCl, 2 mM KCl, 1.5 mM KH_2PO_4, 8 mM Na_2HPO_4.
3. Ribonuclease A (10 mg/mL) boiled 10 min to inactivate DNase (store at −20°C).

4. Proteinase K: 10 mg/mL (store at –20°C).
5. 20% Sodium dodecyl sulfate (SDS).
6. Extraction buffer: 10 mM Tris-HCl, pH 7.5, 150 mM NaCl, 10 mM EDTA.
7. 3M Sodium acetate, pH 5.2.
8. Phenol saturated with 0.5M Tris-HCl.
9. Chloroform:isoamyl alcohol (24:1).
10. Tris-EDTA (TE): 10 mM Tris-HCl, pH 7.5, 1 mM EDTA.
11. Ethanol.

2.2. Restriction Enzyme Digestion

1. Restriction endonucleases (store at –20°C).
2. 10X restriction buffer: Most enzyme suppliers will also provide you with the appropriate 10X buffer.
3. 3M Sodium acetate.
4. Ethanol.

2.3. Agarose Gel Electrophoresis

1. Electrophoresis grade agarose.
2. Ethidium bromide: 10 mg/mL.
3. 1X TBE Electrophoresis buffer: 90 mM Tris-borate, 90 mM boric acid, 2 mM EDTA.
4. 10X loading buffer: 1% bromophenol blue, 1% xylene cyanol FF, 15% Ficoll, 100 mM EDTA.
5. DNA size markers.
6. 254 nm UV transilluminator.

2.4. DNA Transfer

1. Denaturing transfer solution: 0.5M NaOH, 1.5M NaCl.
2. Neutralizing solution: 0.5M Tris-HCl, pH 7.5, 1.5M NaCl.
3. 20X SSC: 3M NaCl, 0.3M Na citrate.
4. Nylon membrane (Hybond N, Amersham, Arlington Heights, IL).
5. Quick Draw blotting paper (Sigma, St. Louis, MO).
6. UV crosslinker (Stratalinker 1800, Stratagene).

2.5. Labeling of DNA Probes by Random Priming

1. ^{32}P-dCTP.
2. DNA Polymerase I: large fragment, Klenow enzyme (store at –20°C).
3. 10X dNTP solution: 0.5 mM dATP, 0.5 mM dGTP, and 0.5 mM dTTP (store at –20°C).
4. 10X hexanucleotide mixture (Boehringer Mannheim [Indianapolis, IN] cat. no. 1277 081) (store at –20°C).

5. Sephadex G-50 spin column.
6. Spin column buffer (TSE): 10 mM Tris-HCl, pH 8, 0.15% SDS, 1 mM EDTA, pH 8.

2.6. Hybridization and Autoradiography

1. 65°C Shaking water bath.
2. Seal-A-Meal bags.
3. 20X SSC: 3M NaCl, 0.3M Na citrate.
4. 100X Denhardt's: 2% Ficoll 400 (Sigma), 2% polyvinyl pyrrolidone (Sigma), 2% BSA (store at –20°C).
5. Hybridization solution: 6X SSC, 5X Denhardt's, 0.5% SDS, 5% dextran sulfate, 100 µg/mL denatured salmon sperm DNA.
6. Saran Wrap™.
7. Darkroom with safelight.
8. Kodak X-Omat AR X-ray film.
9. Exposure cassettes with intensifying screens.

3. Methods

3.1. Isolation of High-Molecular-Weight DNA (See Note 1)

1. Peripheral blood and bone marrow samples used for DNA extraction are collected in sterile tubes containing citrate, EDTA, or heparin anti-coagulant. Excessive amounts of heparin may interfere with restriction endonuclease activity.
2. To separate buffy coat cells; dilute blood 1:1 with PBS and spin in a table-top centrifuge at 1800 rpm for 20 min in a 15-mL conical tube. Remove the buffy coat from the top of the red cell pellet. Resuspend in PBS, and spin at 1500 rpm for 6 min in a table-top centrifuge. Aspirate and discard the supernatant. It is not necessary to remove residual red cells.
3. To separate mononuclear cells; add 5 mL of Ficoll-Hypaque to a 15-mL conical tube. Dilute blood and bone marrow 1:1 with PBS, and layer onto the gradient. Spin at 1800 rpm for 20 min in a table-top centrifuge. Mononuclear cells will form a visible interface between the plasma and the Ficoll-Hypaque. Remove the interface cells, resuspend in PBS, and spin at 1500 rpm for 6 min in a table-top centrifuge. Aspirate and discard the supernatant. Cells can now be stored at –70°C or used immediately for DNA isolation.
4. Resuspend cells in 10 mL of DNA extraction buffer, and add 250 µL of 20% SDS (final concentration = 0.5%) in a 50-mL polypropylene tube and mix gently by inverting.

5. Add 50 μL of 10 mg/mL Ribonuclease A (final concentration = 50 μg/mL), and incubate at 37°C for 30 min.
6. Add 100 μL of 10 mg/mL proteinase K (final concentration = 100 μg/mL), mix gently by swirling, and incubate at 50°C for 3 h.
7. Extract the DNA by adding an equal vol of phenol and inverting the tube for 10 min. Wear gloves when handling phenol to avoid skin burns.
8. Spin at 2400*g* for 10 min at room temperature.
9. Remove the upper, aqueous phase with a wide-bore pipet, and repeat steps 6 and 7.
10. Add an equal vol of chloroform:isoamyl alcohol, and mix by inverting the tube.
11. Centrifuge at 2400*g* for 10 min and remove the aqueous phase.
12. Repeat the chloroform extraction.
13. Precipitate the DNA by adding 0.1 vol of 3*M* Na acetate and 2.5 vol of cold 100% ethanol.
14. The DNA can then be spooled onto a glass rod and washed by dipping into 70% ethanol.
15. Air-dry for 5 min, and then resuspend in 0.5 mL of TE in a 1.5-mL microfuge tube.
16. Dissolve the DNA by placing the tube on a rotating platform for 24 h.
17. Determine the concentration of the DNA with a UV spectrophotometer. An absorbance (A) reading of 1.0 at 260 nm corresponds to a DNA concentration of 50 μg/mL. A pure DNA sample should give an A_{260}/A_{280} ratio of 1.6–2.0.

3.2. Restriction Enzyme Digestion (See Note 2)

1. To a 1.5-mL microfuge tube, add 10 μg of DNA, 10 μL of the appropriate 10X restriction buffer, and sterile distilled water to make up the final reaction vol to 100 μL. Mix gently.
2. Add 30 U of restriction endonuclease, and incubate at the appropriate temperature for 2–4 h. Most enzymes exhibit the maximum activity at 37°C.
3. At this point, an aliquot of the reaction mixture can be run on a gel containing ethidium bromide (0.5 μg/mL) to determine if the DNA digestion has been complete. Ethidium bromide is carcinogenic, so gloves should be worn.
4. Precipitate the DNA with 10 μL of 3*M* sodium acetate and 250 μL of cold ethanol. Mix well, and put at –70°C for 15 min.
5. Spin for 10 min in a microcentrofuge, and remove the ethanol.
6. Allow the DNA to air-dry for 15 min.
7. Dissolve the DNA in 45 μL of TE buffer. The sample can be stored at –20°C or used immediately for gel electrophoresis.

3.3. Agarose Gel Electrophoresis (See Note 3)

1. To separate DNA fragments in the range of 0.5–20 kilobases (kb), use a 0.8% horizontal agarose gel.
2. Tape the ends of the gel plate with adhesive tape. A comb is fixed in place at one end of the plate.
3. For a 20 × 12 cm gel, add 250 mL of 1X TBE buffer to 2 g of agarose and melt in a microwave oven. Add ethidium bromide to a final concentration of 0.5 μg/mL, swirl to mix evenly, and let cool to 60°C before pouring. Ethidium bromide is carcinogenic, so gloves should be worn.
4. The gel is allowed to harden for 45 min, the tape and the comb are removed, and the gel is submerged in an electrophoresis tank filled with 1X TBE.
5. Add 5 μL of 10X loading buffer to the 45 μL of digested DNA, mix, and then load each sample into the wells. DNA mol-wt marker (*Hind*III cut λ phage) should be loaded onto the same gel.
6. The gel is run at a voltage gradient of 1.5 V/cm for 16 h at room temperature. The DNA can be visualized and photographed using a UV transilluminator (254 nm) (Fig. 1). A protective visor or goggles should always be worn when working with UV light in this range.

3.4. DNA Transfer (See Note 4)

1. After electrophoresis, the gel is submerged in denaturing solution and placed on a gently rotating platform for 1 h.
2. Pour off the denaturing solution, replace with neutralizing solution, and rotate for 30 min.
3. Repeat step 2.
4. To transfer the DNA from the gel to a membrane, place a 21 × 21 cm sponge in a tray, and add 20X SSC until the sponge is saturated and immersed in SSC 0.5 cm below the top.
5. Place a 20 × 20 cm piece of blotting paper on the sponge. Wet the paper with 20X SSC, and smooth out any air bubbles.
6. Trim away any unused areas of the gel with a scalpel blade. Flip the gel over onto the blotting paper, and smooth out any air bubbles between the paper and the gel.
7. Cut a piece of nylon membrane to fit the gel, and lay it on top. It is not necessary to wet Hybond N nylon membranes before placing on the gel. Wear gloves when handling membrane to avoid contact with finger oils.
8. Smooth out any air bubbles between the membrane and the gel. Cover the blotting paper next to the gel with Saran Wrap™ to prevent wicking of the membrane directly from the sponge.

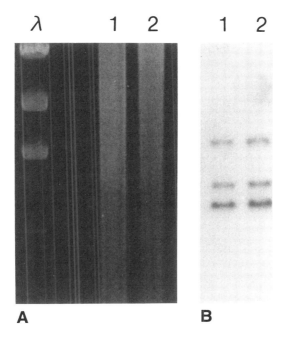

Fig. 1. **A.** Ethidium bromide stained gel of *Hind*III cut λ phage markers (lane 1) and genomic DNA (lanes 2 and 3) prior to transfer to a nylon membrane. **B.** Autoradiograph of the membrane hybridized to a ^{32}P-labeled probe and exposed for 24 h.

9. Layer 10 cm of blotting paper onto the membrane. Place a 500-g weight on top of the blotting paper.
10. Transfer the DNA overnight. After the transfer, remove the blotting paper, and mark the positions of the wells with a ballpoint pen.
11. Remove the membrane from the gel, and rinse in 2X SSC for 2 min.
12. Dry the membrane between two pieces of blotting paper.
13. Place the membrane DNA side up in the UV crosslinker, and expose to 0.15 J/cm^2, or bake at 80°C in a vacuum oven for 1–2 h.

3.5. Labeling of DNA Probes by Random Priming (See Note 5)

1. In a sterile microfuge tube place 25–100 ng of linear DNA.
2. Add distilled water to 18.5 μL.
3. Boil for 5–10 min, put on ice for 5 min, and pulse in a microfuge. The remaining steps are performed in an area approved for handling ^{32}P.

4. Add to the tube: 3 µL of 10X dNTP solution and 3 µL of 10X hexanucleotide mixture.
5. Add 5 µL of ^{32}P-dCTP(10 µCi/µL).
6. Add 0.5 µL of Klenow enzyme.
7. Mix gently, pulse in the microfuge, and incubate at 37°C for 30 min.
8. To remove unincorporated nucleotides, add 170 µL of TSE buffer, load onto a Sephadex G-50 spin column that has been equilibrated with TSE, spin at 1600*g* for 4 min, and collect the effluent. The incorporation of ^{32}P-dCTP into the probe can be assessed by comparing the radioactivity of the effluent to the column with a minimonitor. Discard the column in a designated radioactive waste container.

3.6. Hybridization (See Note 6)

1. Wet the nylon membrane with 2X SSC, and put it into a Seal-A-Meal bag.
2. Boil the sonicated salmon sperm DNA (100 µg/mL of hybridization solution) for 10 min, and cool on ice for 5 min.
3. Add 0.2 mL of hybridization solution for each cm^2 of membrane to the bag, squeeze out the air bubbles, heat seal the bag, and incubate 65°C for 4 h in a shaking water bath.
4. Denature the labeled probe by boiling for 10 min. Cool on ice for 5 min.
5. Cut one corner of the bag containing the membrane, and add the probe. Heat seal the bag. Check with a minimonitor to make sure that the probe is evenly distributed in the bag.
6. Hybridize for 16 h at 65°C.
7. Following the hybridization, the membrane is removed from the bag and washed in 2X SSC, 0.1% SDS at room temperature for 10 min; 2X SSC, 0.1% SDS at 65°C for 15 min; and 0.2X SSC, 0.1% SDS at 65°C for 15 min × 2. If a higher stringency is required, an additional wash in 0.1X SSC, 0.1% SDS at 65°C for 15 min may be done. Wash solutions can be heated in a microwave oven just prior to washing.
8. After the final wash, the membrane is wrapped in Saran Wrap™ while damp, being careful to avoid trapping air bubbles.
9. For the detection of single-copy sequences, expose the membrane at −70°C for 24–72 h using a cassette with an intensifying screen and Kodak X-Omat AR film.
10. The probe can be stripped from the membrane by immersing in 0.05X SSC, 0.5% SDS at 100°C on a rotating platform. Let the wash cool to room temperature, and repeat one time. The membrane can now be rehybridized starting at step 1 (Fig. 2).
11. Membranes that are not reused immediately are air-dried, wrapped in Saran Wrap™, and stored at room temperature in the dark.

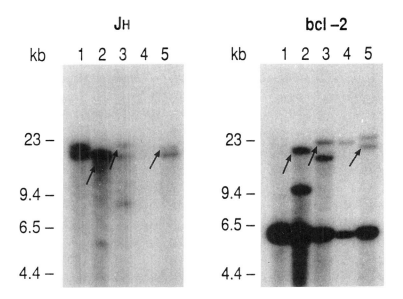

Fig. 2. Autoradiographs of a membrane hybridized sequentially with two different probes. Lane 1 is control placental DNA, and lanes 2–5 contain DNA from four cases of follicular lymphoma digested with *Eco*RI. The bcl-2 probe was a 2.8-kb *Eco*RI–*Hind*III genomic fragment from the major breakpoint region of chromosome 18. The J$_H$ probe was a 2.5-kb *Eco*RI–*Bgl*III genomic fragment from the immunoglobulin heavy chain joining region of chromosome 14. The arrows indicate comigrating fragments that confirm juxtaposition of chromosome 14q32 and chromosome 18q21 DNA sequences. The t(l4:18)(q32:q21) can be detected by Southern hybridization in over 80% of follicular lymphomas and in 30% of diffuse large-cell lymphomas.

4. Notes

1. This procedure can be modified to allow the extraction of high-mol-wt DNA from lymph nodes and other soft tissues *(5)*. Samples are cut into smaller pieces with a scalpel blade and immersed in liquid nitrogen. The sample is placed in a Waring blender, and the tissue is blended into a powder. Allow the liquid nitrogen to evaporate, suspend the powder in extraction buffer, and start the DNA isolation procedure at step 3.
2. One of the most important factors that determines effective enzyme cleavage is the purity of the DNA. High concentrations of NaCl, residual protein, phenol, chloroform, or SDS will inhibit the enzyme reaction. The volume of restriction enzyme should never be >10% of the total

volume of the reaction, because the activity of the enzyme may be inhibited by the glycerol in which the endonucleases are stored. Spermidine is recommended in some digestion protocols, but will result in the precipitation of DNA if used with low-salt buffers. The choice of restriction enzymes will be dependent on the organization of the genomic sequence of interest. The prior knowledge of germline restriction fragments and possible polymorphisms is essential for the correct interpretation of Southern hybridization results. Nongermline fragments that are detected with only one enzyme suggest there is a restriction-site polymorphism.

3. The loading of >1.3 μg/cm^2 of high-mol-wt DNA may result in the distortion of bands *(6)*. It should be possible to detect single-copy sequences using 5–15 μg of DNA. Alternative gel buffers, such as Tris acetate, can be substituted for Tris borate. All buffers should be recirculated if gels are run at a high voltage, but this is probably not necessary at lower voltage gradients for gels that are run for 16 h.

4. The rate of transfer of DNA out of the gel will depend on the percentage of agarose, the thickness of the gel, and the size of the DNA fragments. The movement of DNA fragments >10 kb may be enhanced by partial depurination in dilute acid *(7)*. The time of transfer can be reduced to under an hour by using a vacuum transfer apparatus *(8)*. The vacuum draws buffer from above the gel and elutes the DNA onto an underlying membrane. Either nitrocellulose or nylon membranes can be used for immobilization of DNA. Nylon membranes have the advantage of being more durable, and can be stripped of probe and reused more easily than nitrocellulose. The transfer of DNA to nylon membranes can be carried out under alkaline conditions *(9)*. After electrophoresis, gels are denatured and transferred in an alkaline solution (0.5N NaOH, 1M NaCl).

5. Random hexanucleotide priming is the method of choice in most laboratories for labeling probes to a high specific activity *(10)*. There are now several commercial kits available that utilize bacterophage T7 polymerase. Using this method, probes can be labeled to a high specific activity in 5–10 min at 37°C. Biotin- and digoxigenin-labeled probes can also be used to detect single-copy DNA sequences by Southern hybridization *(11)*. After hybridization to complementary nucleic acids, the labeled probes are detected by enzyme-linked immunoassay using either streptavidin or antidigoxigenin conjugated to alkaline phosphatase. Most DNA probes used in the detection of chromosome aberrations by Southern hybridization will be complementary to single-copy sequences. Genomic and cDNA clones that are used as probes may contain repeti-

tive elements. Hybridization of these probes to genomic DNA results in a smear or multiple bands that may obscure fragments of interest. The hybridization of repeats can be reduced by preannealing denatured labeled probe with unlabeled sonicated human DNA at 65°C *(12)*.

6. It is important to use hybridization conditions and buffers recommended for the specific membranes. For example, Genescreen nylon membranes (Dupont, Boston, MA) require hybridization buffers with a high concentration of SDS to reduce the level of background *(13)*. The addition of formamide to the hybridization mixture will reduce the melting temperature of the DNA and will permit stringent hybridizations at 42°C. The kinetics of hybridization are reduced in the presence of formamide, so longer hybridization times are recommended *(14)*. The addition of dextran sulfate can substantially increase the rate of hybridization. The background will tend to be higher on membranes when using dextran sulfate, but can be reduced by limiting the amount of labeled probe and performing stringent posthybridization washes. The volume of hybridization solution and posthybridization washes can be reduced by using roller bottles (Robbins Scientific, Sunnyvale, CA). Membranes are hybridized to labeled probes and washed in the same rotating glass tubes. Radioisotope contamination of the work area tends to be minimized with this system compared to hybridizations performed in polythene bags.

The most common problem associated with Southern hybridization is the failure to detect the DNA fragment of interest. A probe with a low specific activity may not detect a single-copy sequence in 10 μg of genomic DNA. The contamination of labeled probe with RNA and bacterial genomic DNA will also result in a weak hybridization signal. This problem can be obviated by checking the purity of your probe on a minigel prior to labeling. The hybrization of an excess amount of labeled probe will result in a high background. It is recommended that 10–20 ng of labeled probe (SA = 10^9 cpm/μg) be used/mL of hybridization solution to detect single-copy sequences in genomic DNA *(15)*. The posthybridization washes will also influence the signal intensity and the background. The stringency and the frequency of the washes will depend on the amount of contiguous homology between the labeled probe with the target sequence. Membranes can be checked with a minimonitor in between washes to assess the level of background.

Acknowledgments

We would like to thank Mike Lovett for his comments and Rick Cuevas for his help preparing the manuscript.

References

1. Nowell, P. C. and Hungerford, D. A. (1960) A minute chromosome in human granulocytic leukemia. *Science* **132,** 1497.
2. Heim, S. and Mitelman, F. (1987) *Cancer Cytogenetics.* Liss, New York.
3. Davey, M. P., Bongiovanni, K. F., Kaulfersh, W., Quertemous, T., Seidman, J. H., Hersfield, M. S., Kurtzberg, J., Haynes, B., Davis, M. M., and Waldmann, T. A. (1986) Immunoglobulin and T-cell receptor gene rearrangement and expression in human lymphoid leukemia cells at different stages of maturation. *Proc. Natl. Acad. Sci. USA* **83,** 8759–8763.
4. Southern, E. M. (1975) Detection of specific sequences among DNA fragments separated by gel electrophoresis. *J. Mol. Biol.* **98,** 503–517.
5. Blin, N. and Stafford, D. W. (1976) Isolation of high molecular weight DNA. *Nucleic Acids Res.* **3,** 2303–2308.
6. Johnson, P. H., Miller, M. J., and Grossman, L. I. (1980) Electrophoresis of DNA in agarose gels. II. Effects of loading mass electroendosmosis on electrophoretic mobilities. *Anal. Biochem.* **102,** 159–162.
7. Wahl, G. M., Stern, M., and Stark, G. R. (1979) Efficient transfer of large DNA fragments from agarose gels to DBM paper and rapid hybridization using dextran sulfate. *Proc. Natl. Acad. Sci. USA* **76,** 3683–3687.
8. Medveczky, P., Chang, P. C., Oste, C., and Mulder, C. (1987) Rapid vacuum driven transfer of DNA and RNA from gels to solid supports. *BioTechniques* **5,** 242–246.
9. Church, G. and Gilbert, W. (1984) Genomic sequencing. *Proc. Natl. Acad. Sci. USA* **81,** 1991–1995.
10. Feinberg, A. P. and Vogelstein, B. (1983) A technique for radiolabeling DNA restriction endonuclease fragments to a high specific activity. *Anal. Biochem.* **136,** 6–13.
11. Leary, J. J., Brigati, D. J., and Ward, D. C. (1983) Rapid and sensitive colormetric method for visualizing biotin-labeled DNA probes hybridized to DNA or RNA immobilized on nitrocellulose: Bio-blots. *Proc. Natl. Acad. Sci. USA* **80,** 4045–4049.
12. Sealy, P. G., Whittaker, P. A., and Southern, E. M. (1985) Removal of repeated sequences from hybridization probes. *Nucleic Acids Res.* **13,** 1905–1922.
13. Church, G. and Gilbert, W. (1984) Genomic sequencing. *Proc. Natl. Acad. Sci. USA* **81,** 1991–1995.
14. Casey, J. and Davidson, N. (1977) Rates of formation and thermal stabilities of RNA:DNA and DNA:DNA duplexes at high concentrations of formamide. *Nucleic Acids Res.* **4,** 1539–1552.
15. Sambrook, J., Fritsch, E. F., and Maniatis, T. (1989) *Molecular Cloning: A Laboratory Manual.* Cold Spring Harbor Laboratory, Cold Spring Harbor, NY.

CHAPTER 25

Molecular Analysis of Chromosome Aberrations

In Situ *Hybridization*

Peter Lichter and Thomas Ried

1. Introduction

In situ hybridization provides a means of analyzing chromosomal aberrations in a very direct way. Nucleic acid probes are hybridized to chromosomal preparations, and the site of specific hybridization is detectable by various procedures. Although in the 1970s and 1980s isotopic detection was the preferred technique, new developments in the protocols of nonisotopic *in situ* hybridization resulted in an increasing popularity of this procedure since the late 1980s. This development is owing to the distinct advantages of nonradioactive *in situ* hybridization techniques, such as increased speed of the procedure, higher signal resolution, and most of all the potential to combine several nonisotopic techniques to delineate a number of chromosomal target regions simultaneously. These developments have been discussed in more detail elsewhere (*see,* e.g., refs. *1–3*).

The visualization of many target sites by combining different detection procedures can currently be best performed by using fluorescent dyes, which can be differentiated by their different spectral ranges of emitted light. The protocol described below will focus only on fluorescence *in situ* hybridization, which is also referred to as "FISH" technique in the literature. Other nonisotopic *in situ* hybridization procedures

From: *Methods in Molecular Biology, Vol. 29: Chromosome Analysis Protocols*
Edited by: J. R. Gosden Copyright ©1994 Humana Press Inc., Totowa, NJ

require different posthybridization treatments. For introduction to protocols of these techniques, we refer to the literature *(2,4,5)*.

When nucleic acid probes are to be hybridized to metaphase chromosomes, banding of these chromosomes might be required for analyzing a particular karyotype or for assessing the chromosomal regions to which the nucleic acid probes hybridize. High-quality banding of chromosomes prior to the hybridization can be carried out with various banding techniques using Giemsa dyes (*see,* e.g., refs. *6,7*). However, these prebanding procedures require documentation of banded metaphase chromosomes, destaining and possibly postfixation, and—following *in situ* hybridization—the relocation of the documented chromosomes. With posthybridization banding procedures, excellent banding patterns can be achieved, too. For many applications, simultaneous detection of hybridized probe and chromosomal banding patterns are preferred. Chromomycin/Hoechst 33258, DAPI, or quinacrine banding are easily performed and have proven to be very useful (for discussion, *see,* e.g., refs. *2,8*). These procedures, however, may suffer from variabilities of the procedure of chromosome denaturation prior to the *in situ* hybridization. Simultaneous banding of high quality can be performed by replication banding with propidium iodide following BrdU incorporation (for protocols *see* e.g., refs. *9–11*). However, when clinical material has to be analyzed, it might be difficult to obtain preparations after BrdU incorporation. Alternatively, distinct chromosomal banding can be achieved by hybridization of nucleic acid probes containing interspersed repetitive sequences (IRS). Cohybridization of *Alu* sequences to human chromosomes or of L1 sequences to mouse chromosomes results in simultaneous R-banding-like or G-banding-like patterns, respectively (*see* refs. *2,12,13*).

For the analysis of chromosomal aberrations by *in situ* hybridization, specific probes or probe sets are used. They are carefully selected on the basis of their ability to delineate chromosomal regions, which are involved in structural aberrations or which are flanking chromosomal break points (*see* Figs. 1–3). Thus, the genomic localization of these probes has been established prior to the use as a diagnostic tool. Most diagnostic approaches are based on the number of signals or on the spatial relation of signals, and do not require chromosomal banding. Therefore, we do not include banding protocols in this chapter,

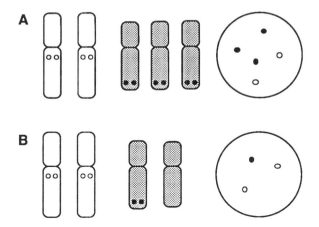

Fig. 1. Schematic illustration of the detection of a trisomy (**A**) and a deletion (**B**) in metaphase and interphase by *in situ* hybridization. In case of a monosomy, signals would be according to (B). For further explanations, *see* text.

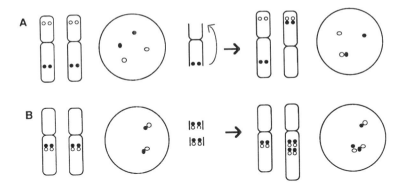

Fig. 2. Schematic illustration of the detection of an inversion (**A**) and a duplication (**B**) in metaphase and interphase by *in situ* hybridization using suitable (local) probes. For further explanations *see* text.

but refer, for chromosomal banding, to other chapters of this book and to the literature cited above.

The first probe sets used for detecting chromosomal aberrations by *in situ* hybridization were chromosome-specific repetitive DNAs, which occur in clusters mainly in centromeric or other heterochromatic regions, such as alphoid and satellite DNAs. They are hybrid-

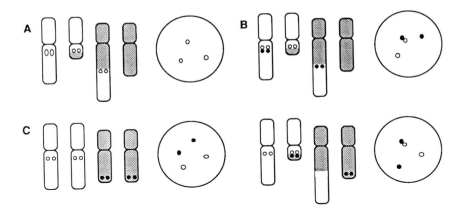

Fig. 3. Schematic illustration of the detection of translocations in metaphase and interphase by *in situ* hybridization using suitable probes. The translocation can be detected by the splitting of a signal generated from a probe covering the whole breakpoint area (**A**), by the separation of two signals from probes flanking the breakpoint area (**B**), or by the juxtaposition of two signals from chromosome areas that are joined by a specific translocation event (**C**). For further explanations, *see* text.

ized to human chromosomes according to Protocol A (*see* Section 3.5.1.). For some members of the family of alphoid DNA sequences, cross-homologies to other centromeres result in the labeling of a number of chromosomes. To achieve a chromosome-specific signal with such probes, a higher stringency of the hybridization reaction or the posthybridization washes is needed. In general, changing of the hybridization conditions is preferred. The stringency can be easily adjusted by varying the temperature, the formamide concentration, or the salt concentration in the hybridization reaction. We prefer to increase the formamide concentration (from 50 to, e.g., 60 or 70%) for higher stringencies, to obtain chromosome-specific signals with alphoid probes.

Whereas for cDNAs and genomic fragments known to be entirely single copy Protocol A can be used, most genomic DNA fragments of higher eukaryotes cannot be hybridized to chromosomes using this protocol, since they contain ubiquitously occurring interspersed repetitive sequences (IRS), such as SINE (small interspersed repetitive elements, e.g., *Alu*-elements) and LINE (large interspersed repetitive elements, e.g., L1-elements) sequences. The IRSs result in various background stainings of the chromosomes (e.g., the predominant *Alu*

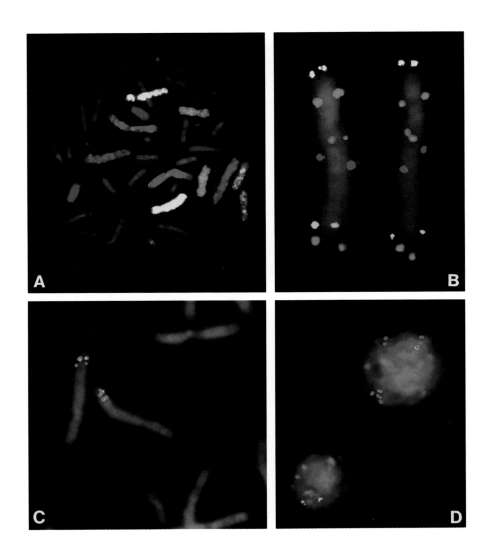

elements result in a R-banding-like pattern) that can more or less strongly correspond to the IRSs present in the probe. Protocols have been developed that suppress the signals from IRSs within probe sets by a competition reaction *(14–16)*. This protocol has also been termed "Chromosomal In Situ Suppression hybridization" or CISS hybridization *(15)* and is given in Section 3.5.2. (Protocol B). It can be used to delineate larger chromosomal regions when sets of pooled probes are used. Individual chromosomes can be visualized by using the library DNA from sorted chromosomes *(15,16)*, a procedure that has also been termed "chromosome painting" *(16)*. Very useful painting tools are the sorted chromosome DNA libraries cloned in bluescribe vectors *(17)*. Examples of multiple-chromosome painting with such libraries are shown in Fig. 4, panel A. Chromosome painting is a powerful tool to

---

Fig. 4. (previous page) **A.** Simultaneous hybridization of six chromosome-specific DNA libraries to human metaphase chromosomes. The libraries for chromosomes 1, 2, 4, 8, 14, and X were labeled with three different reporter molecules singly or in combination, and detected with three antibody or avidin conjugated fluorochromes. Images were acquired with a cooled CCD camera. The hybridization signals were pseudocolored in green (1), violet (2), white (4), yellow (8), red (14), and orange (X). **B.** Mapping of six cosmid clones to chromosome 5. The clones were labeled singly or combinatorially, and hybridized to a metaphase spread. The pseudocolors were chosen arbitrarily. The clones are dispersed over the entire length of chromosome 5, resulting in a hybridization banding pattern. **C.** Hybridization of a pool of phage clones specific for the c-*myc* gene and clones mapping to the centromeric and telomeric sites of c-*myc* in 8q24 to normal human chromosomes. The probe set for the c-*myc* gene was labeled with FITC-dUTP (green), the flanking clones were labeled with digoxigenin, and detected with antidigoxigenin TRITC (red). Some probes used in this experiment were previously published *(34)*. **D.** Hybridization of the same set of clone as in 3 to a mixture of interphase nuclei from a healthy male and a female patient with Burkitt lymphoma carrying a t(2;8) translocation. In addition to the single-copy probes, a centromeric repeat clone specific for the X chromosome is hybridized and visualized in violet. The male nucleus (one violet signal, lower nucleus) shows twice a colocalization of red and green signals, indicating the normal chromosome 8 homologs. In the aberrant female nucleus (two violet X-centromere-specific signals, upper nucleus), one colocalization of the green signal with the two flanking red signals is observed indicating the normal homolog. Two additional green signals occur, both colocalized with only one red colored flanking clones, specifically displaying the breakpoint within the c-*myc* target area. The images in panel A–D were generated in the laboratory of David C. Ward (Yale University). The images are part of publications by Ried et al. Panels A and B: ref. *40;* Panels C and D: ref. *54.*

detect chromosomal aberrations rapidly and has been applied in many areas (for review, *see* ref. *1,* including clinical and tumor cytogenetics [*see,* e.g., refs. *16,18–20*]). CISS hybridization can be applied to genomic DNA fragments from all sources, cloned in plasmid, phage, cosmid, or YAC vectors, or after chromosome dissection or chromosome sorting. If only small amounts of uncloned probe material are available, it is often useful to amplify first by a PCR strategy. When the probe sequences homologous to the chromosomes to be hybridized are a small portion of the whole DNA probe preparation (e.g., the human DNA in a human/rodent hybrid cell DNA, or a YAC in a corresponding yeast preparation), IRS-PCR or protocols derived from this approach are a useful alternative. These more advanced protocols can be found in the literature *(21–23)*.

Delineation of target sequences is not only achieved on metaphase chromosomes, but also in interphase nuclei. The first interphase analyses were performed by visualization of the X and Y bodies in cell nuclei *(24,25)*. The concept of interphase cytogenetics by *in situ* hybridization with defined probes was introduced by Cremer and coworkers *(26)*. The possibility of analyzing chromosome aberrations in interphase is of particular interest for cases where chromosomes are difficult, if at all possible to prepare, such as in many solid tumors. This approach is increasingly used not only in clinical cytogenetics, but also for the analysis of tissues in the pathology laboratory. Chromosomal aberrations are detected in nuclei by the number or the spatial relation of hybridization signals as outlined in the rest of this section.

The various hybridization probes or probe sets have different advantages that have been discussed extensively (*see,* e.g., refs. *8,27*). For the clinical diagnosis of numerical and, especially, structural chromosome aberrations, probes generating focal signals are often preferred. An ideal probe used as a diagnostic tool must be balanced between two criteria: The hybridization signal should be as strong as possible, but (in particular for interphase analysis) the signal should be as focal as possible. According to the first criterion, it seems optimal to use larger probes, such as cosmids, YACs, pools of contiguous cosmids or YACs, or even bigger probe sets (such as libraries from microdissected chromosomes). However, when target areas of more than, e.g., 100 kb in length (other than condensed heterochromatin visualized by repetitive probes) are delineated, the interphase signal might become dispersed. This may result in difficulties in assessing the number of interphase signals. The diagnostic potential of local probes is illustrated in Fig. 1–3.

When numerical aberrations are to be analyzed, any probe specifically staining the chromosome of interest is suitable (*see* Fig. 1, panel A for trisomy, panel B for monosomy). For this kind of analysis, chromosome-specific repetitive DNAs are mostly used as probes. However, in some diseases based on chromosome aneuploidies, it might also be better to use probes of specific chromosomal subregions. For example, Down syndrome can be generated not only by the trisomy of chromosome 21, but—in rare cases—also by partial trisomies of 21q22.3. Therefore, it seems much better to use probes from 21q22.3, in order to cover all chromosome 21 aberrations found in this disease. The feasibility of this approach for the diagnosis of Down syndrome has been demonstrated *(19,28)*.

One of the most challenging tasks of cytogenetics is the identification of microdeletions. Such deletions can be detected by *in situ* hybridization (*see* Fig. 1B) with a much a higher resolution than conventional cytogenetic methods *(29–31)*. The resolution is basically determined by the size of the target area delineated by the hybridization probe. However, the probe must be efficient in order to distinguish the hybridization to one allele from an insufficient hybridization. A minimum of 50%, but preferably more than 90%, of the target regions should be visible. When mixed cell populations or even residual diseases are to be analyzed, the efficiency must be higher than 90% (*see,* e.g., ref. *32*). This is of course an important criterion for any probe used to detect chromosomal aberrations in residual diseases and in cases of genetic mosaicisms.

The number of signals also changes in case of a duplication as outlined in Fig. 2B. The detection of specific duplication events using suitable probes has been demonstrated *(33)*.

The breakpoint of structural aberrations can in principle be detected in three ways:

1. A signal from a hybridized probe covering the whole breakpoint area of a specific translocation/inversion/and so forth, is split by the break resulting in three instead of two signals (Fig. 3A) (*see,* for example, ref. *31* for a translocation);

2. Signals from areas flanking a possible breakpoint lead to the detection of the breaking event by a change in the spatial relation of the signals: instead of two adjacent signals, the signals are on other chromosomes (or in other chromosomal regions in case of intrachromosomal rearrangements); accordingly, interphase signals are clearly separated (Fig. 3B) (*see,* e.g., refs. *2,34*) for translocations; and

3. Vice versa, two distant areas of the genome are becoming closely linked by a specific structural chromosome aberration, which is detected by the juxtaposition of the signals generated by appropriate probes. This is illustrated in Fig. 2A for an inversion and Fig. 3C for a translocation. Corresponding references include *35* for the detection of a specific inversion of chromosome 16 and *36,37* for the detection of the Philadelphia chromosome translocation.

The potential of detecting chromosomal aberrations by *in situ* hybridization greatly increases with the availability of multicolor detection protocols (*see below*). When the number of signals is crucial for a diagnosis, the number of aberrations that can be analyzed simultaneously corresponds to the number of available "colors" to detect distinguishable hybridization sites. When the spatial relation of signals is the indicator for an aberration, in principle, one color would be sufficient for detecting both probes involved in the analysis. However, for better resolving the juxtaposed signals, the application of two-color protocols is generally preferred (*see* Figs. 2A and 3C). Many investigators use two differentially labeled probes (e.g., biotin and digoxigenin) for a simultaneous detection via two common fluorochromes that can be distinguished by conventional fluorescence microscopy (e.g., FITC and rhodamine). A third probe labeled in both ways (e.g., biotin *and* digoxigenin) could be differentiated by a new color that was generated by the overlap of two fluorochromes (e.g., the overlay of FITC [green] and rhodamine [red] results in a yellow signal). After protocols for three-color *in situ* hybridization were established using a blue coumarine dye *(38,39),* the potential of simultaneous visualization of different chromosomal areas has considerably increased. By the various combinations of three colors, seven target areas can be detected in the same preparation as indicated in the following listing:

Probe 1	Fluorochrome A
Probe 2	Fluorochrome B
Probe 3	Fluorochrome C
Probe 4	Fluorochromes A + B

Probe 5	Fluorochromes A + C
Probe 6	Fluorochromes B + C
Probe 7	Fluorochromes A + B + C
Counterstain	Fluorochrome D

Examples for multicolor detection are given in Fig. 4, panels A and B. *See also* ref. *40.*

2. Materials

2.1. Materials for Pretreatment of Cellular Preparations

1. Phosphate-buffered saline (PBS), pH 7.0.
2. Pepsin-solution: 30–100 µL of 10% pepsin solution is diluted in 100 mL 10 mM HCl immediately before use. Stock solution: Dissolve 10% pepsin in ddH$_2$O at 37°C for 30 min. Store at –20°C.
3. Postfixation solution: 1% acid-free formaldehyde, in PBS, containing 50 mM MgCl$_2$.
4. Series of cold ethanol: 70, 90, and 100% ethanol.
5. Coplin jars and water bath.

2.2. Materials for Nick Translation

1. 10X Nick translation buffer: 0.5M Tris-HCl, pH 8.0, 50 mM MgCl$_2$, and 0.5 mg/mL bovine serum albumin (BSA).
2. β-mercaptoethanol (0.1M): Dilute 0.1 mL of β-mercaptoethanol with 14.4 mL ddH$_2$O. Store up to 2 wk at 4°C.
3. 10X nucleotide stock: 0.5 mM dATP, 0.5 mM dGTP, 0.5 mM dCTP, and 0.4 mM modified dTP. Examples for the modified dNTP are: biotin-11-dUTP; dinitrophenol-11-dUTP; FITC-11-dUTP (or other conjugated fluorochromes); and digoxigenin-11-dUTP. When the modified nucleotide is not a dUTP, substitute the nucleotides accordingly. Linker arms longer than 11 C-atoms (e.g., biotin-14-dXTP or biotin-16-dXTP) are also suitable for *in situ* hybridization probes.
4. Template DNA: The DNA should be free of RNA and should be concentrated to 50–2000 µg/mL.
5. DNA polymerase 1 from *Escherichia coli.*
6. DNase I solution: 1 µL stock solution is diluted in 1 mL cold water immediately before use. Stock solution: 1–3 mg DNase I in 0.15M NaCl, add glycerol to 50%, and store at –20°C. For each DNase I stock solution, the volume to be used in the nick-translation reaction must be tested in a series of reactions with, e.g., 1, 2.5, 5, or 10 µL of the DNase I dilution. After 2 h at 15°C, aliquots with 200 ng of probe are tested on

a gel as described below (*see* Note 4). Choose the volume of DNase that resulted in probe fragments of 100–500 nucleotides in length.

7. 10X stop mix: 0.1M EDTA, pH 8.0, 1% SDS.
8. Column buffer: 50 mM Tris-HCl, pH 8.0, 1 mM EDTA, and 0.1% SDS.
9. Sephadex G-50 (medium): Equilibrate 30 g of Sephadex G-50 in 300 mL of column buffer, and autoclave or incubate at 95°C for several hours.
10. One-milliliter syringes and clinical centrifuge for spin columns.

2.3. Materials for Dot Assay

1. Filter membrane (e.g., nylon filter).
2. DNA dilution buffer: 6X SSC, and 0.1 mg/mL sheared salmon sperm DNA.
3. Dilutions of labeled standard DNA: Dilute well-labeled probe at a concentration of, e.g., 1, 3, 10, 20 pg/μL in DNA dilution buffer.
4. Washing buffer: PBS.
5. AP-buffer 9.5: 0.1M Tris-HCl, pH 9.5, 0.1M NaCl, 50 mM MgCl$_2$.
6. Preincubation buffer: PBS containing 3% BSA.
7. Streptavidin-conjugated alkaline phosphatase (for biotinylated probe) or antidigoxigenin antibody-conjugated alkaline phosphatase (for digoxigenin-labeled probe).
8. Substrate buffer: Add 44 μL nitroblue tetrazolium (NBT) (75 mg/mL in dimethylformamide) to 10 mL AP-buffer 9.5, mix gently, add 33 μL 5-bromo-4-chloro-3-indolyl phosphate (BCIP) (50 mg/mL in dimethylformamide), and mix again gently. Attention: NBT and BCIP are hazardous. Wearing gloves is recommended when handling these solutions.
9. Plastic bags and bag sealer for small-volume incubations, plastic Petri dishes for washing steps, and 37 and 80°C incubators.

2.4. Materials for Denaturation of Cellular Preparations

1. Denaturation solution: 70% deionized formamide, 2X SSC, 50 mM sodium phosphate, pH 7.0. Adjust pH carefully after mixing the solutions.
2. Series of 70, 90, and 100% ice-cold ethanol.
3. Coplin jars and heating water bath.

2.5. Materials for Probe Hybridization

1. Labeled probe DNA: Probes are commonly labeled with biotin, digoxigenin, dinitrophenol, or directly with fluorochromes.
2. Competitor and carrier DNA: Total human DNA or the Cot1 fraction of human DNA (*see* Note 5) is used as competitor for human DNA probes. For probes of other species, the corresponding genomic DNA should be used. Salmon sperm DNA is an appropriate carrier DNA, which can

be supplemented by yeast t-RNA (optional). Competitor and carrier DNA must be sheared, chemically treated, or enzymatically digested to be in the size range of 300–500 bp in length.

3. 3M Sodium acetate, pH 5.
4. Ice-cold ethanol.
5. 70% Ethanol.
6. Deionized formamide.
7. 2X Hybridization cocktail: 4X SSC, 20% dextran sulfate, 100 mM sodium phosphate, pH 7.0. Alternatively, 2X SSC is used for hybridization at higher stringency. When formamide is not used at a final concentration of 50%, the hybridization cocktail has to be adjusted accordingly; for example, for 70% formamide (*see* Section 1.): 3.3× hybridization cocktail containing 6.6X SSC, 33% dextran sulfate, 165 mM sodium phosphate, pH 7.0.
8. Cover slips, rubber cement, incubators for –70°C or –20°C (freezer), 75°C (water bath or heating block), 37°C (water bath or heating block, and incubator), and 42°C (water bath or heating block), vacuum concentrator, and moist chamber (*see* Scheme 1).

2.6. Materials for Probe Detection

1. Wash buffer I: 50% formamide, 2X SSC, prewarmed to 42°C.
2. Wash buffer II: 0.1X SSC (for lower stringency, use 0.3X SSC or 1X SSC), prewarmed to 60°C.
3. Blocking solution: 3% BSA, 4X SSC, 0.1% Tween 20.
4. Detection solution: 1% BSA, 4X SSC, 0.1% Tween 20, and detection reagent.
5. Detection reagents: Detection reagents are offered by several suppliers, and the concentration of reagents varies considerably among the different preparations. When the probe is biotinylated, avidin- or streptavidin-conjugated fluorochromes are used, whereas all the other indirect methods require antibodies. Recommendations by the manufacturer are usually helpful in finding the optimal concentration for this histochemical detection procedure. As a rule of thumb, avidin/streptavidin is usually used at a final concentration of 5 ng/mL, and most antibodies are diluted between 1:100 and 1:1000.
6. Wash buffer III: 4X SSC, 0.1% Tween 20.
7. Counterstain: 2X SSC, 200 ng/mL propidium iodide and/or 200 ng/mL DAPI (less DAPI yields in a better chromosome banding).
8. Poststaining wash: 2X SSC and 0.05% Tween 20.
9. Mounting medium: 0.233 g (1,4-diazobicyclo [2.2.2.] octane) (DABCO) is dissolved in 800 μL ddH$_2$O; add 200 μL 1M Tris-HCl, pH 8.0, and 9

Moist Chamber

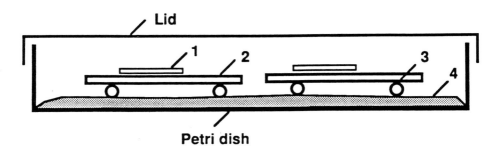

Scheme 1. 1: Cover slide; 2: microscope slide; 3: glass pipet, fixed with tape; 4: water-soaked paper towels.

mL glycerol; mix by inverting. Store in the dark at 4°C. Application of DABCO decreases the bleaching of fluorochromes after excitation (good quality mounting/antifading media are also commercially available).
10. Coplin jars, heatable shaking water bath, cover slips, moist chamber, and 37°C incubator.

2.7. Materials for Signal Amplification

1. Same as Section 2.6., steps 4–10.
2. Amplification reagents for amplification of biotin-mediated signals: Detection solution (*see* step 4 in Section 2.6.) with 2.5 ng/mL biotinylated antiavidin antibodies.

2.8. Materials for Microscopic Evaluation

1. Conventional microscope equipped for epifluorescence. Filter sets must be according to the fluorochromes used. For many applications, three filter combinations are sufficient. Examples of the three most used colors are given below.

Color	Conjugate	Counterstain
Blue	Coumarines (e.g., AMCA)	DAPI, Hoechst 33258
Green	FITC	Quinacrine
Red	Rhodamines, Texas Red, Cy3	Propidium iodide

Recently, more fluorochrome "colors" in the far red and infrared spectral range (e.g., specific cyanin dyes, such as Cy5) are used in combination with the above-listed classical spectral ranges for multicolor hybridization (*see* Fig. 4) *(40)*.

Whereas for some applications, filter sets that are very selective for a given fluorochrome are preferred, in other applications, filter sets are used that allow the simultaneous detection of two fluorochromes. Changing of filter sets generally leads to more or less pronounced shifts of images, which are detectable, e.g., after double exposure for photographic documentation (registration problem). However, double-band pass filter sets are available, which allow the simultaneous recording of fluorochromes (such as FITC and rhodamine). Such filter sets become very important when the geometric relation of two differentially stained sites has to be recorded as precisely as possible (as, e.g., in two-color mapping experiments).

2. More sophisticated evaluations (fine localization of signals, visualization of weak signals and multiple colors, ratio imaging) are facilitated by digital imaging microscopy. Digitized images can be generated by using specialized camera systems or by confocal laser scanning microscopy. Camera systems are combined with conventional microscopes, allowing the detection of a broad range of fluorochromes differentiated by their excitation/emission ranges. In contrast, laser-scanning microscopy is limited to the use of fluorochromes that can be excited by the available lasers. Most commercial instruments allow excitation of one or two fluorochromes (green and red fluorochromes), and in particular, equipment with a UV laser for an efficient excitation of blue fluorochromes is very costly. The most sensitive camera system to date is the so-called cooled CCD (charged coupled device) camera. Its sensitivity is superior to the commercially available laser-scanning microscopes, and it costs considerably less than the laser microscope. However, with the laser microscope, the registration problem can be overcome by parallel excitation/emission of different fluorochromes in the dual- or triple-channel mode. The confocal laser microscope can greatly reduce the out of focus fluorescence, allowing the generation of high-quality optical sections through labeled specimen. Therefore, this instrument is used for three-dimensional analyses. Sections from different focal planes of an object obtained by camera systems can also be used for three-dimensional analysis. However, the out-of-focus fluorescence has to be reduced by deconvolutions after generating the images. This is achieved by algorithms comparing the gray images from neighboring sections, which requires considerable computer work. Currently, it seems that if three-dimensional recording of fluorescent cellular specimens is needed, a

confocal laser-scanning microscope is the instrument of choice (regarding commercially available instruments), whereas the cheaper camera systems seem preferable when only two-dimensional work—such as mapping of signals on metaphase chromosomes or detection of chromosome aberrations—is carried out. Further developments in devices for digital imaging microscopy are discussed below (*see* Section 3.8.).

3. Methods

3.1. Preparation of Specimen

For gene mapping, chromosomes from primary cell cultures are preferred. Metaphase chromosomes are easily prepared from short-term (48 or 72 h) cultures of peripheral blood lymphocytes. The preparation scheme follows the protocols given in Chapters 1 and 2. In clinical cases where chromosome aberrations are to be diagnosed on metaphase chromosomes of primary cells, peripheral blood might not be the source of choice. Adherently growing fibroblasts from biopsy material comprise an often-used alternative.

For many clinical applications—e.g., in cytogenetic analyses of many solid tumors—it is very difficult, if not impossible, to prepare metaphase chromosomes. However, interphase analysis can circumvent some of these difficulties. In hematological malignancies, interphase analyses can be performed on nucleated blood cells prepared the same way as metaphase chromosomes. It is also possible to use blood or bone marrow smears for interphase cytogenetics. However, when solid tissue has to be analyzed, sections of frozen or paraffin-embedded tissue are still very difficult to use. Such an analysis is often hampered by autofluorescence of the tissue and insufficient probe penetration, thus limiting the potential of visualizing genomic DNA to relatively large regions (e.g., the centromeric regions delineated by a repetitive DNA probe). So far, no satisfying standard procedure can be given for preparation of tissue sections for *in situ* hybridization to genomic DNA. Each tissue type still requires a lot of effort to optimize the preparation procedure. For starting *in situ* hybridization of tissue sections, the reader is advised to look at more specialized literature *(41–43)*. A promising alternative is to isolate nuclei from the tissue and perform interphase analysis on these nuclei. For the protocol, the reader is referred to ref.*44*.

Methanol/acetic-acid-fixed metaphase chromosomes and nuclei are prepared as described in Chapters 1–3. After dehydration and air-drying, slides are directly used, stored for up to 4 wk at room temperature, or stored in a dry box (sealed in a plastic bag) at –70°C for up to 2 yr. Refreezing of slides that were once thawed might decrease the quality of the preparations for *in situ* hybridization.

Although optimal specimen preparations yield signals of high quality in hybridization, it is in practice often helpful to perform protease pretreatment, which improves probe accessibility. The protocol below is derived from Raap and Wiegant (personal communication).

1. Wash slides in PBS (Coplin jar) for 5 min at 37°C.
2. Incubate slides in pepsin solution for 10 min at 37°C. For variation of the digestion reaction, adjust pepsin concentration or incubation time.
3. Wash slides in PBS for 5 min at room temperature.
4. Incubate in formaldehyde postfixation solution for 10 min at room temperature.
5. Wash slides in PBS for 5 min at room temperature.
6. Incubate in a series of 70, 90, and 100% ethanol for 5 min each followed by air-drying.

3.2. Probe Labeling

Enzymatic incorporation of modified nucleotides is preferred over labeling by incubation with reactive compounds owing to the higher labeling efficiency. An important requirement for a good *in situ* hybridization is the size of the probe molecules obtained after the labeling reaction. The molecules should not be much longer than 500 (!), but more than 100 nucleotides in length. The labeling efficiency of primer extension and nick-translation is comparable, but the desired size range of molecules can be more easily obtained in a nick-translation reaction by adjusting the DNase concentration. This is particularly important when long genomic fragments are used as template, since they often result in probe molecules of a higher size range in primer extension reactions. Other specialized labeling reactions using modified nucleotides include in vitro transcription-generating riboprobes (*see Focus,* vol. 7:4, p. 12, 1985), end tailing of, e.g., oligonucleotides *(45),* and the polymerase chain reaction *(46,47).* Based on the size of the templates used for these procedures, probe molecules usually have an adequate size for *in situ* hybridization.

A standard nick-translation reaction is carried out with a template DNA concentration of 20 µg/mL. The protocol is according to Langer et al. *(48)*.

1. Make up the following reaction mixture: 10 µL 10X nick-translation buffer, 10 µL 0.1*M* β-mercaptoethanol, 10 µL 10X nucleotide stock containing modified-dNTPs (use the modified nucleotide of your choice), 2 µg template DNA, 20 U DNA polymerase 1, empirically determined volume of DNase I solution (*see* Section 2.2.), and ddH$_2$O to a final vol of 100 µL.
2. Incubate for 2 h at 15°C, and then store on ice.
3. Remove aliquot of 6–10 µL to test the actual probe size by gel electrophoresis (*see* Section 4.).
4. If the labeled probe molecules are more than 500 nucleotides in length (up to 10,000 nt), add DNAse I solution, and incubate longer at 15°C to cut the maximal probe length to 500 nucleotides. Thereafter, test aliquot again by agarose gel electrophoresis. If the labeled probe is shorter than 100 nucleotides or bigger than 10,000 nucleotides, clean up template (e.g., perform phenol extraction and ethanol precipitation), and start labeling reaction again.
5. Add 1/10 volume of 10X stop mix, and incubate for 15 min at 68°C.
6. Prepare spin columns: Fill the barrel of a 1-mL syringe (silianized glass wool is used to plug the bottom) with equilibrated Sephadex G50, put it in a 15-mL plastic tube, and spin in a swing-out rotor at 1600*g* for exactly 5 min.
7. Remove flow through, load 100 µL of column buffer, and repeat centrifugation.
8. Repeat step 7 two more times (after the last spin, the flow through should be exactly 100 µL.
9. Pipet the nick-translation mixture onto the center of the Sephadex column, and spin again as before.
10. The flow through contains the labeled probe. It can be stored at –20°C for long periods (even for years) without affecting the probe quality.

3.3. Test of Labeling Efficiency by Dot Assay

When the conditions for probe labeling are established in a laboratory, it might not be necessary to check the labeling efficiency. However, when the procedure is still new or when the hybridization experiments are negative, it might be wise to perform such an analysis. Kits for this assay are commercially available.

1. Prepare a series of dilutions from the labeled probe in DNA dilution buffer (e.g., 1, 3, 10, and 20 pg/μL).
2. Spot 1 μL of each dilution along with the standard DNA dilutions on a filter membrane.
3. Incubate filter for 30 min at 80°C.
4. Wash filter in a dish in PBS for 1 min at room temperature.
5. Seal filter in plastic bag with, e.g., 10 mL preincubation buffer and incubate for 30 min at 37°C.
6. Remove preincubation buffer, add 1 μg/mL streptavidin-conjugated alkaline phosphatase in PBS (or antireporter [e.g., digoxigenin] antibody-conjugated alkaline phosphatase according to the recommendation by the suppliers), seal again, and incubate as before.
7. Wash two times in a dish with PBS for 5 min each at room temperature.
8. Wash in AP-buffer 9.5 for 10 min at room temperature.
9. Seal filter in a bag with, e.g., 10 mL substrate buffer, and incubate in the dark at room temperature for 10–30 min or until the color reaction is complete (longer incubations might lead to higher background).
10. Wash filter in PBS for 5 min at room temperature.
11. The colored spots of the probe should have the same intensity as the comparable spots of the standard DNA. As a rule of thumb, 1 pg of labeled DNA should be visible in this assay for good hybridization results to be expected.

3.4. Denaturation of Cellular Preparations

1. Select the area on the slide to be hybridized, and label it from the reverse by scratches.
2. Preincubate the slides at 60°C to avoid dropping of the temperature during the denaturation step.
3. Put slides into prewarmed denaturation solution (it is important that the temperature of solution is at exactly 70–72°C) and incubate for 2 min at 70°C.
4. Put slides through a series of 70, 90, and 100% ice-cold ethanol, 3 min each, and air-dry.

3.5. In Situ *Hybridization of Probes*

The amount of probe DNA used varies with the kind of probe material. In a typical 10 μL hybridization mixture, 2–20 ng of repetitive DNA, or 30–80 ng of cDNA or average genomic DNA (e.g., plasmid, phage, or cosmid probes) are used. More probe DNA is hybridized when pools of fragments are used; e.g., from the chromosome

DNA libraries cloned in bluescribe vectors, 150–500 ng of labeled DNA are used in a 10 μL vol. When the percentage of DNA to be hybridized specifically is small within a labeled DNA preparation, such as a YAC in the total yeast DNA or human sequences in a human/rodent hybrid DNA, 0.5–2 μg of labeled probe are used (in 10 μL).

For repetitive probes, as well as cDNAs or genomic sequences known to consist entirely of single copy sequences, follow Protocol A (Section 3.5.1.). This protocol has evolved from the long experience of a number of laboratories including ourselves. Some references are mentioned for further information *(5,49–53)*. For probes known (or unknown) to contain IRS to be suppressed (most cloned genomic DNA and some cDNAs), follow Protocol B (Section 3.5.2.), which is based on previously published work *(12,15)*.

3.5.1. Protocol A (Standard Hybridization)

1. Pipet the chosen amount of labeled probe in a vial. As an option, 1–5 μg of carrier DNA can be added. If the volume of labeled probe is 3 μL or smaller, dry the probe in a vacuum concentrator. If the volume is bigger, ethanol precipitation is preferred: Adjust volume with ddH$_2$O to at least 10 μL, add $^1/_{20}$ vol 3M sodium acetate, and 2 vol cold ethanol, vortex, incubate at –70°C for 30 min, spin in table-top centrifuge for 10 min at high speed, discard supernatant, add 100 μL 70% ethanol, spin as before, discard supernatant, and dry pellet in a vacuum concentrator.
2. Dissolve pellet first in 5 μL deionized formamide, add 5 μL 2X hybridization cocktail, and mix well (variation for some alphoid repetitive DNA probes: dissolve in 7 μL formamide and add 3 μL 3.3X hybridization cocktail).
3. For denaturation, incubate probe for 5 min at 75°C.
4. Chill on ice for 3 min.
5. Apply the 10-μL hybridization volume to the slide (marked area) with denatured cellular preparations (*see* Section 3.4.), add 18-mm^2 coverslip, and seal with rubber cement.
6. Incubate slides in moist chamber (*see* Scheme 1) overnight (see Note 7) at 37°C.

3.5.2. Protocol B (CISS Hybridization)

The main difference from the standard protocol is the addition of competitor DNA and an additional preannealing step after probe denaturation.

1. Combine the labeled probe DNA (e.g., 50 ng) with 1–3 µg competitor DNA, and adjust with carrier DNA to a total of 10 µg DNA (the concentration of total DNA could be increased to 30 µg and more). When multiple differentially labeled probes are used, the amount of competitor DNA is increased. For example, when hybridizing seven cosmid probes simultaneously, combine, e.g., 7×50 ng labeled probe, 15 µg competitor DNA, and 10 µg carrier DNA.
2. Add $^1/_{20}$ vol 3*M* sodium acetate and 2 vol cold ethanol, vortex, incubate at –70°C for 30 min, spin in table-top centrifuge for 10 min at high speed, discard supernatant, add 200 µL 70% ethanol, spin as before, discard supernatant, and dry pellet in a vacuum concentrator.
3. Dissolve pellet first in 5 µL deionized formamide, add 5 µL 2X hybridization cocktail, and mix well (e.g, by agitating the tubes for 5–10 min on a vortex shaker at high speed).
4. Prewarm slides with denatured cellular preparations to 42°C.
5. For denaturation, incubate probe cocktail for 5 min at 75°C.
6. Transfer the tube quickly to 37°C to allow preannealing for 5–10 min. The preannealing time can be considerably increased (*see* Note 6).
7. Apply the 10 µL hybridization vol to the prewarmed slide (marked area), add 18-mm^2 cover slip, and seal with rubber cement.
8. Incubate slides in moist chamber overnight (*see* Note 7) at 37°C.

3.6. Detection of Hybridized Probes

The slides should not get dry at any time during the detection procedure!

1. Remove rubber cement and incubate slides (Coplin jar in shaking water bath) in prewarmed (42°C) wash buffer I for 5–10 min at 42°C.
2. Transfer slides to new jar with prewarmed wash buffer I (during this process the cover slip falls off), and incubate for 5 min at 42°C (agitation).
3. Substitute two times with new prewarmed (42°C), wash buffer I, and incubate for 5 min at 42°C each time.
4. Substitute three times with new prewarmed (60°C) wash buffer II and incubate for 5 min at 42°C each time. Choose salt concentration of buffer II for the desired stringency (*see* Section 2.6.).
5. When directly fluorochrome-labeled probes are used, no further detection is needed. Proceed with step 13.
6. Take one slide out of the jar, drain as much as possible (but do not let it dry!) by touching the slide edges with a paper towel, add 200 µL blocking buffer, add large cover slip (22×40 mm), and transfer to moist chamber. Then continue this procedure with the next slide.
7. Incubate in moist chamber for ca. 30 min at 37°C.

8. Tilt slides to let coverslip fall off, drain as much as possible, add 200 µL detection solution containing detection reagents (e.g. 5 ng/mL avidin-conjugated FITC to detect biotinylated probes), add large cover slip.

9. Incubate in moist chamber for ca. 30 min at 37°C.

10. Tilt slides to let cover slip fall off, transfer slides in jar with prewarmed (42°C) wash buffer III, and incubate for 5 min at 42°C (agitation).

11. Substitute two times with new prewarmed (42°C) wash buffer III, and incubate for 5 min at 42°C each time.

12. Whereas for many applications one detection step is sufficient (fluorochrome-conjugated avidin or antibodies), some detection protocols require two or more detection steps (for example, antireporter molecule antibodies of one species during the first step [e.g., sheep antidigoxigenin] and fluorochrome-conjugated antibodies directed against the antibodies from that species [e.g. rhodamine-conjugated rabbit antisheep] during the second step). For each additional detection step, repeat steps 8–11. In general, the more layers of detection reagents are added, the more fluorochromes are bound and therefore the stronger the signal. However, background fluorescence is also increased (*see* Notes 10–12 for discussion).

13. Incubate slides in Coplin jar with suitable counterstain (*see* Section 2.8.) for 15 min at room temperature (agitation).

14. Substitute with poststaining wash and incubate for 2 min at room temperature.

15. Take one slide out of the jar, drain as much as possible, add 30 µL mounting medium, add large cover slip (22 × 40 mm), and transfer to dark box for storage. Then continue this procedure with the next slide.

3.7. Signal Amplification

When the target is of low complexity (e.g., 0.5–2 kb) or when the microscopic inspection reveals only weak signals, it is helpful to perform a signal amplification procedure. A technique to amplify avidin-mediated signals with a sandwich technique was published by Pinkel et al. *(52)* and is described below. Similar procedures with one or two antibody layers can be carried out for other detection methods (*see* Note 11).

1. When amplification is carried out immediately, proceed as in Section 3.6. steps 8–11 with detection solution containing amplification reagents (e.g., biotinylated antiavidin antibodies) and a second time steps 8–11 with the first detection solution (e.g., fluorochrome-conjugated avidin).

2. When amplification should be carried out after mounting; carefully remove cover slip with forceps, incubate with agitation in Coplin jar in wash buffer III for 10 min at 42°C, repeat three more times with new wash buffer III, proceed as described in step 1.

3.8. Microscopic Evaluation

1. Fluorochromes for probe detection and counterstain should be selected based on the list in Section 2.8., step 1. For choosing the appropriate counterstain, the fluorochromes for probe detection must be considered to avoid overlap of the emission ranges; for example, do not combine FITC and quinacrine, rhodamine (or Texas red) and propidium iodide, or AMCA and DAPI.

   For the visualization of one hybridized probe, a fluorochrome-mediated probe detection (typically via FITC) is combined with one or two counterstains (DAPI and/or propidium iodide). For the visualization of two differentially labeled probes, two different fluorochromes are used for probe detection (typically via FITC and rhodamine or Texas red) combined with one counterstain (e.g., DAPI). More than three probes could be differentially labeled by including combinations of fluorochromes for single probes as outlined above (*see* Section 1.).

2. With filter sets that are very selective for a given fluorochrome, documentation by conventional photography might be very difficult when signals are small. For example, documentation of two dot-like FITC signals on a black background requires overexposure for most photographic films, resulting in a disproportionally strong visualization of, e.g., chromosomal background. However, simultaneous visualization of such a signal with propidium iodide counterstain using a suitable filter set usually provides enough light for adequate photographic documentation. For recording of multicolor experiments by conventional photography, shifting of the images owing to changing of filter sets leads to the abovementioned registration problem. This can be overcome in part by using pass filters.

   In general, signal documentation and data handling are facilitated by digital imaging microscopy. With sensitive detection devices, even very weak signals can be documented in a sufficient way. Application of optical filtering, such as thresholding, might improve the quality of a digitized image. For recording multicolor experiments, usually digitized gray scale images are generated for each fluorochrome, the images are overlayed electronically, and a pseudocolor is assigned to each layer. We find it very helpful to assign to each layer the same color that is exhibited by the actual imaged fluorescent dye. However, when dyes invisible to the human eye are used or when hybridization probes are differentiated by using a combination of fluorochromes for one signal (*see* Section 1.), new pseudocolors will be assigned. For a more advanced image analysis of, e.g., seven probes on DAPI counterstained chromosomes, the reader is referred to the literature *(40)*.

The problem of image shifting with the various devices for digital imaging microscopy has been discussed above (*see* Section 2.8.). To overcome this obstacle, the advent of commercially available colored CCD camera systems provides promising alternatives, since multiple colors are recorded without the need for filter change. The development of filter-changing devices designed to minimize an image shifting is also an area of active research. If electronically overlayed gray level images are not in alignment, the shift can be corrected by moving each layer electronically pixel by pixel. However, for this correction, the criteria for a correct alignment must be carefully defined. One solution is to include the use of multiple-band pass filters to present the signals from several fluorochromes in one gray level image, and this image is then used to align the images of single fluorochromes by matching the signal spots. Alternatively, background fluorescence or the addition of reagents that emit fluorescence in all spectral ranges used in an experiment (e.g., beads with conjugated fluorescent dyes or cohybridized probes detected simultaneously with several dyes) can be used for realignment. The advantage of confocal laser scanning microscopy with regard to image shifting is discussed above.

3. It should be mentioned that most nucleic acid probes delineate their target sequence with high specificity and efficiency. Therefore, when probes are mapped to chromosomes, the need for a statistical analysis is considerably reduced as compared to conventional isotopic *in situ* hybridization mapping approaches. For example, cosmid probes generally label more than 90% of their target sites, i.e., both chromatids of both chromosome homologs are stained on metaphase chromosomes, and unspecific fluorescent spots are greatly reduced. Thus, probe mapping can be easily performed by analyzing 20–30 chromosome homologs. With smaller target sequences, the percentage of delineated target areas might drop (e.g., down to 30–60% for target sites of 1 kb in length or smaller). However, based on the greatly reduced unspecific fluorescence, such probes are still rapidly mapped by analyzing, e.g., 50 chromosome homologs (i.e., 25 metaphases). If background spots are frequent (e.g., after multiple amplifications when small single-copy DNA probes are used), they can in general be distinguished from hybridization signals by counting only fluorescent doublets (on both chromatids) as signals.

4. Notes

1. In general, it is not necessary to isolate inserts from vector sequences. Hybridization signals produced by isolated insert probes are not superior to the ones produced by the corresponding whole DNA probe. Only when certain large probe sets are used, such as pooled phage library DNA with a fraction of ca. 90% vector sequences, the vector sequences might contribute to an increase in background fluorescence.

2. Although it is generally believed that slides should age several days before performing an *in situ* hybridization, we have achieved good results with slides prepared on the same day. However, in these cases, baking of the slides for 2–3 h at 50–60°C might be helpful for the conservation of chromosome morphology.

3. Modification of DNA with biotin, digoxigenin, dinitrophenol, and many other reporter molecules introduces hydrophopic residues to the DNA, and the probe might become very sticky. Therefore, SDS has to be included in the spin column (including spin column buffer and loading volume). Otherwise, more than half of the probe might get stuck in the column (alternatively, the column could be saturated with carrier DNA). For the same reasons, such modified DNA should not become the subject of a phenol extraction, since it will be lost in the interphase or in the phenol phase. Accordingly, such modified DNAs dissolve better in formamide than in aqueous solution. Therefore, the hybridization probe is resuspended first in formamide before adding hybridization buffer (*see* Section 3.5.).

4. We find it very important to test the actual size of the probe molecules after the labeling reaction. Probe DNA from different sources and different preparations vary in their quality (e.g., RNA or protein content, salt concentration, and so forth), and therefore, labeling conditions can often not be standardized to result in probe molecules of the same size range. We add gel running buffer to an aliquot of the probe (ca. 200 ng), heat denature by boiling in a water bath for 3 min, chill on ice for 3 min, quickly load it on a 2% agarose minigel (in TBE-buffer), and run the gel along with a DNA size marker at 15 V/cm. After ethidium bromide staining, the pool of fragments is visible as a smear. The smear should not exceed 500 nucleotides and should not be smaller than 100 nucleotides. With increasing length of the fragments, a pronounced background fluorescence pattern increases: Strong fluorescent spots are found all over the slide and give the impression of a "starry night." When the probes are too small, the signals are often weak, and a general background staining of chromosomes and nuclei might occur.

5. Total genomic DNA is an efficient competitor DNA. It provides an excess of IRS that are also present in the probe sequence. Based on the higher concentration of repetitive sequences, they reassociate much faster than low or single-copy sequences. Therefore, the IRS of the probe becomes double-stranded during the preannealing step, whereas low and single-copy subsequences stay single-stranded. Furthermore, the excess repetitive DNA from the competitor might also compete for the repetitive sequences on the chromosomes. However, when high concentrations of total genomic DNA are used as competitor, the signal intensities might be lowered, based on the increase of (unlabeled) single-copy sequences also present within the competitor DNA. The Cot1 fraction of reassociating DNA of higher eukaryotes is highly enriched in highly repetitive DNA, and therefore, it serves as a perfect competitor. Even with large amounts of Cot1 DNA, signal intensities are not lowered. For special applications when probes are enriched in IRS, competition with Cot1 DNA is essential *(22)*.

6. The preannealing period can be elongated to 1 h and more. Although the signal intensity might decrease, some unwanted crosshybridizations decrease as well. In particular, the staining of all the short arms of the human D-group and G-group chromosomes by almost any library derived from either one of these chromosomes can be diminished by elongated preannealing times.

   A certain probe might be especially rich in IRS, resulting in chromosomal background staining using the standard suppression procedure described above. Although an increase in preannealing time leads to a certain degree to a decrease of such background, it is much more efficient to increase the concentration of competitor DNA.

7. Although most of the *in situ* hybridization reaction takes place in the first few hours of incubation, longer incubation times result in stronger signals. In general, incubation overnight gives excellent results. However, for critical experiments, it might be wise to incubate for longer periods (e.g., 48 or 72 h).

8. During the detection procedure, slides must not be allowed to dry, since this leads to considerable background. For similar reasons, air bubbles that could occur when cover slips are applied should be avoided as much as possible.

9. As soon as slides are incubated with fluorochromes, they should be kept in the dark as much as possible (wrap containers in aluminium foil). Avoid direct exposure to light sources.

10. The more fluorochromes that are located in a particular area, the stronger the signal. Accordingly, the signal strength roughly correlates with

the number of reagent layers used for detection and/or amplification. Currently, directly labeled probes are sufficient for many *in situ* hybridization applications, but the signal intensity is less than that achieved with an indirect detection procedure by which more fluorochromes are bound to a local point.

11. Typical avenues for fluorescent detection are:

Probe	1. Layer	2. Layer	3. Layer
Fluorochrome conjugated	–	–	–
Fluorochrome conjugated	Antifluorochrome antibody	Fluorochrome-conjugated secondary antibody	–
Biotinylated	Avidin/ streptavidin-conjugated fluorochrome	–	–
Biotinylated	Avidin/ streptavidin-conjugated fluorochrome	Biotinylated antiavidin antibody	Avidin/ streptavidin conjugated fluorochrome
Digoxigenin labeled	Fluorochrome-conjugated antidigoxigenin antibody	–	–
Digoxigenin labeled	Fluorochrome-conjugated sheep antidigoxigenin antibody	Fluorochrome-conjugated antisheep antibody	–
Digoxigenin labeled	Sheep antidigoxigenin antibody	Fluorochrome-conjugated antisheep antibody	–
Digoxigenin labeled	Mouse antidigoxigenin antibody	Digoxigenin-labeled antimouse antibody	Fluorochrome-conjugated antidigoxigenin antibody
Dinitrophenol labeled	Rat antidinitro-phenol antibody	Fluorochrome-conjugated antirat antibody	–

Many more combinations are possible, for example:
a. Using antibodies from different species;
b. Using different reagents for signal amplification; and
c. Using different probe labeling systems.

12. Signal amplification increases signal intensity, but it also decreases the difference between signal and noise, i.e., it increases background fluorescence disproportionally (since number of fluorochromes and signal intensity do not relate in a linear way). Therefore, signal amplification should only be carried out where necessary. Slides should be amplified after visual inspection only when the background is low. When very sensitive systems are used for image recording, documentation of weak signals without a further amplification step is recommended.

13. It might be necessary to change the chromosomal counterstain or to destain the chromosomes. This is easily performed by washing the preparation several times in wash buffer III (*see* Section 2.6.). Restaining or refreshing of old (and bleached) counterstain can be performed at any time following the procedure in Section 3.6. (steps 13 and 14), or by adding counterstain to the mounting medium.

14. After histochemical detection, slides are usually stored at 4°C. The quality of the fluorochrome detection can be very good for many months. However, quality might drop at very variable rates (for some preparations within weeks or even days). Usually, weak signals on old slides can be refreshed by applying amplification procedures.

15. A very crucial step for the whole procedure is the adequate preparation of cellular specimen. This includes a careful fixation procedure. For example, standard methanol/acetic acid fixation of peripheral blood lymphocytes should be repeated at least seven times.

Acknowledgments

We would like to thank Thomas Cremer and David C. Ward for discussion, and the Verein zur Förderung der Krebsforschung in Deutschland as well as the Deutsche Forschungsgemeinschaft (postdoctoral fellowship to T. Ried) for support.

References

1. Lichter, P. and Ward, D. C. (1990) Is non-isotopic in situ hybridization finally coming of age? *Nature* **345,** 93–95.
2. Lichter, P., Boyle, A. L., Cremer, T., and Ward, D. C. (1991) Analysis of genes and chromosomes by non-isotopic in situ hybridization. *Genet. Anal. Techn. Appl.* **8,** 24–35.

3. Raap, A. K., Dirks, R. W., Jiwa, N. M., Nederlof, P. M., and van der Ploeg, M. (1990) In situ hybridization with hapten-modified DNA probes, in *Modern Pathology of AIDS and Other Retroviral Infections* (Racz, P., Haase, A. T., and Gluckman, J. C., eds.) Karger, Basel, pp. 17–28.

4. Narayanswami, S. and Hamkalo, B. A. (1991) DNA sequence mapping using electron microscopy. *Genet. Anal. Techn. Appl.* **8,** 14–23.

5. Manuelidis, L. (1985) In situ detection of DNA sequences using biotinylated probes. *Focus* **7,** 4–8.

6. Klever, M., Grond-Ginsbach, C., Scherthan, H., and Schroeder-Kurth, T. M. (1991) Chromosomal in situ suppression hybridization after Giemsa banding. *Hum. Genet.* **86,** 484–486.

7. Arnold, N., Bhatt, M., Ried, T., Ward, D. C., and Wienberg, J. (1992) Fluorescence in situ hybridization on banded chromosomes, in *Techniques and Methods in Molecular Biology: Non-Radioactive Labeling and Detection of Biomolecules* (Kessler, C., ed.) Springer Verlag, Berlin, in press.

8. Lichter, P. and Cremer, T. (1991) Chromosome analysis by non-isotopic in situ hybridization, in *Human Cytogenetics: A Practical Approach* (Rooney, D. E. and Czepulkowski, B. H., eds.) IRL, Oxford, pp. 157–192.

9. Cherif, D., Julier, C., Delattre, O., Derré, J., Lathrop, G. M., and Berger, R. (1990) Simultaneous localization of cosmids and chromosome R-banding by fluorescence microscopy: application to regional mapping of human chromosome 11. *Proc. Natl. Acad. Sci. USA* **87,** 6639–6643.

10. Fan, Y.-S., Davis, L. M., and Shows, T. B. (1990) Mapping small DNA sequences by fluorescence in situ hybridization directly on banded metaphase chromosomes. *Proc. Natl. Acad. Sci. USA* **87,** 6223–6227.

11. Takahashi, E., Hori, T., O'Connell, P., Leppert, M., and White, R. (1990) R-banding and nonisotopic in situ hybridization: precise localization of the human type II collagen gene (COL2A1). *Hum. Genet.* **86,** 14–16.

12. Lichter, P., Tang, C. C., Call, K., Hermanson, G., Evans, G. A., Housman, D., and Ward, D. C. (1990) High resolution mapping of human chromosome 11 by in situ hybridization with cosmid clones. *Science* **247,** 64–69.

13. Boyle, A. L., Ballard, S. G., and Ward, D. C. (1990) Differential distribution of LINE and SINE sequences in the mouse genome: chromosome karyotyping by fluorescent in situ hybridization. *Proc. Natl. Acad. Sci. USA* **87,** 7757–7761.

14. Landegent, J. E., Jansen, in de Wal, N., Dirks, R. W., Baas, F., and van der Ploeg, M. (1987) Use of whole cosmid cloned genomic sequences for chromosomal localization by non-radioactive in situ hybridization. *Hum. Genet.* **77,** 366–370.

15. Lichter, P., Cremer, T., Borden, J., Manuelidis, L., and Ward, D. C. (1988) Delineation of individual human chromosomes in metaphase and interphase cells by in situ suppression hybridization using recombinant DNA libraries. *Hum. Genet.* **80,** 224–234.

16. Pinkel, D., Landegent, J., Collins, C., Fuscoe, J., Segraves, R., Lucas, J., and Gray, J. W. (1988) Fluorescence in situ hybridization with human chromosome-specific libraries: detection of trisomy 21 and translocations of chromosome 4. *Proc. Natl. Acad. Sci. USA* **85,** 9138–9142.

17. Collins, C., Kuo, W. L., Segraves, R., Fuscoe, J., Pinkel, D., and Gray, J. (1991) *Genomics* **11,** 997–1006.

18. Cremer, T., Lichter, P., Borden, J., Ward, D. C., and Manuelidis, L. (1988) Detection of chromosome aberrations in metaphase and interphase tumor cells by in situ hybridization using chromosome specific library probes. *Hum. Genet.* **80,** 235–246.

19. Lichter, P., Cremer, T., Tang, C. C., Watkins, P. C., Manuelidis, L., and Ward, D. C. (1988) Rapid detection of human chromosome 21 aberrations by in situ hybridization. *Proc. Natl. Acad. Sci. USA* **85,** 9664–9668.

20. Jauch, A., Daumer, C., Lichter, P., Murken, J., Schroeder-Kurth, T., and Cremer, T. (1990) Chromosomal in situ suppression hybridization of human gonosomes and autosomes and its use in clinical cytogenetics. *Hum. Genet.* **85,** 145–150.

21. Lengauer, C., Riethman, H., and Cremer, T. (1990) Painting of human chromosomes generated from hybrid cell lines by PCR with Alu and L1 primers. *Hum. Genet.* **86,** 1–6.

22. Lichter, P., Ledbetter, S. A., Ledbetter, D. H., and Ward, D. C. (1990) Fluorescence in situ hybridization with Alu and L1 polymerase chain reaction probes for rapid characterization of human chromosomes in hybrid cell lines. *Proc. Natl. Acad. Sci. USA* **87,** 6634–6638.

23. Lengauer, C., Green, E. D., and Cremer, T. (1992) Fluorescence in situ hybridization of YAC clones after Alu-PCR amplification. *Genomics,* 826–828.

24. Barr, M. L. and Bertram, E. G. (1949) A morphological distinction between neurons of the male and female, and the behaviour of the nuleolar satellite during accelerated nuleioprotein synthesis. *Nature* **163,** 676–677.

25. Pearson, P. L., Bobrow, M., and Vosa, C. G. (1970) Technique for identifying Y chromosomes in human interphase nuclei. *Nature* **226,** 78–80.

26. Cremer, T., Landegent, J., Brückner, A., Scholl, H. P., Schardin, M., Hager, H. D., Devilee, P., Pearson, P., and van der Ploeg, M. (1986) Detection of chromosome aberrations in the human interphase nucleus by visualization of specific target DNAs with radioactive and nonradioactive in situ hybridization techniques: diagnosis of trisomy 18 with probe L1.84. *Hum. Genet.* **74,** 346–352.

27. Tkachuk, D. C., Pinkel, D., Kuo, W.-L., Weier, H.-U., and Gray, J. W. (1991) Clinical applications of fluorescence in situ hybridization. *Genet. Anal. Techn. Appl.* **8,** 67–74.

28. Lichter, P., Jauch, A., Cremer, T., and Ward, D. C. (1990) Detection of Down syndrome by in situ hybridization with chromosome 21 specific DNA probes, in *Molecular Genetics of Chromosome 21 and Down Syndrome* (Patterson, D., ed.) Liss, New York, pp. 69–78.

29. Lux, S. E., Tse, W. T., Menninger, J. C., John, K. M., Harris, P., Shalev, O., Chilcote, R. R., Marchesi, S. L., Watkins, P. C., Bennett, V., McIntosh, S., Collins, F. S., Francke, U., Ward, D. C., and Forget, B. G. (1990) Hereditary spherocytosis associated with deletion of human erythrocyte ankyrin gene on chromosome 8. *Nature* **345,** 736–739.

30. Ried, T., Mahler, V., Vogt, P., Blonden, L., van Ommen, G. J. B., Cremer, T., and Cremer, M. (1990) Carrier detection by in situ suppression hybridization

with cosmid clones of the Duchenne/Becker muscular dystrophy (DMD/BMD)-locus. *Hum. Genet.* **85,** 581–586.

31. Rowley, J. D., Diaz, M. O., Espinosa, R., III, Patel, Y. D., van Melle, E., Ziemin, S., Taillon-Miller, P., Lichter, P., Evans, G. A., Kersey, J. H., Ward, D. C., Domer, P. H., and Le Beau, M. M. (1990) Mapping chromosome band 11q23 in human acute leukemia with biotinylated probes: identification of 11q23 translocation breakpoints with a yeast artificial chromosome. *Proc. Natl. Acad. Sci. USA* **87,** 9358–9362.

32. Stilgenbauer, S., Döhner, H., Bulgay-Mörschel, M., Weitz, S., Bentz, M., and Lichter, P. (1993) Retinoblastoma gene deletion in chronic lymphoid leukemias: a combined metaphase and interphase cytogenetic study. *Blood* **81,** 2118–2124.

33. Lupski, J. R., Montes de Oca-Luna, R., Slaugenhaupt, S., Pentao, L., Guzzetta, V., Trask, B. J., Saucedo-Cardenas, O., Barker, D. F., Killian, J. M., Garcia, C. A., Chakravarti, A., and Patel, P. I. (1991) DNA duplication associated with Charcot-Marie-Tooth disease type 1A. *Cell* **66,** 219–232.

34. Ried, T., Lengauer, C., Cremer, T., Wiegant, J., Raap, A. K., van der Ploeg, M., Groitl, P., and Lipp, M. (1992) Specific metaphase and interphase detection of the breakpoint region in 8q24 of Burkitt lymphoma cells by triple color fluorescence in situ hybridization. *Genes, Chromosomes & Cancer* **4,** 69–74.

35. Dauwerse, J. G., Kievits, T., Beverstock, G. C., van der Keur, D., Smit, E., Wessels, H. W., Hagemeijer, A., Pearson, P. L., van Ommen, G.-J. B., and Breuning, M. H. (1990) Rapid detection of chromosome 16 inversion in acute nonlymphocytic leukemia, subtype M4: regional localization of the breakpoint in 16p. *Cytogenet. Cell Genet.* **53,** 126–128.

36. Arnoldus, E. P. J., Wiegant, J., Noordemeer, I. A., Wessels, J. W., Beverstock, G. C., Grosveld, G. C., van der Ploeg, M., and Raap, A. K. (1990) Detection of the Philadelphia chromosome in interphase nuclei. *Cytogenet. Cell Genet.* **54,** 108–111.

37. Tkachuk, D., Westbrook, C., Andreef, M., Donlon, T., Cleary, M., Suranarayan, K., Homge, M., Redner, A., Gray, J., and Pinkel, D. (1990) Detection of BCR-ABL fusion in chronic myelogeneous leukemia by two-color fluorescence in situ hybridization. *Science* **250,** 559–562.

38. Nederlof, P. M., Robinson, D., Abuknesha, R., Wiegant, J., Hopman, A. H. N., Tanke, H. J., and Raap, A. K. (1989) Three-color fluorescence in situ hybridization for the simultaneous detection of multiple nucleic acid sequences. *Cytometry* **10,** 20–27.

39. Nederlof, P. M., van der Flier, S., Wiegant, J., Raap, A. K., Tanke, H. J., Ploem, J. S., and van der Ploeg, M. (1990) Multiple fluorescence in situ hybridization. *Cytometry* **11,** 126–131.

40. Ried, T., Baldini, A., Rand, T. C., and Ward, D. C. (1992) Simultaneous visualization of seven different DNA probes by in situ hybridization using combinatorial fluorescence and digital imaging microscopy. *Proc. Natl. Acad. Sci. USA* **89,** 1388–1392.

41. Emmerich, P., Jauch, A., Hofmann, M.-C., Cremer, T., and Walt, H. (1989) Interphase cytogenetics in paraffin embedded sections from human testicular

germ cell tumor xenografts and in corresponding cultured cells. *Lab. Investigation* **61,** 235–242.

42. Hopman, A. H. N., Ramaekers, F. C. S., Raap, A. K., Beck, J. L. M., Devilee, P., van der Ploeg, M., and Vooijs, G. P. (1988) In situ hybridization as a tool to study numerical chromosome aberrations in solid bladder tumors. *Histochemistry* **89,** 307–316.

43. Hopman, A. H. N., Poddighe, P. J., Smeets, W. A. G. B., Moesker, O., Beck, J. L. M., Vooijs, G. P., and Ramaekers, F. C. S. (1989) Detection of numerical chromosome aberrations in bladder cancer by in situ hybridization. *Am. J. Pathol.* **135,** 1105–1117.

44. Arnoldus, E. P. J., Noordermeer, I. A., Peters, A. C. B., Voormolen, J. H. C., Bots, G. T. A. M., Raap, A. K., and van der Ploeg, M. (1991) Interphase cytogenetics of brain tumors. *Genes, Chromosomes & Cancer* **3,** 101–107.

45. Baldino, F. and Lewis, M. E. (1989) Non-radioactive in situ hybridization histochemistry with digoxigenin-dUTP labeled oligonucleotides, in *Methods in Neuroscience* (Conn, P. M., ed.) Academic, New York.

46. Lo, Y.-M. D., Mehal, W. Z., and Fleming, K. A. (1988) Rapid production of vector-free biotinylated probes using the polymerase chain reaction. *Nucleic Acids Res.* **16,** 8719.

47. Weier, H.-U. G., Segraves, R., Pinkel, D., and Gray, J. W. (1990) Synthesis of Y chromosome-specific labeled DNA probes by in vitro DNA amplification. *J. Histochem. Cytochem.* **38,** 421–426.

48. Langer, P. R., Waldrop, A. A., and Ward, D. C. (1981) Enzymatic synthesis of biotin-labeled polynucleotides: novel nucleic acid affinity probes. *Proc. Natl. Acad. Sci. USA* **78,** 6633–6637.

49. Albertson, D. G. (1985) Mapping muscle protein genes by in situ hybridization using biotin labeled probes. *EMBO J.* **4,** 2493–2498.

50. Lawrence, J. B. and Singer, R. H. (1985) Quantitative analysis of in situ hybridization methods for the detection of actin gene expression. *Nucleic Acids Res.* **13,** 1777–1799.

51. Lawrence, J. B., Villnave, C. A., and Singer, R. H. (1988) Interphase chromatin and chromosome gene mapping by fluorescence detection of in situ hybridization reveals the presence and orientation of two closely integrated copies of EBV in a human lymphoblastoid cell line. *Cell* **52,** 51–61.

52. Pinkel, D., Straume, T., and Gray, J. W. (1986) Cytogenetic analysis using quantitative, high sensitivity, fluorescence hybridization. *Proc. Natl. Acad. Sci. USA* **83,** 2934–2938.

53. Raap, A. K., Marijnen, J. G. J., Vrolijk, J., and van der Ploeg, M. (1986) Denaturation, renaturation, and loss of DNA during in situ hybridization procedures. *Cytometry* **7,** 235–242.

54. Ried, T., Lengauer, C., Lipp, M., Fischer, C., Cremer, C., and Ward, D. C. (1993) *DNA and Cell Biology,* in press.

Chapter 26

Alu- and L1-Primed PCR-Generated Probes for Nonisotopic *in Situ* Hybridization

John Gosden, Matthew Breen, and Diane Lawson

1. Introduction

Hybrid cells are proving to be an important resource in the genetic analysis of chromosome regions. These hybrids may take the form of fusions between somatic cells from different genera, followed by selection for specific chromosome markers (somatic cell hybrids—*see* Chapter 17), the introduction of individual chromosomes into host cells of a different genus, and selection for the expression of specific genes (chromosome-mediated gene transfer, CMGT—*see* Chapter 20), or the introduction of a fragment of a mouse or human chromosome into a vector that can replicate as a chromosome in yeast cells (yeast artificial chromosomes, YACs—*see* Chapter 21). The donated material carried by the host cell can range from a small fragment of a chromosome (100 kbp to 1 or 2 Mbp) in a YAC to one or more complete chromosomes in the somatic cell hybrids. The donated material is known as a transgenome. In each of these cases, in order for the hybrid cell line to be of value as a resource for studying aspects of the human genome, it is essential that the precise chromosome composition of the transgenome is ascertained. The use of Southern hybridization to identify specific DNA segments carried by the transgenome is relatively straightforward (*see* Chapter 20). However, this method

From: *Methods in Molecular Biology, Vol. 29: Chromosome Analysis Protocols*
Edited by: J. R. Gosden Copyright ©1994 Humana Press Inc., Totowa, NJ

can only answer specific questions; in order to find out precisely which regions of the donor transgenome are present in the host cell, a different approach is needed. Cytogenetic analysis is of limited use, since host and donor chromosome material may be involved in complex translocations. In some cases, it has proven possible to answer the question by using the whole hybrid genome as a probe for *in situ* hybridization to normal chromosomes from the donor species. In many cases, the transgenome forms a very small part of the hybrid cell, and the concentration of transgenome DNA sequences is often too low to give efficient hybridization kinetics. In such cases, it is possible to use the polymerase chain reaction (PCR) *(1)* to amplify the transgenome sequences independently of the host DNA, by using primers derived from dispersed repeated DNA sequences present only in the donor genome. The most valuable of these sequences in the analysis of human transgenomes have proven to be the *Alu (2)* and L1 or *Kpn (3)* families.

The *Alu* and L1 sequences are the major representatives of the short interspersed repeat (SINES) and long interspersed repeat (LINES) sequences, respectively. The *Alu* family consists of approx 10^6 copies of a 300-bp sequence spaced approximately every 4 kb in the human genome *(4)*. Although repetitive sequences homologous to the human *Alu* repeats are found in rodent genomes, they are sufficiently diverged to permit the design of human-specific primers for PCR. The L1 family consists of 10^4–10^5 copies of either complete or truncated versions of a 6-kbp sequence *(5)*. Because the *Alu* and L1 sequences are interspersed with unique sequences, primers located near the ends of the repeated sequence and initiating replication through the end of the sequence (*see* Table 1) will amplify those unique sequences in the template DNA that are adjacent to *Alu* or L1 sequences. Using a number of different primers for each type of interspersed repeat sequence in single primer reactions gives the greatest chance of amplifying the majority of the unique sequences. Of course, part of the repeated sequences will be amplified as well, and it is necessary to compete these out of any hybridization reaction before the unique, chromosome-specific signal can be detected.

The product of each PCR will be detected on an agarose gel as one or more bands, each band representing a different initiation and termination site for the polymerase enzyme (and thus a different annealing site for the primer). Although each band may be only one or a few

Table 1
Sequences of Oligonucleotide Primers Used in *Alu* and L1 PCR

Name	Origin	Sequence
450 (19-mer)	*Alu*, 5' end of consensus	AAAGTGCTGGGATTACAGG
153 (21-mer)	*Alu*, 5' end of consensus	GTGGCTCACGCCTGTAATCCC
451 (26-mer)	*Alu*, 3' end of consensus	GTGAGCCGAGATCGCGCCACT GCACT
154 (21-mer)	*Alu*, 3' end of consensus	TGCACTCCAGCCTGGGCAACA
B201 (30-mer)	L1 (L1H, ref. *9*)	CATGGCACATGTATACATAT GTAAC(AI')AACC
B390 (21-mer)	Human L1(A)	CACAGGAAGCGGAACATCACA
B392 (21-mer)	Human L1(B)	GGGGAG(3GATAGCATTAGGAG

hundred base pairs in length, the sum of all the different primed reactions will be several kilobase pairs in length, and, even after eliminating the repeated sequences by competition, there will be enough unique sequences left to provide an easily detected signal in an *in situ* hybridization. This interspersed repeated sequence PCR (IRS-PCR; *6*) is proving the method of choice for analyzing the human chromosome composition of all sorts of hybrid cell lines, from those that contain a tiny fraction of a human chromosome (as in YACs) to those that contain a number of different human chromosome fragments. Design of the primers for the PCR process is critical, and we have found the OLIGO program *(7,8)* invaluable for this.

2. Materials

2.1. Polymerase Chain Reaction

1. 2'-Deoxyadenosine 5'-triphosphate (dATP) (Pharmacia, Brussels, Belgium).
2. 2'-Deoxycytosine 5-triphosphate (dCTP) (Pharmacia).
3. 2'-Deoxyguanosine 5'-triphosphate (dGTP) (Pharmacia).
4. 2'-Deoxythymidine 5-triphosphate (TTP) (Pharmacia).
5. 5-(*N*-[*N*-biotinyl-ε-amino-caproyl]-3-amino-allyl)uridine 5'-triphosphate (Bio-dUTP) (Sigma) (*see* Note 1).
6. The products of the PCR reaction may be labeled with biotin in one of two ways: either by nick translation of the pooled PCR products (*see* [a]), or by direct incorporation of Bio-dUTP in the PCR reaction mix (*see* [b]). (*See* Note 2).

   Either (a) mix equimolar amounts of the first four dNTPs to make a 10 m*M* dNTP stock, and label the products by nick translation (*see* Section 2.2.), or (b) mix equimolar amounts of the first three dNTPs with a mixture of TTP and Bio-dUTP (2:1) to make a 10 mM dNTP stock, which will produce a biotin-labeled product. Store at −20°C.

7. *Taq*I DNA polymerase (Promega, Madison, WI) (store at −20°C).
8. 10X *Taq* buffer (Promega) (store at −20°C).
9. Template DNA at 100 ng/μL.
10. Oligonucleotide primer DNA at 250 ng/μL (*see* Note 3 and Table 1).
11. Deionized, double-distilled water.
12. PCR Machine (programs are given for the Cetus and Hybaid machines. Other machines will need calibration to compare temperature response profiles).

2.2. Labeling PCR Products with Biotin by Nick Translation

1. 10X nick buffer; 0.5M Tris-HCl, pH 7.8, 0.05M MgCl$_2$, 0.01M β-mercaptoethanol, 50 μg/mL BSA.
2. 0.5 mM dATP, dCTP, dGTP (diluted from same stock as used for PCR).
3. Bio-16 dUTP (BCL, Mannheim, Germany).
4. DNase I (electrophoretically pure) 1 mg/mL.
5. DNA Polymerase 1.
6. Stop buffer, 300 mM Na$_2$EDTA, pH 8, 1 μL 5% SDS.
7. TNE; 0.2M NaCl, 10 mM Tris-HCl pH 8.0, 1mM EDTA.
8. Nick column (Pharmacia).

2.3. Assay for Biotin Incorporation

1. Buffer A: 0.1M Tris-HCl, pH 7.5, 1X SSC (diluted from 20X SSC stock—*see* Section 2.4.1.).
2. Buffer B: 0.1M Tris-HCl, pH 7.5, 1X SSC, 3% BSA fraction V.
3. Buffer C: 0.1M Tris-HCl, pH 9.5, 1X SSC, 50 mM MgCl$_2$.
4. Stop buffer: 0.01M Tris-HCl, pH 7.5, 1 mM EDTA.
5. Streptavidin-alkaline phosphatase (Streptavidin-AP).
6. Alkaline phosphatase substrate kit IV (Vector Labs, Burlingame, CA).

2.4. In Situ *Hybridization*

1. 20X SSC: 3M NaCl, 0.3M trisodium citrate.
2. Ribonuclease A: 10 mg/mL in 2X SSC, boiled 5 min to inactivate DNase (Store at 4°C).
3. Formamide (Analar) deionized with Amberlite resin (BDH, Poole, Dorset, UK). Shake 500 mL formamide with 20 g Amberlite. Allow to settle and carefully decant off, leaving resin as a precipitate.
4. Dextran sulfate.

5. Hybridization mix:
    50% Formamide;
    10% Dextran;
    10% 20X SSC;
    0.1% Tween 20;
6. Proteinase K: 1 mg/mL in 2 mM CaCl, 20 mM Tris-HCl, pH 7.5 (Store at 4°C).
7. Sonicated salmon sperm DNA: 10 mg/mL (Store at 4°C).
8. Cot-1 human DNA (Life Technologies Inc., Gaithersburg, MD).
9. Rubber solution (e.g., Tip-Top, Stahlgruber, D-8011 Poing, Germany) (*see* Note 4).
10. Constant temperature annealing environment at 37°C (water bath or incubator).
11. Slides carrying human metaphase chromosome spreads, made as described in Chapter 1, not more than 2 wk old (*see* Note 5).
12. Water bath at 70°C.
13. Water bath at 45°C.

2.5. Detection

1. Wash buffer: 4X SSC, 0.05% Triton X-100. Make fresh as required.
2. Blocking buffer: wash buffer plus 5% skimmed milk powder. Make fresh each time.
3. Avidin DCS-FITC (Vector Labs).
4. Biotinylated anti-Avidin (Vector Labs).
5. Propidium iodide.
6. 4',6-Diamidino-2-phenylindole (DAPI).
7. Citifluor AF3 (Citifluor).
8. Glycerol for fluorescence microscpy (Merck, Poole, Dorset, UK).
9. Microscope equipped for epi-illumination with UV, and filters suitable for FITC (fluorescein) and propidium iodide.

3. Methods

3.1. Polymerase Chain Reaction

All materials and equipment must be scrupulously clean and sterile. It is as well to keep a separate set of micropipets, microcentrifuge tubes, and so on, for PCR, to reduce the risk of contamination. In each 0.5-mL microcentrifuge tube (Sigma), put 5 μL 10X *Taq* buffer, 1 μL 10 mM dNTP mix, 100 ng hybrid cell DNA, and 250 ng of one oligonucleotide primer (*see* Table 1). Mix and add 1 U *Taq* I DNA polymerase and sterile deionized, double-distilled water to a total of 50 μL. Mix again, and overlay with two drops of

Table 2
Programs for *Alu* and L1 PCR on Cetus or Hybaid Machines

Denature	Anneal	Extend
Cetus:		
94°C, 3 min	60°C, 1 min	72°C, 1 min × 1 cycle
92°C, 45 s	60°C, 1 min	72°C, 1 min + 6 s each cycle × 35 cycles
92°C, 45 s	60°C, 1 min	72°C, 10 min
Hybaid:		
94°C, 2.5 min	65°C, 1 min	72°C, 1 min × 1 cycle
92°C, 20 s	65°C, 1 min	72°C, 1 min × 5 cycles
92°C, 20 s	65°C, 1 min	72°C, 1.5 min × 5 cycles
92°C, 20 s	65°C, 1 min	72°C, 2 min × 5 cycles
92°C, 20 s	65°C, 1 min	72°C, 2.5 min × 5 cycles
92°C, 20 s	65°C, 1 min	72°C, 3 min × 5 cycles
92°C, 20 s	65°C, 1 min	72°C, 3.5 min × 5 cycles
92°C, 20 s	65°C, 1 min	72°C, 4 min × 7 cycles

heavy white mineral oil (Sigma). Place in the PCR machine, and set program for the appropriate temperature cycle as shown in Table 2. The products of typical reactions are shown in Figs. 1 and 2. The products of all the PCR reactions from one hybrid cell DNA are pooled, and precipitated by the addition of 2 vol of absolute ethanol and incubation at –20°C for at least 1 h. The suspension is then centrifuged for 5 min to collect the DNA precipitate, the excess ethanol decanted (carefully), and the residue evaporated to dryness. The DNA is then dissolved in 20 µL of 100 m*M* Tris-HCl, pH 7.5, and 10 m*M* EDTA; 1 µL of the dissolved DNA is run on an agarose gel, together with a dilution series of a standard DNA to measure the concentration of the pooled PCR products.

3.2. Biotin Labeling PCR Products by Nick Translation

1. In a 1.5-mL microcentrifuge tube place:
   2 µL 10X nick buffer;
   2.5 µL 0.5 m*M* dATP, dCTP, dGTP (Pharmacia) (diluted from 100 m*M* stock);
   2.5 µL bio-16-dUTP (BCL);
   0.5–1.0 µg DNA;
   1 µL DNase I (1 mg/mL diluted 1 µL/500 µL H₂O); and
   H₂O to 19 µL.

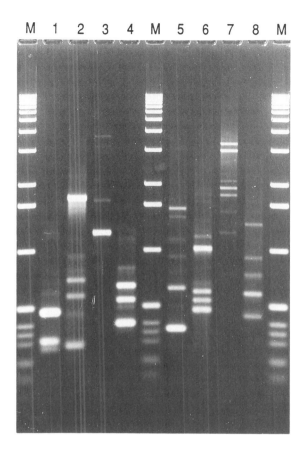

Fig. 1. Agarose gel electrophoresis of amplification products obtained by *Alu* PCR of two YAC recombinants, E5 (lanes 1–4) and E3 (lanes 5–8), each with four different *Alu* primers. Lanes 1 and 5, primer 450, lanes 2 and 6, primer 153, lanes 3 and 7, primer 451, lanes 4 and 8, primer 154. For details of the primers, *see* Table 1. M denotes size markers.

2. Whirlimix briefly and centrifuge to collect.
3. Add DNA Polymerase 1 1.0 μL.
4. Mix by hand and centrifuge to collect.
5. Incubate 1.5 h + at 15°C (can be left overnight at 4°C if more convenient).
6. Add 5 μL stop buffer (300 m*M* Na$_2$EDTA, pH 8), 1 μL 5% SDS, and 25 μL TNE. Whirlimix briefly, spin to collect, and load onto a "NICK" column (Pharmacia) developed in TNE. Elute with 2X 400 μL TNE and collect second fraction.

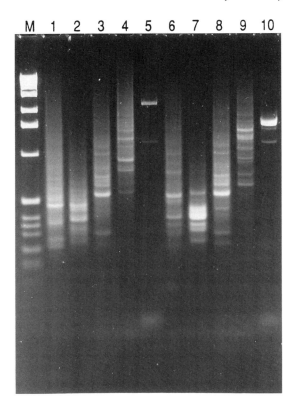

Fig. 2. Agarose gel electrophoresis of amplification products obtained by *Alu* and L1 PCR of two hybrid cell-lines, EJNAC (lanes 1–5) and E67-1 (lanes 6–10). Lanes 1 and 6, primer 153, lanes 2 and 7, primer 154, lanes 3 and 8, primer 450, lanes 4 and 9, primer 451, lanes 5 and 10, primer B201. For details of the primers *see* Table 1. M denotes size markers.

7. Add 10 µL sonicated salmon sperm DNA (10 mg/mL), 50 µL 3*M* ammonium acetate, mix, and fill Eppendorf tube with EtOH. Chill for 1 h at –20°C, spin for 5 min, decant supernatant, and dry precipitate in lyophilizer. Dissolve in 100 µL TE (TE: 10 m*M* Tris-HCl, pH 7.5, 1 m*M* EDTA). Assay for incorporation as described in Section 3.3. Store frozen at –20°C.

3.3. Assay for Biotin Incorporation

1. Make serial 10-fold dilutions of biotin-labeled DNA in 10X SSC, spot 1 µL of each on nitrocellulose filter (**Not nylon!**), and bake 2 h at 80°C in vacuum oven. Store dry in sealed plastic bag until convenient. Run similar dilutions of nick-translated biotin-labeled salmon sperm DNA in parallel to provide a standard.

2. Soak filter for 5 min in buffer A.
3. Incubate in buffer B for 30 min at room temperature.
4. Dilute Streptavidin-AP 1:1000 (5 µL/5 mL) in buffer B, seal filter in plastic bag with SV-AP, and reincubate for 30 min at room temperature, squeezing occasionally.
5. Wash 3 × 5 min in buffer A.
6. Wash 1 × 5 min in buffer C.
7. Make up substrate from Vector AP substrate kit IV in 5 mL buffer C.
8. Incubate in sealed bag in dark. Color develops for up to 3 h (can be left overnight if convenient).
9. Wash in 20 mL stop buffer for 5 min. Wrap filter in Clingfilm, and photocopy. Store filter in refrigerator in dark.

3.4. In Situ *Hybridization*

3.4.1. Slides

1. Slides should be between 1 and 2 wk old. Older slides may need to be treated with RNase and Proteinase K as detailed below (steps 2–5), but slides <2 wk old need only be passed through an alcohol series before denaturation (i.e., start at step 6).
2. RNase 1 h at 37°C in 100 µg/mL RNase in 2X SSC.
3. Pass through ethanol series (70, 90, 100%), 3 min each step. Dry.
4. Prewarm on tray for 5 min at 37°C before putting into Proteinase K.
5. Proteinase K 60 ng/mL for 2 min at 37°C.
6. Pass through ethanols (70, 90, 100%). Dry.
7. Prewarm at 70°C for 5 min in metal rack on tray before denaturing.
8. Denature 3 min in 70% Formamide, 2X SSC at 70°C.
9. Into **ice-cold** 70% EtOH, then 90 and 100% room temperature. Dry.

3.4.2. Probe

1. Make up reaction mixes by putting an appropriate amount of each of three DNAs (labeled probe [pooled PCR products], competitor [human Cot1 DNA], and salmon sperm DNA) in a 1.5-mL microcentrifuge tube, mixing, and adding 2.5–3 vol EtOH, chilling quickly, spinning down, and drying on a spin drier. Add 10 µL of hybridization mix (*see* step 2) to each tube, and then let stand for at least 1 h at room temperature to ensure that the probe has dissolved.
2. The precise ratio of competitor to probe DNA can only be determined empirically. However, a reasonable starting point is 10:1, and a typical hybridization would contain (in 10 µL): 150 ng labeled pooled PCR DNA; 1.5 µg Cot1 DNA; 5 µg sonicated salmon sperm DNA in 2X SCC; 50% formamide.

3.4.3. Preannealing

Dissolved probe is denatured at 75°C for 5–10 min, and incubated at 37°C for 15 min. Other probes (e.g., chromosome-specific alphoid) can be denatured and added after this stage.

3.4.4. Hybridization

1. Slides and coverslips are prewarmed at 37°C for 5 min.
2. Transfer dissolved, preannealed probe to a prewarmed coverslip (20 × 20 mm), pick up on a prewarmed slide, seal with rubber solution, and put in hybridization tray *immediately* (without waiting for rubber solution to dry).
3. Incubate overnight at 37°C.

3.4.5. Washes

1. Washes are in 50% formamide, 2X SSC at 45°C, 4 × 3 min; 2X SSC 4 × 3 min. Use 250 mL of wash solution in a stain dish (or 50 mL in a Coplin jar if there are only one or two slides), prewarmed to 45°C, for each wash. Be careful **not** to remove coverslip before first wash. Peel off rubber solution, but let coverslip soak off in first wash.
2. Transfer slides to 4X SSC, 0.05% Triton X-100.

3.5. Detection

1. Treat with blocking buffer, 40 µL/slide for 5 min at room temperature under 20 × 40 mm coverslips.
2. Remove coverslips, drain excess fluid, and apply first antibody: FITC-avidin DCS from Vector. Stock concentration is 2 mg/mL. Make 4 µg/mL in blocking buffer (i.e., 2 µL in 1.0 mL). Use 40 µL/slide. Replace same coverslips. Incubate 30 min at 37°C in moist chamber.
3. Wash 3 × 2 min in 4X SSC, 0.05% Triton X-100 at 45°C.
4. Drain excess fluid and apply second antibody: biotinylated goat antiavidin (Vector) diluted to 5 µg/mL in blocking buffer. Stock is 0.5 mg/mL, so dilute 1:100. Use 40 µL/slide. Use fresh coverslips, and incubate 30 min at 37°C in moist chamber.
5. Remove coverslips. Wash 3 × 2 min in 4X SSC, 0.05% Triton X-100 at 45°C.
6. Drain excess fluid, and apply third antibody, using fresh coverslips. This is the same as step 2: FITC-avidin DCS from Vector diluted 2 µL in 1.0 mL. Use 40 µL/slide. Incubate 30 min at 37°C.
7. Remove coverslips. Wash 3 × 2 min in 4X SSC, 0.05% Triton X-100 at 45°C.
8. There may be adequate signal at this stage, but we find that it is usually worth adding a third layer of FITC by repeating steps 4–7.
9. Drain excess fluid and mount in Citifluor AF3:Glycerol (1:1) containing 750 ng/mL propidium iodide and 3.75 µg/mL DAPI; blot and seal with rubber solution.

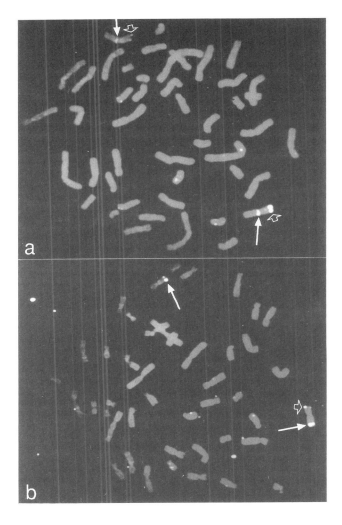

Fig. 3. *In situ* hybridization of pooled *Alu* PCR products of YAC recombinants shown in Fig. 1. **a.** E5. **b.** E3. Open arrows mark site of hybridization of cosInsulIGF2, a marker located at 11p1.5, used to confirm the identity of chromosome 11. Filled arrows mark the site of hybridization of YAC recombinant.

10. Slides are examined under UV fluorescence with appropriate filters for FITC and propidium iodide. The signal is visible as a greenish white dot, band, or region, whereas the chromosomes are R-banded (*see* Chapter 8) by the propidium iodide/DAPI in bright and dull red. The results of *in situ* hybridizations are shown in Figs. 3 and 4.

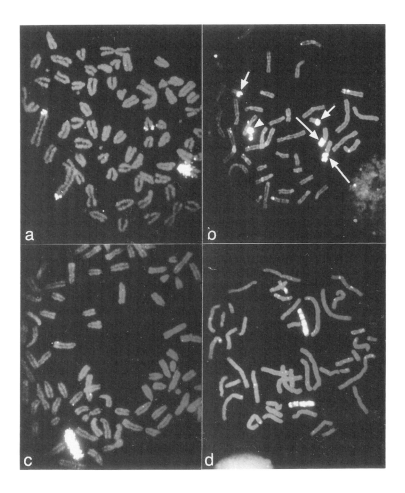

Fig. 4. *In situ* hybridization of (**a** and **c**) biotinylated human Cot-1 fraction DNA to chromosomes of hybrid cell lines; (**b** and **d**) pooled *Alu* PCR products of hybrid cell lines shown in Fig. 2. **a** and **b** show the cell line EJNAC, with four human chromosome fragments detected in the hybrid by Cot-1 hybridization (a) and three distinct chromosomes identified as the source of the fragments by hybridization of the *Alu* PCR products (b), including 11p (large arrow), 19p (small arrow), and the Y (arrowhead). c and d show the cell line E67-1, with a single fragment detected by Cot-1 hybridization (c), which is shown to be derived exclusively from chromosome 11 by *Alu* PCR hybridization (d).

4. Notes

1. Bio-dUTP from Sigma may be dissolved in sterile, deionized, double-distilled water at a concentration of 20 mM (1 mg in 55 μL).
2. Where PCR reactions have previously been carried out, and the products characterized, it is possible to eliminate one step by incorporating the biotin label in the PCR mix (*see* Section 2.1., step 6). However, until the parameters of the specific PCR have been established, it is better to perform the PCR, characterize the products by running an aliquot on a 1.5% agarose minigel, pool the successful reaction products, and label them by nick translation (*see* Sections 2.2. and 3.2.).
3. Oligonucleotides can be synthesized on an Applied Biosystems DNA Synthesizer Model 381A according to the manufacturer's instructions. Details of the sequences that we have used successfully are given in Table 1.
4. The type of rubber solution is important. Some leave a residue on the slide, which is spread across it by later treatments and can affect the result of the hybridization reaction. It is worth persevering to find a make that gives a good seal and is removed cleanly.
5. As in the PRINS reaction (Chapter 18), the age of the slides is critical. Slides should be between 1 and 2 wk old. Chromosome suspensions may be stored in methanol:acetic acid (3:1) at –20°C for 2 or 3 mo, and fresh slides made as required. After dropping the suspensions on acid:alcohol cleaned slides, they are incubated for 1 h in methanol:acetic acid (3:1), air-dried, and treated for 10 min in acetone. They are then air-dried again and stored in an evacuated dessicator for up to 2 wk. Older slides may need to be treated with RNase and Proteinase K as detailed in refs. *2–5,* but slides <2 wk old need only be passed through an alcohol series before denaturation.

References

1. Saiki, R. K., Scharf, S. J., Faloona, F., Mullis, K. B., Horn, G. T., Ehrlich, H. A., and Arnheim, N. (1985) Enzymatic amplification of beta-globin genomic sequences and restriction site analysis of diagnosis of sickle cell anemia. *Science* **230,** 1350–1354.
2. Bains, W. (1986) The multiple origins of human Alu sequences. *J. Mol. Evol.* **23,** 189–199.
3. Scott, A. F., Schmeckpeper, B. J., Abdelrazik, M., Comey, C. T., O'Hara, B., Rossiter, J. P., Cooley, T., Heath, P., Smith, K. D., and Margolet, L. (1987) Origin of the human L1 elements: proposed progenitor genes deduced from a consensus sequence. *Genomics* **1,** 113–125.

4. Britten, R. J., Baron, W. F., Stout, D. B., and Davidson, E. H. (1988) Sources and evolution of human Alu repeated sequences. *Proc. Natl. Acad. Sci. USA* **85,** 4770–1774.

5. Singer, M. F. and Skowronski, J. (1985) Making sense out of LINES: long interspersed repeat sequences in mammalian genomes. *Trends Biochem. Sci.* **10,** 119–122.

6. Lichter, P., Ledbetter, S. A., Ledbetter, D. H., and Ward, D. C. (1990) Fluorescence *in situ* hybridization with *Alu* and L1 polymerase chain reaction probes for rapid characterization of human chromosomes in hybrid cell lines. *Proc. Natl. Acad. Sci. USA* **87,** 6634–6638.

7. Rychlik, W. and Rhoads, R. E. (1989) A computer program for choosing optimal oligonucleotides for filter hybridization, sequencing and *in vitro* amplification of DNA. *Nucleic Acids. Res.* **17,** 8543–8551.

8. Rychlik, W., Spencer, W. J., and Rhoads, R. E. (1990) Optimization of the annealing temperature for DNA amplification in vitro. *Nucleic Acids Res.* **18,** 6409–6412.

9. Ledbetter, S. A., Nelson, D. L., Warren, S. T., and Ledbetter, D. H. (1990) Rapid isolation of DNA probes within specific chromosome regions by interspersed repetitive sequence polymerase chain reaction. *Genomics* **6,** 475–481.

CHAPTER 27

Chromosome Substructure Investigation

Telomeres

Robin C. Allshire and Howard J. Cooke

1. Introduction

Telomeres are the specialized structures that define chromosome ends and have been the subject of several recent reviews *(1–5)*. Telomeres allow a linear replication unit to be maintained as a linear molecule and overcome the end replication problem. The telomere must also distinguish a bona fide chromosome end from ends derived from an interstitial chromosome break, since broken chromosome ends are unstable. Most telomeres isolated to date are composed of tandem repetitive sequence arrays that are generally rich in T and G residues, for example, the vertebrate repeat is $(TTAGGG)_n(6)$ and that of many plants appears to be $(TTTAGGG)_n(7)$. Telomeres are synthesized by telomerase, identified in ciliates and mammalian cells, which adds on additional terminal repeats to a preexisting telomere (reviewed in *2–5*). It is these repetitive sequences that form a functional telomere.

Because telomeres have been found to terminate with a 3' overhanging end they must first be treated with exonucleases, such as *Bal*31 to give clean, blunt, clonable ends. The repetitive nature of telomeres makes them difficult substrates for cloning in *E. coli,* since they are prone to deletion and rearrangement, although telomeres have been cloned in *E. coli (8)*. However, for genome-mapping purposes, it is advantageous to isolate sizable fragments of DNA adjacent to telomeres.

From: *Methods in Molecular Biology, Vol. 29: Chromosome Analysis Protocols*
Edited by: J. R. Gosden Copyright ©1994 Humana Press Inc., Totowa, NJ

An alternative method of cloning telomeres from an organism where they have not previously been characterized is by functional complementation in the budding yeast *Saccharomyces cerevisiae*. This strategy is based on the observation that telomeric repeats from several organisms function as telomeres when placed at the end of a linearized episome in yeast *(9)*. Indeed, the original YAC vectors for cloning large DNA in yeast utilize arrays of $(TTGGGG)_n$ terminal repeats from *Tetrahymena thermophila* as seeds for the addition of the yeast telomere repeat $(TG_{1-3})_n$ *(10)*. Here we present protocols used for the cloning of human telomeres. This method should be applicable to cloning telomeres from most organisms. The method is often referred to as "half YAC" or "one armed YAC" cloning. There have been several recent publications that report the cloning of human telomeres on half YACs. These should be referred to in conjunction with this chapter *(11–15)*.

The scheme for cloning a telomere on a half YAC can be divided into three parts, as shown in Fig. 1:

1. Enrichment for telomeres and ligation to vector;
2. Transformation of *S. cerevisiae* spheroplasts and screening for telomere clones; and
3. Recovery of telomere subclone from yeast and analyses.

The exact details of the enrichment strategy will vary depending on the size of telomeric arrays in an organism and on how much telomere flanking DNA one wishes to clone. Here we present an enrichment strategy suitable for isolating short regions of telomere-flanking DNA from human telomeres. However, several other enrichment strategies have been reported *(11–15)*.

2. Solutions and Media

1. YEPD: Yeast extract 10 g, peptone 20 g, glucose 20 g: Make up to 1 L for routine growth under nonselective conditions. For plates, add agar 20 g/L.
2. CAS-MM (–Trp – Ura): Yeast nitrogen base (without amino acids): 1.7 g, glucose 20 g, casamino acids 11 g, ammonium sulfate 5.0 g, tyrosine 0.1 g, adenine 0.1 g: Make up to 1 L. This is a supplemented minimal medium used for the selection of Trp⁺Ura⁺ transformants. For Sorbitol plates, add agar 20 g/L and sorbitol 182 g/L.
3. Top –Trp –Ura agar: CAS-MM (*as above*), sorbitol 182 g, and agar 30 g/L. For Top +Trp + Ura agar, add 150 µL of 10 mg/mL trytophan and uracil to 15 mL item 2.

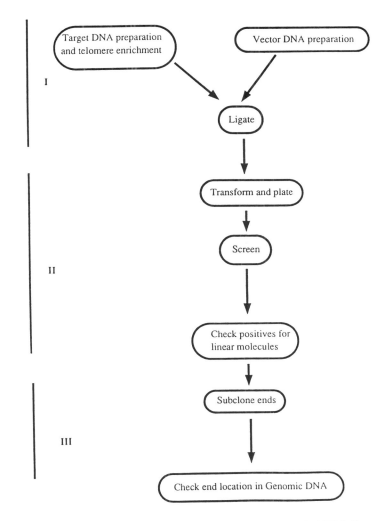

Fig. 1. Scheme for closing a telomere on a half YAC.

4. Sorbitol (1.0*M*): 182 g/L.
5. PEG: Polyethyleneglycol 4000: 44 g/L.
6. STC: 2*M* Sorbitol 100 mL, 100 m*M* CaCl₂ 20 mL, 100 m*M* Tris-HCl, pH 7.6, 20 mL, dH₂O 80 mL.
7. Lyticase (Sigma, St. Louis, MO): Resuspend at 50,000 U in 2 mL of TE.
8. SOS: YEPD 25 mL, 2*M* sorbitol 55 mL, 100 m*M* CaCl₂ 10 mL, 100 μg/mL tryptophan 10 mL, and 100 μg/mL uracil 10 mL.
9. SCE: 1*M* Sorbitol, 100 m*M* sodium citrate, 60 m*M* EDTA, pH 7.0.

10. Lipofectin: This was purchased from Gibco BRL (Paisley, Scotland) as a 1 mg/mL suspension.
11. Quick Hyb: Bovine serum albumin 0.5 g, polyvinylpropylene 0.5 g, Ficoll 0.5 g, SDS 1.0 g, pyrophosphate 1.0 g, and 20X SSC 250 mL. Make up to 1 L.
12. Calf intestinal phosphatase: This was purchased from Boehringer (Mannheim, Germany).
13. *Bal*31 exonuclease: This was purchased from Gibco BRL, 1X *Bal*31 buffer is 0.65M NaCl, 20 mM Tris-HCl, pH 8.1, 10 mM MgCl$_2$, 10 mM CaCl$_2$, 1 mM EDTA.

3. Methods

3.1. Preparation of Target Genomic DNA and Size Fractionation of Telomeres

1. Prepare genomic DNA from mammalian cells by standard methods, which give high-mol-wt DNA (*16* and *see* vol. 4 of this series).
2. Digest DNA to completion with the enzyme chosen under appropriate conditions. *See* Note 1 for a discussion of enzyme choice.
3. Southern blot an aliquot of this digested DNA after gel electrophoresis under suitable conditions (*see* Chapters 14, 20, and 24). The size of the terminal-repeat-containing fragments is determined by hybridization with a γ–[^{32}P]-labeled oligonucleotide probe prepared by standard methods, hybridized by standard methods in "Quick Hyb" at 55°C, and washed in 4X SSC at 65°C.
4. Where the bulk of the DNA migrates in a different size range from the fragments that hybridize to the telomeric-repeat probe, size fractionation can be used. Cut the region from a preparative low-melting-point agarose gel, and recover DNA from the gel using a standard method.

3.2. Vector DNA Preparation

1. Prepare vector plasmid DNA from bacterial cultures by normal CsCl/EtBr gradient methods (*16* and *see* vol. 2 of this series).
2. Digest 50 μg of vector DNA with the appropriate restriction enzyme under recommended conditions, and check digestion on an agarose gel. Inactivate enzyme, and recover DNA by ethanol precipitation.
3. Dephosphorylate DNA with calf intestinal phosphatase according to the manufacturer's instructions (*see* ref. *16*).
4. Inactivate the phosphatase by adding SDS to 1% and proteinase K to 50 μg/mL.
5. Incubate at 50°C for 60 min, and phenol extract once. Ethanol precipitate the DNA from the supernatant, and dry under vacuum. Redissolve and determine the concentration of the solution.

3.3. Ligation

1. Determine the concentration of the target DNA, and add a five-to 10-fold molar excess of digested vector to it. The final DNA concentration for a 20-kb fragment should be 100 μg/mL.
2. Add T4 ligase and ligase buffer as recommended by the manufacturer, and incubate for 16 h at 15°C.
3. Heat inactivate the reaction at 65°C for 15 min, and freeze at –20°C prior to transformation.

3.4. Transformation
of S. cerevisiae Spheroplasts

3.4.1. Strains

The *S. cerevisiae* strain AB1380 (*MAT* α, Φ⁺ *ura*3 *trp*1 *ade*2-1 *can*1-100 *lys*2-1 *his*5; ref. *10*) can be used to clone telomeres on half YACs.

3.4.2. Preparation and Transformation
of Spheroplasts

This method is based on that described by Burgers and Percival *(17)*, but *see* McCormick et al. *(18)* for another variation.

1. Inoculate 100 mL of YEPD with a single colony of yeast strain (AB1380). Grow to a density of approx 3×10^7 cells/mL (OD 660 nm = 24 OD U). Overgrowth of cells will inhibit spheroplast formation.
2. Harvest cells in sterile 50-mL Falcon tubes by centrifugation at 1250*g* for 5 min. Wash the pellets in a total of 50 mL 1.0*M* sorbitol. Resuspend final pellets in a total of 10 mL of 1.0*M* sorbitol (3×10^8 cells/mL).
3. Add 1000 U of Lyticase to 10 mL of cells. Incubate at 30°C for up to 2 h. Monitor the extent of the cell-wall digestion by placing 100-μL samples from the digestion reaction every 20 min into 1 mL of water and 1.0*M* sorbitol. The spheroplasts are ready when the water suspension is clear, whereas the sorbitol suspension remains cloudy. These suspensions should also be inspected by microscopy. High-quality spheroplasts are obtained when >95% of cells lyse in water and between 5–10% lyse in sorbitol (there should be some lysis in sorbitol). The above assay indicates when most of the cell wall has been removed without excessive lysis.
4. Pellet the spheroplasts at 150*g* for 5 min. Wash in 20 mL of STC and pellet. Resuspend in 1 mL of STC.
5. Place 100-μL aliquots of spheroplasts into 4-mL Falcon tubes. Add DNA from ligations and control plasmids. Add 4 μg of sterile calf thymus DNA as carrier. Mix and incubate for 10 min at room temperature (*see* Note 2).

6. Optional step: Transformation efficiency can be increased approx 10-fold by the addition of lipofectin (BRL) *(19)*. Add 100 μL of STC containing 4 μg of lipofectin to the transformation. Incubate at room temperature for an additional 10 min.

7. Add 2 mL of 44% PEG 4000. Mix by invertion. Incubate at room temperature for 15 min.

8. Spin spheroplasts at 150g for 10 min. Remove as much of the PEG solution as possible. Gently resuspend pellet in 150 μL of SOS. Incubate at room temperature for 30 min.

9. Add all (or part of) SOS cell suspension to 10–15 mL aliquots of molten Top – Trp agar preheated to 47.5°C in individual tubes. Mix and pour onto a –TRP sorbitol plate immediately.

10. When top agar has set, incubate plates at 30°C. Colonies should be visible after 2–4 d.

3.4.3. Picking, Replica-Plating, and Hybridization of Yeast Transformants

1. Once all colonies have grown to a reasonable size (3–4 d), they are ready to be picked. Patch colonies onto a CAS-MM –Trp –Ura plates. Incubate at 30°C for 1–2 d. Replica plate patches to sterile nitrocellulose (or other) filters on fresh CAS-MM –Trp –Ura plates. Incubate at 30°C for 16–24 h.

2. Remove filters from plates, and place on 3MM paper soaked in 2 mL of SCE containing 500 U of lyticase and 5 μL of β-mercaptoethanol in a Petri dish. Seal the Petri dishes with Parafilm, and incubate overnight at 37°C.

3. Lyse, denature, and neutralize the yeast cells by placing the filters on 3-mm disk soaked in the following solutions: 10% SDS for 3 min, $0.5M$ NaOH, $1.5M$ NaCl for 10 min, $1.0M$ Tris-HCl, pH 7.5, $1.5M$ NaCl for 5 min, 2X SSC for 5 min.

4. Air-dry the filter, and bake at 80°C for 2 h.

5. The filters are now ready to hybridize with the telomeric-repeat oligonucleotide $(TTAGGG)_n$. The filters are initially prehybridized in Quick Hyb at 55°C for 30 min. Subsequently, the labeled oligonucleotide is added and hybridized at 55°C for 1–4 h. Filters are then washed 4 × 15 min in 4X SSC and 0.1% SDS at 60°C, and autoradiographed. Positive clones are then picked, grown in selective medium, and stored at –70°C as a 25% glycerol stock. For further analyses, DNA should be prepared from positive clones.

3.5. Preparation
of S. cerevisiae *Chromosomal DNA*
in Agarose Plugs

1. Inoculate 10 mL of CAS-MM –Trp –Ura with two colonies. Grow to late-log phase, 20–24 h at 30°C.
2. Harvest cells, and wash pellet twice with 50 mM EDTA, pH 8.
3. Resuspend in 500 µL of SCE + 0.7M β-mercaptoethanol + 1 mg/mL Zymolyase 100T.
4. Mix 500 µL of cell suspension warmed to 37°C with 500 µL of 1.6% low-melting-temperature agarose (prepared in 125 mM EDTA and equilibrated to 42°C).
5. Pour mixture into plug molds, and place on ice.
6. When set, push plugs out of molds directly into a tube containing 2 mL of 450 mM EDTA, pH 9, 10 mM Tris-HCl, pH 8, and 7.5% β-mercaptoethanol. Incubate overnight at 37°C.
7. Remove the above solution, and add 2 mL of 450 mM EDTA, pH 9, 10 mM Tris-HCl, pH 8, 1% N-Lauryl Sarcosine, and 1 mg/mL proteinase K. Incubate for 1–2 d at 50°C.
8. Store blocks at 4°C in above solution without proteinase K.
9. These plugs can the be used to separate all *S. cerevisiae* chromosomes by pulsed-field gel electrophoresis. The YAC containing a cloned telomere from the target DNA can be visualized after Southern blotting by hybridization with the telomere-repeat oligo in Quick Hyb, as described above.

3.6. Yeast DNA Preparation

1. Grow yeast in 500 mL selective medium to A_{600} of about 1.0.
2. Wash by centrifugation 2X 50 mL in dH_2O.
3. Resuspend in 20 mL 1M sorbitol and pellet.
4. Resuspend in 10 mL SCE, add Zymolyase to 0.5 mg/mL, and incubate at 30°C.
5. Sample 0.1 mL at 15 min, and dilute into 0.9 mL 0.5% SDS. When adequately spheroplasted for DNA preparation, the cell suspension will clear. Continue incubation and sampling if the suspension does not clear in 15 min.
6. When sample clears, pellet cells and wash in 1M sorbitol, pellet again, and resuspend in 5 mL 0.05M EDTA, pH 8, 1% SDS, and 200 µg/mL proteinase K. Incubate overnight at 50°C.
7. Phenol extract once, and make the supernatant 0.3M NaOAc. Precipitate the DNA by dropwise addition of 0.6 vol propan-2-ol.

8. Dry the pellet and redissolve in TE.
9. Add RNase to 50 mg/mL, and incubate for 30 min at 37°C. Repeat the propan-2-ol precipitation (*see* Note 3).

3.7. Recovery of Target Telomere End of YAC into E. coli

Strategies for the recovery of the ends of YAC clones all depend on converting the telomeric structure into one that can be ligated. The protocol given below is based on circularization, but other approaches are possible based on adapter oligonucleotide addition and production of a library from the yeast cells. Circularization is possible with all commonly used YAC vectors.

1. Digest yeast DNA with *Bal*31 nuclease. Fifty micrograms of DNA in 200 µL 1X *Bal* buffer (*see below*) are digested with 5 U of *Bal*31, and 5-µg aliquots sampled at 2 min intervals and made 20 m*M* EGTA. Heat to 70°C for 15 min to ensure enzyme inactivation (*see* Note 4).
2. Dilute *Bal* treated DNA to 1 mL in T4 ligase buffer. Add T4 ligase to 5 U/mL, and incubate overnight at 15°C. Recover the DNA by ethanol precipitation, and wash carefully in 70% ethanol to remove any traces of salts.
3. Dissolve in 2–4 µL dH$_2$O, and introduce into *E. coli* either by electroporation *(16)* or by transformation of competent cells (Sure cells, Stratagene, La Jolla, CA).
4. Plate the bacteria, and select on appropriate plates. A single yeast strain should give rise to plasmids that contain the vector used and additional DNA. Early in the time-course of digestion, this additional DNA may contain terminal repeats, both yeast, tetrahymena, and from the species whose telomeres are being cloned. Later time-points should contain the same more proximal sequence but will have less or no terminal repeats.

3.8. Confirmation that "End" Clone Is from a Telomere in Target DNA by Bal31 Time-Course

To test that isolated clones are indeed telomeric in the DNA from which they were isolated, a time-course with *Bal*31 exonuclease can be preformed—*see* Note 4 on *Bal*31. With increasing length of digestion, telomeric-located restriction fragments should be degraded, whereas interstitially located restriction fragments will remain intact (*see* refs. *11–15* for examples).

1. Genomic DNA is treated with *Bal*31 exonuclease. With mammalian DNA, at least 10 μg should be digested/time-point. Make up one reaction mix containing all DNA at a concentration of 200 μg/mL in 1X *Bal*31 buffer. Preincubate at 30°C for 10 min, and then add *Bal*31 to a final concentration of 15 U/mL. An aliquot of the reaction is removed at each time-point and added to 1/10 vol of 200 m*M* EGTA, pH 8.0, to stop the reaction.

2. Each aliquot is then extracted twice with phenol/chloroform and the DNA recovered by ethanol precipitation. The DNA is resuspended in TE and treated with the appropriate restriction endonuclease. The resulting digested DNA is separated by agarose gel electrophoresis, Southern blotted, and hybridized sequentially with putative telomeric clones and control interstitial probes.

4. Notes

1. The choice of restriction enzyme used to cut the genomic DNA determines the amount of subtelomeric sequence that will be cloned, the vector that can be used for cloning, and the possibility of using size-based enrichment protocols. Enzymes that cut infrequently in genomic DNA give telomeric fragments that do not differ appreciably in size from other fragments, whereas enzymes that cut frequently often give rise to telomeric fragments that are much larger than the vast majority of nontelomeric ones.

2. Transformations with an undigested control plasmid, such as pYAC4, and with no plasmid should always be performed. To assess background, the cut but unligated vector fragment from pYAC4NEO should be used. Controls for spheroplast survival and regeneration are also useful. Dilute spheroplasts, after resuspension in 150 μL of SOS, 1:100,000 in SOS, and plate 150 μL (approx 3×10^3) in Top +Trp +Ura Agar. Approximately 10% of cells should survive in high-efficiency transformation. Less than 10% survival suggests too much lysis. Higher survival indicates that spheroplasting reaction was stopped too soon. It is important to ensure that all spheroplasting and transformation solutions are free of contamination with detergents. All glassware used for growth of cells and preparation of spheroplasts and solutions should be rinsed thoroughly with distilled water.

3. Many enzymes used to modify DNA structure are inhibited by RNA. *Bal*31 is one such enzyme, which is frequently used for telomere analysis. If yeast DNA is refractory to such enzymes, an additional step of CsCl/ethidum bromide centrifugation can be used. Protocols used for plasmid DNA centrifugation are applicable.

4. The unit definition and quality of this enzyme are variable. If possible, obtain a subtelomeric probe with which you can check out your particular enzyme. If this is not available, use a defined molecule to test the extent of unwanted side reactions.

References

1. Blackburn, E. H. and Szostak, J. W. (1984) The molecular structure of centromeres and telomeres. *Ann. Rev. Biochem.* **53,** 163–194.
2. Zakian, V. A. (1989) Structure and function of telomeres. *Ann. Rev. Genet.* **23,** 579–604.
3. Greider, C. W. (1990) Telomeres, telomerase and senescence. *BioEssays* **12,** 363–369.
4. Greider, C. W. (1991) Telomeres. *Curr. Opinion Cell Biol.* **3,** 444–451.
5. Blackburn, E. H. (1991) Structure and function of telomeres. *Nature* **350,** 569–573.
6. Meyne, J., Ratliff, R. L., and Moyzis, R. K. (1989) Conservation of the human telomere sequence (TTAGGG)n among vertebrates. *Proc. Natl. Acad. Sci. USA* **86,** 7049–7053.
7. Richards, E. J. and Ausubel, F. M. (1988) Isolation of a higher eukaryotic telomere from *Arabidopsis thaliana. Cell* **53,** 127–136.
8. de Lange, T., Shiue, L., Myers, R. M., Cox, D. R., Naylor, S. L., Killery, A. M., and Varmus, H. E. (1990) Structure and variability of human chromosome ends. *Mol. Cell Biol.* **10,** 518–527.
9. Shampay, J., Szostak, J. W., and Blackburn, E. H. (1984) DNA sequences of telomeres maintained in yeast. *Nature* **310,** 154–157.
10. Burke, D. T., Carle, G. F., and Olson, M. V. (1987) Cloning of segments of exogenous DNA into yeast by means of artificial chromosome vectors. *Science* **236,** 806–812.
11. Cross, S. H., Allshire, R. C., McKay, S. J., McGill, N. I., and Cooke, H. J. (1989) Cloning of human telomeres by complementation in yeast. *Nature* **338,** 771–774.
12. Brown, W. R. A. (1988) Molecular cloning of human telomeres in yeast. *Nature* **338,** 774–776.
13. Reithman, H. C., Moyzis, R. K., Meyne, J., Burke, D. T., and Olson, M. V. (1989) Cloning human telomeric DNA fragments into *Saccharomyces cerevisiae* using a yeast-artificial-chromosome vector. *Proc. Natl. Acad. Sci. USA* **86,** 6240–6244.
14. Cheng, J.-F., Smith, C. L., and Cantor, C. R. (1989) Isolation and characterization of a human telomere. *Nucleic Acids Res.* **17,** 6109–6127.
15. Bates, G. P., MacDonald, M. E., Baxendale, S., Sedlacek, Z., Youngman, S., Romano, D., Whaley, W. L., Allitto, B. A., Poustka, A., Gusella, J. F., and Lehrach, H. (1990) A yeast artificial chromosome telomere clone spanning a possible location of the Huntingdon disease gene. *Am. J. Hum. Genet.* **46,** 762–775.

16. Sambrook, J., Fritsch, E. F., and Maniatis, T. (1989) *Molecular Cloning: A Laboratory Manual,* 2nd ed. Cold Spring Harbor Laboratory, Cold Spring Harbor, NY.

17. Burgers, P. M. J. and Percival, K. J. (1987) Transformation of yeast spheroplasts without cell fusion. *Anal. Biochem.* **163,** 391–397.

18. McCormick, M. K., Shero, J. H., Connelly, C. J., Antonarakis, S. E., and Hieter, P. A. (1990) Methods for cloning large segments as artificial chromosomes in *S. cervisiae. Technique* **2,** 65–71.

19. Allshire, R. C. (1990) Introduction of large linear minichromosomes into *Schizosaccharomyces pombe* by an improved transformation procedure. *Proc. Natl. Acad. Sci. USA* **87,** 4043–4047.

Index